Healthcare in Northern Ireland, 1921–73

Manchester University Press

SOCIAL HISTORIES OF MEDICINE

Social Histories of Medicine is concerned with all aspects of health, illness and medicine, from prehistory to the present, in every part of the world. The series covers the circumstances that promote health or illness, the ways in which people experience and explain such conditions, and what, practically, they do about them. Practitioners of all approaches to health and healing come within its scope, as do their ideas, beliefs, and practices, and the social, economic and cultural contexts in which they operate. Methodologically, the series welcomes relevant studies in social, economic, cultural, and intellectual history, as well as approaches derived from other disciplines in the arts, sciences, social sciences and humanities. The series is a collaboration between Manchester University Press and the Society for the Social History of Medicine.

To buy or to find out more about the books currently available in this series, please go to: https://manchesteruniversitypress.co.uk/series/social-histories-of-medicine/

Healthcare in Northern Ireland, 1921–73

Politics, policies and management

Donnacha Seán Lucey

MANCHESTER UNIVERSITY PRESS

Published by Manchester University Press
Oxford Road, Manchester, M13 9PL

www.manchesteruniversitypress.co.uk

British Library Cataloguing-in-Publication Data
A catalogue record for this book is available from the British Library

ISBN 978 1 5261 1980 3 hardback

First published 2026

Typeset
by Deanta Global Publishing Services, Chennai, India

To Michelle and Vivienne, the lights of my life

Contents

Maps and figures

Maps

Figures

Tables

Acknowledgements

I would like to acknowledge the Arts and Humanities Research Council (UK), which funded the project 'Welfare and public health in Belfast and its region, 1800–1973' [Grant AH/J003816/1] which funded much of the research for this monograph. I would also like to thank this project's Principal Investigator and Co-Investigator, Prof. Peter Gray and Prof. Olwen Purdue, respectively, and my former colleague Dr Georgina Laragy. I would also like to thank Prof. Matthias Beck, Prof. Eoin McLaughlin and Dr Ida Milne for reading and commenting on earlier drafts. Thank you also to colleagues in University College Cork including Prof. Ursula Kilkelly, Prof. Thia Hennessy and Colman Quain, and the College of Business and Law Office, for providing me with time and support to complete this work. I would also like to thank the staff of the following archives and libraries: the Public Record Office of Northern Ireland, The National Archives (Kew), Newspaper Library (Belfast Central Library), Queen's University Belfast Library and the National Library of Ireland. I would like to thank the anonymous reviewers for their valuable feedback and suggestions on how to enhance the work. I would particularly like to thank the Manchester University Press editorial team, including Meredith Carroll and Humairaa Dudhwala, for their never-ending patience, assistance and advice in getting this book published.

Abbreviations

BHA	British Hospitals Association
BMA	British Medical Association
BMJ	*British Medical Journal*
BN	*Belfast News-Letter*
BO	*Ballymena Observer*
BT	*Belfast Telegraph*
BWT	*Ballymena Weekly Telegraph*
DIB	*Dictionary of Irish Biography*
EHS	Emergency Hospital Service
FS	*Frontier Sentinel*
GP	General Practitioners
HMC	Hospital Management Committee
HMSO	His/Her Majesty's Stationery Office
IHS	*Irish Historical Studies*
IMR	Infant Mortality Rate
IN	*Irish News*
LDS	*Londonderry Sentinel*
LGB	Local Government Board
LT	*Larne Times*
MCW	Maternity and Child Welfare
MHA	Ministry of Home Affairs
MHLG	Ministry of Health and Local Government
MHSS	Ministry of Health and Social Services
MOH/MOsH	Medical Officer/Officers of Health
MUM	*Mid-Ulster Mail*
NDHCDI	*North Down Herald and County Down Independent*

NHS	National Health Service
NIHA	Northern Ireland Hospitals Authority
NIHoC	Northern Ireland House of Commons
NILP	Northern Ireland Labour Party
NIRHC	Northern Ireland Regional Hospitals Council
NPHT	Nuffield Provincial Hospitals Trust
NW	*Northern Whig*
PRONI	Public Record Office of Northern Ireland
PT	*Portadown Times*
QUB	Queen's University Belfast
RUC	Royal Ulster Constabulary
RVH	Royal Victoria Hospital
SC	*Strabane Chronicle*
SMA	Socialist Medical Association
SMSA	Socialist Medical Service Association
UH	*Ulster Herald*
UMJ	*Ulster Medical Journal*

Introduction

Northern Ireland's modern health services have long been viewed as characterised by an unusually high degree of managerialism and centralised government authority. Multiple experts, academics and reports have called for greater local control and enhanced clinical power in decision-making.[1] While Northern Ireland's overly centralised health system is a modern-day policy concern, there is little understanding of its long-term development. This book focuses on the policies, politics and management of healthcare in Northern Ireland during the period from 1921 to 1973. These years were bookended by two significant political events: the partition of Ireland and the establishment of Northern Ireland in 1921 under a devolved government, and the proroguing of that parliament in 1972 and its dissolution in 1973, which led to the introduction of direct rule from Westminster. This period witnessed a complete transformation in the management of Northern Ireland's health services, evolving from a highly fragmented system marked by differentiated providers and weak centralisation to the most integrated and centrally managed organisation in the United Kingdom. The overall aim of this study is to explain how this change came about and, in doing so, to uncover the role played by the major stakeholders in Northern Ireland's health policy, politics and management, and the dynamic tensions to which these gave rise. At the core of this analysis is an exploration of the actors and interest groups that were progenitors of change or, conversely, obdurately resisted reform and shaped health policy. These included medical professionals, hospitals, medical voluntarism, local interests, central government and political and religious groupings. This examination provides new insights into healthcare, as well as politics and policy-making in Northern Ireland during these critical years.

This book is structured into three sections. Section I includes Chapters 1, 2 and 3 and examines the interwar mixed economy of healthcare and the three main providers of health provision: the poor law, municipal and voluntary sectors. Section II explores the changes of the 1940s, leading to the creation of the National Health Service (NHS) in Northern Ireland. Section III, comprising the final two chapters, explores hospital policies under the NHS and describes the rise of the central state and its managerialist approaches. While these three sections are organised chronologically, the work's central themes of politics, policy and management run through the analysis of each chapter. In doing so, much is also revealed about many facets of healthcare in Northern Ireland, such as the development of services.

In the first section, Chapter 1 focuses on the poor law and workhouse infirmaries in the 1920s and 1930s. During this period, health policy was not driven centrally and was marked instead by localism. At one level, this led to progress and innovation through the transformation of workhouses into district hospitals in some areas. Meanwhile, in other regions, there was a lack of reform and continued reliance on the stigmatising poor law; this was predominantly the case in largely nationalist and Catholic areas. Nationalist and unionist political tensions are highlighted as key to the continuation of workhouses in many areas. Local and institutional loyalties are also identified as key drivers for the creation of district hospitals. These dynamics were combined with a wider commitment to investment in modern hospitals for acute patients, with little incentive to enhance care for the long-term chronically sick, the enduring workhouse patient. Chapter 2 complements the focus on poor law provision in Chapter 1 by looking at municipal health services. The key theme examined is the politics surrounding the failure to develop maternity and child welfare. Through a case study of Belfast Corporation, this policy failure is attributed to political, class and gender divisions in local health policies, especially between the city's labour movement, epitomised by the Northern Ireland Labour Party, and socially conservative Ulster Unionists, and the inherent fissures of medical cultures, which both represented. This failure was compounded by the weakness and parsimony of central government. The observations about the attenuation of poor law hospital provision and municipal maternity and child welfare are contrasted with the buoyant medical voluntary sector in Chapter 3. Politically tied to the ruling Ulster Unionist Party, medical voluntarism was intertwined with the social elite of industrialists and landed gentry, backboned by the skills of the professional and middle classes and financed mainly by working-class contributions. Medical voluntarism was further strengthened by its alignment with medical education and research on the back of a political consensus that favoured a socially and fiscally conservative unionist-governed state. The chapter argues that medical voluntarism's vitality was reflective of the wider political, ethnic, social and economic makeup of the new Northern Irish state and intertwined with the interests of the medical profession, academia and the unionist elite and establishment.

Overall, this section depicts a developing health system characterised by multiple providers, or a mixed economy of healthcare, which witnessed increased organisation, medical sophistication and expansion. This picture challenges widely held perceptions among historians about the limitations of interwar healthcare in Northern Ireland.[2] However, health policy and the management of services were undermined by multiple factors. The strength of unionist-backed voluntarism in Northern Ireland weakened other visions of healthcare, specifically rate-aided municipal provision favoured by the labour movement. Catholic-managed healthcare, as represented by the Mater Infirmorum Hospital, also became increasingly isolated from the wider hospital system, which was unionist and implicitly Protestant in outlook. Furthermore, the different sectors were disparate, disjointed and marked by scant central government control or policymaking. It is argued that powerful interests – notably medical voluntarism and embedded localism – emerged during these years, and that they would later resist the emergence of the NHS and come into conflict with an increasingly centralised state in the 1940s and post-war period. The role of politics also emerges as a central theme in this section, with a focus on divisions between nationalism, unionism and the labour movement, which are all key to the shape and organisation of healthcare that prevailed.

The second section comprises Chapter 4 and focuses on the 1940s and the introduction of the NHS in Northern Ireland. Describing these years as a transitional period, it explores how the central state was forced into action by circumstances such as war, rising societal discontent and Westminster's post-war social policies. It is argued that while the Health Services Act of 1948 succeeded in introducing the universal, free-at-the-point-of-contact NHS, this was also a political and policy settlement between the Stormont central government, medical elite, voluntary hospitals and local interests.[3] This settlement blocked direct state command, solidified existing medical power bases and sectoral divisions in hospital care and diluted consolidation. This was born out of extensive conflict between stakeholders and vested interests in Northern Irish medicine, primarily the voluntary sector and the emerging central state, now thrust to the centre of health policymaking and management; the latter was forced into making significant concessions, little understood in the historiography, which baked fragmentation into the new structures. This attenuated many of the founding principles and values of the NHS, which sought integrated planning to meet need. Yet, the new management structure introduced in 1948 in the form of the Northern Ireland Hospitals Authority was an important, albeit partial, stage in the increased centralisation of hospital and health services and the road to greater state power.

The final section of the book explores the tensions between modernisation and older medical power structures identified in the previous two sections. Here, the encroachment of the central state on Northern Ireland's deep-rooted policy of health provision is explored. In this context, the central state's focus shifted to new technocratic and modernising themes, such as medical planning, efficiency and administrative reform. Further change was driven by an extensive hospital-building programme, growth of consultant services and emergence of new specialisms and academic disciplines, such as social medicine and gerontology, which created new dynamics in health policy and significantly impacted management in the sector. Returning to the theme of politics, this section shows how these new trends drew political support from the modernising strands in the Ulster Unionist Party, spearheaded by the premiership of Terence O'Neill. This trajectory toward greater modernisation, however, was resisted by medical power brokers, which contributed to a new fragmentation of unionist health policy and politics that led up to the outbreak of the Northern Irish Troubles.

Nationalist fears over discrimination and alienation were also deepened by aspects of the new services' management, which led to further divisions and tensions. Finally, it argues that the need to address long-standing nationalist and Catholic grievances to quell the Troubles created a window of opportunity to reform healthcare radically. Entrenched stakeholder objections were finally overcome, leading to significant reforms of the health services implemented in 1973, which went further than similar changes in Britain. It is argued that these reforms were motivated not just by the need to address Catholic and nationalist disadvantage but also by a longer trajectory dating back to the 1940s, when modernising forces began to challenge stakeholder power. These reforms created a remarkable paradox: the modernisation of health services combined with managerialism in a Northern Irish society torn apart by political, ethnic and violent upheaval.

Accordingly, this analysis questions academic understandings of acquiescence among stakeholders in Northern Irish healthcare. Academic work has claimed that Northern Irish health policymaking in this era was atrophied by political and social conservatism, a desire to maintain the status quo and a reliance on London's funding and policies.[4] Instead, a picture of largely involuntary change – shifting from fragmentation, localism and weak managerialism to centralisation and stronger managerialism – is depicted. Conflict between the ruling unionist factions and multiple stakeholders is posited as central to shaping Northern Ireland's healthcare. At the same time, less surprisingly, nationalist–unionist political divisions are also identified as important. The exploration of such tensions allows for a more nuanced, though complex, understanding of the history of Northern Ireland's healthcare than has been previously provided.

No other published work has attempted to explore healthcare in Northern Ireland from partition until the dissolution of the Stormont parliament in 1973. The published literature on hospitals in Northern Ireland remains limited, mainly focusing on institutional and educational histories.[5] Important research on the impact of the Troubles on healthcare, family planning and some diseases, such as tuberculosis and venereal disease, reveals much about Northern Irish medicine and provision but does not offer an analysis of the history of health politics, policy or management.[6]

Certain aspects of Northern Irish healthcare politics are examined in the wider literature. The failure of the Mater Infirmorum Hospital to come into the post-1948 health services and its subsequent tense relationship with the Northern Irish state has been the focus of historical work, revealing the political and religious tensions underpinning this facet of policy.[7] However, the focus on the Mater Hospital by historians has distracted from other aspects of Northern Irish healthcare. As a result, the Mater Hospital is not a major feature of this book. Political tensions between conservative-minded Ulster unionism and Clement Attlee's post-war Labour government, as well as within unionism regarding the welfare state, have been well documented. Historians John Privilege and Greta Jones have argued that crises in local health politics metamorphosed into a broader political emergency, which was a critical factor in bringing about health reform in Northern Ireland.[8] Elsewhere, Privilege has also emphasised the role of William Grant, the Minister of Health and Local Government, in implementing reform in the face of internal unionist opposition.[9] However, this wider literature does not identify or explore the tensions between powerful stakeholders, particularly medical voluntarism and the state, which this book argues were key dynamics in shaping Northern Ireland's health services. Furthermore, this book's analysis of the trajectory of Northern Ireland's healthcare from partition to the early 1970s provides long-term insights that are not achievable through the more discrete studies which have characterised much of the literature to date on Northern Irish healthcare. The post-war Hospitals Authority has been examined in Ann Marie Gray's unpublished D.Phil thesis from 1993. Based largely on official publications and some interviews, the work provides important insights into the Hospitals Authority from its establishment in 1948 to its dissolution in 1973. This study provides much relevant detail and information on the Hospitals Authority while also highlighting the difficulties in bringing about rationalisation and embedding of planning principles in the post-1948 system. However, as Gray highlights, this study is limited by the lack of access to many of the archives located in the Public Record Office of Northern Ireland related to the creation and running of the Hospitals Authority, due to time restrictions on consultation in place at that time.[10] In contrast, this monograph draws on previously inaccessible sources, allowing for original material and analysis of the development of healthcare.

This work also addresses significant gaps in the general understanding of Northern Irish history. Despite healthcare's centrality to Northern Irish society (as in the present day, health services were the biggest source of employment and public expenditure during much of the period under examination), the sector barely features in wider historical work on the region's politics. Traditionally, the focus has been on constitutional matters, political violence and the politics of nationalism and unionism, with some emphasis on the labour movement. This book's exploration of Northern Ireland's healthcare addresses this significant historiographical gap. It sheds new light on interwar Northern Irish healthcare, the coming of the welfare state in the region and the relationship between health and politics, including nationalist disenchantment and fragmentation of unionist health policy in the lead-up to the Troubles. It also identifies health policy as a central plank of the modernising policies of the Terence O'Neill administration in the 1960s, offering original insights into this key juncture in Northern Irish politics and history.[11] Many of these topics have received little, if any, attention from historians.

This study of Northern Irish healthcare also adds much to the wider literature on the history of the subject in Britain and Ireland. In the UK context, few comparable works tease out the long-term trajectory of healthcare from the interwar years to the reforms of the early 1970s. Since the start of the twenty-first century, there has been a revised historiographical focus on the interwar period, which presents an increasingly positive picture of healthcare than the older, more negative depictions allow.[12] Drawing on this wider historiography, this book also argues that Northern Ireland, too, witnessed progress during these years, but that significant shortfalls persisted. Yet, much of this literature does not expand beyond the interwar years. Instead, a separate, older literature explores the coming of the NHS and its subsequent political, bureaucratic, organisational and clinical history.[13] More recent histories of the NHS in Britain have focused on multiple topics and themes, such as cultural histories, health consumerism, management of certain diseases and emergence of management consultants in health policymaking.[14] This monograph is one of the few in-depth studies that covers the interwar years, 1940s and early decades of the NHS in any part of the UK. This analysis of the pre- and post-1948 years illustrates that the creation of the NHS was not the *tabula rasa*, as is often assumed. Interwar power structures continued to shape healthcare in the post-war era, which ultimately came into conflict with a modernising and centralising state. Such policy inheritance or path dependency – in which earlier policies and structures conditioned later trajectories – has received some attention in the British historiography, with some regional studies focusing on areas such as the north-east and south-west of England.[15] This book's examination of Northern Ireland offers a deeper historical analysis than these works and allows for a fuller, more detailed exploration of how older forces shaped post-1948 structures.

There is a lack of historical understanding of how health services and the NHS developed outside England. Historiographical focus on the NHS has been overly marked by Klien's 'reluctant little Englander' approach, and there has been muted exploration of the historical development of the system in the other countries of the UK.[16] The dearth of scholarly country-specific studies is evident in a leading historiographical review of the NHS, which does not mention Scottish, Welsh or Northern Irish experiences.[17] Some work on Wales and Scotland has identified differences in the governance, culture and ethos of the NHS.[18] The NHS in Wales and Scotland have been the focus of some surveys and general studies, but these are circumscribed in scope.[19] Work comparing the historical development of the NHS across the UK's constituent nations is even more scarce, although research on the continued place of voluntarism in the early NHS illustrates that hospital services differed between countries.[20] The need for sustained and substantial historical research on the NHS's comparative development across the UK is even more pressing, considering that historical contexts shape modern-day health systems in the constituent countries.[21] This monograph's examination of Northern Ireland addresses a significant lacuna in understanding the NHS. It reveals crucial differences in funding, management and politics in Northern Ireland compared to other UK countries, which shows that the system was marked as much by variance as continuity across national contexts.

The focus on Northern Ireland also informs wider historiographical debates about the NHS. The exploration of tensions in Northern Irish healthcare substantiates Charles Webster's argument that conflict between progressive forces, including the broad labour movement, and more conservative and reactionary influences ultimately weakened NHS organisational structures in Britain.[22] This challenges competing perspectives that consensus among various medical professionals, government officials and hospitals – influenced by an increasingly apolitical, rational and technocratic health planning – lay behind the new service.[23] The tensions and divisions identified in Northern Ireland indicate that health policy was characterised more by conflict than consensus. Unlike in Britain, where the role of the labour movement was instrumental, hospital policy in Northern Ireland was shaped to a greater degree by the interests of powerful stakeholders, primarily medical voluntarism, which sought to protect their many advantages in the new service.

Several aspects of Northern Ireland's health system are not covered in this monograph. The focus is primarily on hospital provision, with meagre attention given to general practice, personal health services of local authorities (except Chapter 3's emphasis on maternity and child welfare) and environmental health. These are all important aspects of Northern Ireland's health history. Still, the approach taken here is justified by the centrality of hospitals in policymaking, which is reflected in the large budgets allocated to secondary care. The story of Northern Irish medicine in the twentieth century is, by and large, the story of hospitals.

The work focuses on Northern Ireland, although in places there is a natural concentration on Belfast due to the city's political, economic and social importance and predominate role in hospital and academic medicine. Yet this study is not a narrow parochial Northern Irish account, and, where possible, developments are viewed through a comparative lens. Comparisons with Great Britain and south of the Irish border are made, helping to provide more profound and comprehensive understandings of healthcare in UK and island of Ireland contexts. Northern Ireland's healthcare is also presented as being shaped by circumstances brought about by the creation of new, small political entities that emerged across Europe in post-First World War imperial changes, often within the context of nationalist movements and violent political frameworks.

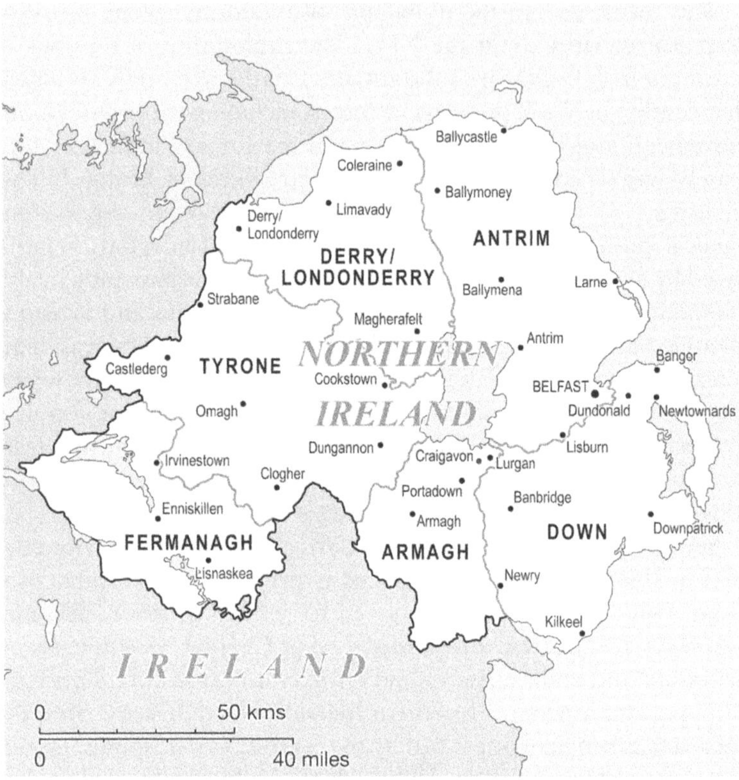

Map 0.1 Counties, cities and towns in Northern Ireland

Overview of Northern Ireland's healthcare

At partition in 1921, Northern Ireland's hospital system was run by a mixed economy of healthcare provided by multiple charitable and rate-aided local authorities in a complex, differentiated, and often overlapping system. These providers included voluntary hospitals, the poor law system, and municipal authorities. The Ministry of Home Affairs was responsible for health services provided by the poor law and county and city councils. The largest provider of hospital beds was the poor law system. Established originally in 1838 for the relief of destitution, the poor law is traditionally synonymous with the horrors of the Great Irish Famine (1845–52), when workhouses were sites of disease and death. Irish workhouses had become increasingly medicalised during the late nineteenth and early twentieth century, and workhouse infirmaries had emerged as central to hospital provision for much of the Irish poor. Workhouse infirmaries provided a range of services, including some general medical and surgical treatment, while also catering for long-term chronic illness and infectious diseases, often in fever hospitals ancillary to the main workhouse. Such provision remained stigmatising and suffered from the 'taint' of the poor law. At their worst, workhouses were mixed institutions that relieved not just the sick poor but also multiple other categories of patients and inmates, including the destitute able-bodied, children, many born out of wedlock and considered 'illegitimate' and people suffering from disabilities, both physical and cognitive. In lieu of the Northern Irish government's reform of the poor law, local boards of guardians, which managed workhouses, could use permissive legislation to transform workhouses into district hospitals. Some local authorities undertook this reform, often along with significant rebuilding projects, which helped to greatly enhance this tier of healthcare and now catered for a wider social spectrum beyond the poor. Institutions that remained workhouses were considered to provide low-quality medical provision. The system was mostly funded out of local rates and received no central government financial support. By the early 1940s, there were twelve district hospitals and eleven workhouse infirmaries in Northern Ireland.

Northern Ireland's six county councils and two county boroughs also had public health responsibilities. Local government was further democratised with the 1898 Local Government (Ireland) Act, modelled on the British 1888 legislation, which introduced county councils and boroughs. By the time of the Irish partition, they had multiple medical functions, including mental health and infectious disease provision. Edwardian public health legislation bestowed further responsibilities on these bodies, including maternity and child welfare, school medical service and provision for venereal disease and tuberculosis. Largely known as personal health services, these new responsibilities differed from local authorities' long-standing role in sanitary public health. Funding was based on a combination of local rates and central government grants, while tuberculosis provision was partly funded through National Insurance payments. County councils and boroughs in Northern Ireland were responsible for six sanatoria. Belfast Corporation was the largest provider of tuberculosis beds; the 285-bed Whiteabbey and 58-bed Municipal Hospital for Tuberculosis (TB) Children were under its remit. Smaller local authority sanatoria, ranging from eighteen to thirty-three beds, were also run by the Armagh, Down and Tyrone County Councils. Only Belfast Corporation had a fever hospital, the large 585-bed Purdysburn Hospital. Infectious disease outside Belfast was mostly the responsibility of poor law fever hospitals and the semi-voluntary county fever infirmaries. There were also five mental institutions run by Belfast Corporation and Armagh, Down, Londonderry and Tyrone County Councils, respectively, totalling 3,581 beds in 1930.[24] This monograph largely avoids focusing on infectious disease, tuberculosis, venereal disease or mental health provision, with excellent works already covering many of these topics.[25] Instead, it concentrates on the failure to develop other areas of county borough provision, particularly Belfast Corporation's unsuccessful maternity and child welfare policies.

Voluntary hospitals, the focus of Chapter 3, were the most prestigious type of medical institutions. This study identified 2,311 beds provided by the numerous types of voluntary hospitals in the early 1940s (for a complete list of voluntary hospitals and bed numbers, see Table 3.1). The most prominent voluntary hospitals were based in Belfast, provided general and specialist care and acted as teaching facilities for the city's Queen's University. These included the Royal Victoria Hospital, Northern Ireland's largest general voluntary hospital. The Mater Infirmorum, also located in Belfast, was the only Catholic general voluntary hospital in Northern Ireland; it provided acute medical and surgical care, along with maternity services. Specialist voluntary hospitals – mostly in Belfast although Derry/Londonderry had a voluntary eye, ear and throat hospital – emerged with the growth in medical specialisation in the mid- to late nineteenth century.[26] Philanthropic sources, including bequests, donations and subscriptions, historically funded these general and specialist voluntary hospitals. By the interwar years, working-class contribution schemes became increasingly important, and patient payment, along with private beds, slowly emerged as a source of income for these hospitals. Medically, voluntary hospitals mostly provided for the acute sick and did not cater for the long-term chronically unwell or infectious disease cases, often overly associated with poverty. These were predominantly cared for in local authority hospitals. Their focus on general and specialist acute and surgical care, as well as their deep relationship with consultants and academic medicine, ensured that voluntary hospitals were prestigious and reputable. They were managed by a combination of lay governors, mostly drawn from the leading subscribers, often representative of Northern Ireland's political and social establishment, and clinicians. Doctors provided their medical services for free in voluntary hospitals, which helped to build their reputations and attract private patients, often from subscribers. The Mater was established and run by the Sisters of Mercy, a religious congregation founded in Dublin in 1831, which also ran the Mater Misericordiae in Dublin and Mercy Hospital in Cork. The Roman Catholic Bishop of Down and Connor chaired its management committee.[27] Voluntary hospital patients were mainly the 'necessitous poor' and working classes. Entitlement was based on multiple factors, including medical condition, concepts of deservingness and membership of a working-class contribution scheme. Meanwhile, means-testing determined patients' capacity to financially contribute to their care. Also, subscribers could grant the sick a ticket to access voluntary hospitals, acting as an essential form of patronage for the former. In the interwar years, more middle-class patients turned to voluntary hospitals for private care in line with medical and technological advances.

Outside Belfast, medical voluntarism mainly was comprised of semi-voluntary county infirmaries and smaller cottage hospitals. Dating from the late eighteenth and early nineteenth century, seven county infirmaries provided general acute and surgical care and served as the main source of consultancy services in provincial Ulster. Two county fever infirmaries provided infectious disease services. County infirmary patients were often poor and working-class in need of acute surgical and medical care. However, like Belfast's voluntary hospitals, better-off patients sought treatment in these facilities by the interwar years. Although typically considered voluntary hospitals, local government county councils contributed to their funding and management. A combination of local authority rates, traditional voluntary funding, patient fees and contributions financed them. At the same time, boards of management were made up of a mixture of governors and county councillors.

The final type of voluntary institution was the cottage hospital. Often ignored by historians of medical voluntarism, cottage hospitals provided an important, if small, form of local voluntary provision. Established in the late nineteenth and early twentieth century and located outside of cities, cottage hospitals were smaller than the large urban voluntary institutions. There were seven cottage hospitals in Northern Ireland, mostly situated in unionist areas, each managed by governors and/or trustees. Unlike their urban counterparts, cottage hospitals were not primarily established to care for the poor and working classes. Instead, they often catered to fee-paying, better-off patients who were slow to turn to local authority provision and were attracted by the consultancy services these hospitals typically provided. Cottage hospitals were usually kept up to date and focused on acute medical, surgical and maternity care, while chronic and infectious cases were not received.

The 1940s brought major organisational and structural reform of Northern Ireland's health services. The Ministry of Health and Local Government was established in 1944 and took responsibility for health services from the Ministry of Home Affairs. This was a significant reform and represented the first government bureaucracy devoted largely to health services – the Ministry of Home Affairs was also responsible for, and often preoccupied with, justice and internal security. In 1944, the Northern Ireland Tuberculosis Authority was established, which took over tuberculosis provision from local authorities until its disestablishment in 1959, when the Northern Ireland Hospitals Authority subsumed it. The 1948 Health Services Act radically restructured health in Northern Ireland. In line with the simultaneously introduced National Health Service Acts (separate legislation existed for Scotland and England and Wales) in Britain, a similar tripartite system was initiated. The General Health Services administered primary care including general practice, dentistry and pharmacy, while the Hospitals Authority was responsible for hospital and specialist provision; local authorities inherited environmental and public health from the pre-1948 structures but were stripped of the hospitals under their jurisdiction. Although part of the overall National Health Service in the UK, the operational delivery of most services was provided by the Hospitals Authority and General Health Services Board. Similarly, today's services are run by Northern Ireland's Health and Social Care system; however, the system is commonly referred to as the NHS in Northern Ireland. This book also refers to the post-war Northern Irish health service as the NHS. The Mater Hospital remained outside the NHS and continued to act as an independent voluntary facility until 1972. As outlined in the final three chapters of this book, until the late 1960s, the Hospitals Authority was not an agent of the Ministry of Health and Local Government or its successor, the Ministry of Health and Social Services, established in 1965. Central government direct power over the Hospitals Authority was limited to approving its annual budget and costly capital projects; otherwise, the Hospitals Authority was free to administer services largely independent of ministerial and parliamentary oversight. Thirty hospital management committees comprised the lower administrative tier of the service. These sought to bring together the management of multiple hospitals in the quest for greater coordination and efficiency in management, a key objective of the new service. A far-reaching reorganisation of the system came about in 1973, when the administration of medical services was merged with social personal services under four area boards and the Hospitals Authority was dissolved. Uniquely, this reform created a highly integrated system which went much further than similar reorganisations in Britain which did not include social services. The post-1948 service was universal and free-at-the-point-of-contact and primarily funded through central taxation.

Notes

1 Department of Health, Northern Ireland, *Systems, Not Structures: Changing Health and Social Care* (Belfast: Department of Health, 2016), p. 16 [popularly known as the Bengoa review after the panel's chair Prof. Rafael Bengoa]; M. Dayan and D. Heenan, *Change or Collapse: Lessons from the Drive to Reform Health and Social Care in Northern Ireland* (London: Nuffield Trust, 2019).

2 A. Jackson, 'Local government in Northern Ireland, 1920–73', in M. E. Daly (ed.), *County and Town: One Hundred Years of Local Government in Ireland* (Dublin: Institute of Public Administration, 2001), pp. 57, 60; D. S. Johnson, 'The Northern Ireland economy, 1914–39', in L. Kennedy and P. Ollerenshaw (eds), *An Economic*

History of Ulster, 1820–1939 (Manchester: Manchester University Press, 1985), p. 213.

3 Throughout this work 'Stormont' refers to the Parliament of Northern Ireland after it relocated to the purposely built building in 1932.

4 S. L. Greer, *Territorial Politics and Health Policy: UK Health Policy in Comparative Perspective* (Manchester: Manchester University Press, 2004), p. 164.

5 For example, see R. S. J. Clarke, *The Royal Victoria Hospital, Belfast: A History, 1797–1997* (Belfast: Blackstaff, 1997).

6 R. Duffy, *Health Care and the Troubles: The Conflict Experience of the Northern Ireland Health Service, 1968–1998* (Liverpool: Liverpool University Press, 2024); G. Jones, '*Captain of All These Men of Death': The History of Tuberculosis in Nineteenth and Twentieth Century Ireland* (Amsterdam: Rodopi, 2001); L. McCormick, *Regulating Sexuality: Women in Twentieth-Century Northern Ireland* (Manchester: Manchester University Press, 2009); G. Jones, 'Marie Stopes in Ireland – The Mother's Clinic in Belfast, 1938–47', *Social History of Medicine*, 5:2 (1992), 255–77.

7 P. Martin, '"Why have a Catholic Hospital at all?": The Mater Infirmorum Hospital Belfast and the state, 1883–1972', in D. S. Lucey and V. Crossman (eds), *Healthcare in Ireland and Britain from 1850: Voluntary, Regional and Comparative Perspectives* (London: Institute of Historical Research, 2014), pp. 101–17.

8 J. Privilege and G. Jones, 'Crisis and scandal: Government, local government and health reform in Northern Ireland, 1939–44', *Irish Economic and Social History*, 42 (2015), 33–52.

9 J. Privilege, 'The Northern Ireland government and the welfare state, 1942–8: The case of health provision', *Irish Historical Studies*, 39:155 (2015), 439–59.

10 A. M. Gray, 'Government and the administration of hospital services in Northern Ireland: The Northern Ireland Hospitals Authority, 1948–73' (University of Ulster: D.Phil Thesis, 1993), pp. 7–8.

11 For the modernising agenda of the O'Neill government, see M. Mulholland, *Northern Ireland at the Crossroads: Ulster Unionism in the O'Neill Years 1960–9* (Basingstoke: Macmillan Press, 2000).

12 This is a large historiography, for key publications see A. Levene, M. Powell, J. Stewart and B. Taylor, *Cradle to Grave: Municipal Medicine in Interwar England and Wales* (Oxford: Peter Lang, 2011); B. M. Doyle, *The Politics of Hospital Provision in Early Twentieth-Century Britain* (London: Pickering and Chatto, 2014); M. Gorsky, '"Threshold of a New Era": The development of an integrated system

in north-east Scotland, 1900–39', *Social History of Medicine*, 17:2 (2004), 247–67.

13 R. Klein, *The New Politics of the NHS: From Creation to Reinvention* (London: CRC Press, 7th ed., 2013); G. Rivett, *From Cradle to Grave: Fifty Years of the NHS* (London: Kings Fund Publishing, 1986); C. Webster, *The National Health Service: A Political History* (Oxford: Oxford University Press, 2nd ed., 2002).

14 P. Begley and S. Sheard, 'From "honeymoon period" to "stable marriage": The rise of management consultants in British health policymaking', *Bulletin of the History of Medicine*, 95:2 (Summer 2021), 227–55; J. Crane and J. Hand (eds), *Posters, Protests and Prescriptions: Cultural Histories of the National Health Service in Britain* (Manchester: Manchester University Press, 2022); A. Mold, *Making the Patient-Consumer: Patient Organisations and Health Consumerism in Britain* (Manchester: Manchester University Press, 2015); M. D. Moore, *Managing Diabetes, Managing Medicine: Chronic Disease and Clinical Bureaucracy in Post-War Britain* (Manchester: Manchester University Press, 2019).

15 J. Mohan, *Planning, Markets and Hospitals* (Abingdon: Routledge, 2002); M. Gorsky, '"To regulate and confirm inequality"? A regional history of geriatric hospitals under the English National Health Service, *c.*1948–*c.*1975', *Ageing and Society*, 33:4 (2013), 620.

16 Klein, *The New Politics of the NHS*, p. vii.

17 M. Gorsky, 'The British National Health Service 1948–2008: A review of the historiography', *Social History of Medicine*, 21:3 (2008), 437–60.

18 J. Stewart, 'The National Health Service in Scotland, 1947–74: Scottish or British?', *Historical Research*, 76:193 (2003), 389–410; J. Stewart, 'Health care systems in Britain and Ireland in the nineteenth and twentieth centuries: The national, international and sub-national contexts', in Lucey and Crossman (eds), *Healthcare in Ireland and Britain from 1850*, pp. 31–60; C. Webster, 'Devolution and the health service in Wales, 1919–69', in P. Michael and C. Webster (eds), *Health and Society in Twentieth-Century Wales* (Cardiff: University of Wales Press, 2006), pp. 240–69.

19 M. McCrae, *The National Health Service in Scotland: Origins and Ideals, 1900–50* (East Lothian: Tuckwell Press, 2003); P. Michael and S. Thompson, *Public Health in Wales (c. 1800–2012): A Brief History* (Cardiff: Welsh Government, 2012).

20 B. Harris and R. Cresswell, 'The legacy of voluntarism: Charitable funding in the early NHS, *The Economic History Review*, 77:2 (May 2024), 554–83.

21 M. Anderson, H. Alderwick, E. Pitchforth, A. McGuire, N. Edwards and E. Mossialos, *Health Systems in Transition: United Kingdom: Health System Review*, 2022, vol. 1 (Copenhagen: World Health Organization, 2022), p. 25.

22 C. Webster, 'Conflict and consensus: Explaining the British health service', *Twentieth Century British History*, 1:2 (1990), 115–51.

23 Klein, *The New Politics of the NHS*; D. M. Fox., 'The National Health Service and the Second World War: The elaboration of consensus', in H. L. Smith (ed.), *War and Social Change: British Society in the Second World War* (Manchester: Manchester University Press, 1986), pp. 32–57; for a brief outline of these historiographical debates see M. Gorsky, 'The British National Health Service 1948–2008', 441–3.

24 H. Burdett, *Burdett's Hospitals and Charities: Being the Yearbook of Philanthropy and the Hospital Annual* (London: Scientific Press, 1930), p. 538.

25 Jones, '*Captain of All These Men of Death*'; McCormick, *Regulating Sexuality*; P. M. Prior, *Mental Health and Politics in Northern Ireland: A History of Service Development* (Aldershot: Avebury, 1993).

26 'Derry/Londonderry' is used throughout this book. 'Londonderry' is used when referring to official bodies such as Londonderry Hospital Management Committee. The dual naming of Derry/Londonderry is used to acknowledge the different perspectives within Northern Ireland's communities. It is not intended to cause offence nor make a political point but to make the work as neutral as possible.

27 Catholic religious sisters were to the forefront of hospitals in Ireland; see B. Casey, 'The Franciscan Missionaries of the Divine Motherhood and the Provision of Healthcare in Provincial Ireland, 1942–1970', *The Historical Journal* (December 2024), 1–21 (First View: https://www.cambridge.org/core/journals/historical-journal/article/franciscan-missionaries-of-the-divine-motherhood-and-the-provision-of-healthcare-in-provincial-ireland–19421970/C5D5F5F953711814116634C33B6EF880#article accessed 30 December 2024).

Section 1

1

Irish partition and poor law reform in Northern Ireland

Introduction

Irish partition in 1921 led to the establishment of two new political entities on the island of Ireland – the nationalist and largely Catholic independent Irish Free State (twenty-six of the island's thirty-two counties) and Northern Ireland with a two-thirds unionist and Protestant majority. The Irish Free State had broken from the United Kingdom. It became an independent country but was bound by the Anglo-Irish Treaty to adopt Dominion status and stay in the Empire. Northern Ireland remained part of the United Kingdom but with a new government, based on the Westminster model, which was devolved from but subordinate to the mother parliament in London.[1] Northern Ireland was an integral part of the political union with Great Britain, yet retained imperial strands. Ireland's two new political structures were reflective of the changing constitutional nature of the British Empire following the First World War. The creation of newer, smaller countries throughout Europe often emanated from nationalist political movements and revolutions. Northern Ireland's experience of poor law and workhouse infirmary reform illustrates the dynamics that both stymied and facilitated healthcare reform in regions that witnessed new political settlements in interwar Europe when older imperial orders were challenged. The focus on small countries such as Ireland adds to an understanding of the history of comparative welfare and health systems, which have tended to explore large, industrialised nations.[2] Welfare and healthcare development in smaller countries that experienced political transformation during transitionary periods in empire has garnered some attention.[3] The post-First World

War years were a key transitionary period in imperial systems when the power of Russia, Austria-Hungary, Germany and Turkey was shattered, and the British Empire was reshaped through political settlements, including the evolution of the Dominions.[4] This was evident in Ireland where the nationalist revolution (1919–23) led to partition. Revolutionaries turned state-builders in the newly independent Irish Free State tied poor law reform to developing notions of citizenship. Northern Ireland's record of reform offers a different perspective. Irreconcilable political and religious divisions between nationalists and unionists, sharpened by turmoil, violence and militarisation surrounding partition and the establishment of Northern Ireland, negatively impacted poor law reform.

Workhouse infirmaries added up to the most numerous and geographically diverse hospital network in Northern Ireland. They exceeded the other types of hospitals, mainly the county and city infirmaries and the Belfast-focused voluntary facilities.[5] On the eve of Irish partition, there were twenty-six workhouses located in the region that would become Northern Ireland. The infirmaries were medically underdeveloped and mixed institutions in which older people, the chronically ill, the young and the disabled poor were relieved. They were the least attractive form of hospital provision in Northern Ireland, where eligibility was confined to the poor and infirmaries' 'pauper taint' ensured that medical relief was stigmatising.[6] Policymakers in Britain and Ireland sought reform of poor law medical services and the separation of healthcare from the ordinary relief of poverty since the time of the Edwardian poor law commissions.[7] By Irish partition, reform of significance had yet to come about anywhere in the United Kingdom. However, the newly independent Free State quickly set about dismantling the system. In 1927, the Northern Irish Departmental Commission on Local Government Administration recommended that district hospitals replace workhouse infirmaries. This was in keeping with wider poor law reform in Britain. In England and Wales, and separately in Scotland, the poor law was eradicated in 1929 when boards of guardians were disbanded, and former workhouse infirmaries came under county councils and boroughs. The formal break-up of the poor law in Northern Ireland, however, was not forthcoming and proved intractable until the major health reforms of the 1940s.

In lieu of central government measures, this chapter analyses locally led reforms, including the replacement of workhouse infirmaries with district hospitals by individual boards of guardians. This was a standard measure, and by the end of the interwar years, twelve out of Northern Ireland's twenty-three workhouses were transformed into district hospitals. In turn, it is argued that a multitiered poor law hospital system emerged. District hospitals were the first tier, providing increasingly modernised and sophisticated acute care with upgraded buildings, new equipment and access to specialist and consultant expertise. These facilities represented a progressive step in hospital development. The second tier consisted of unreformed workhouse infirmaries, characterised by rudimentary care in harsh and stigmatising buildings mostly dating from the mid-nineteenth century. Local communities and patients reliant on workhouse infirmaries by and large suffered from inferior care compared to areas with district hospitals.

Geographical, political and religious trends are identified as key factors in shaping local reform. District hospitals were mostly located in eastern Northern Ireland in areas with majority unionist and Protestant populations. In contrast, many districts with more nationalists and Catholics did not witness poor law reform. Varying levels of social and political collegiality and division are identified as key dynamics in bringing about this dichotomy. Predominantly unionist areas were loyal to Northern Ireland and could rely on pan-class unionist support for district hospitals in genuine attempts to ameliorate local medical provision. In contrast, many nationalist areas politically disavowed the new state, and, in places, nationalists were gerrymandered out of local government power. Political imbroglio enveloped many local authorities in nationalist areas, which diluted the capacity for meaningful hospital reform.

This chapter's exploration of the poor law hospital structure also offers more nuanced interpretations of Northern Irish interwar local authorities than the older, highly pessimistic accounts have allowed. These emphasise the sector's disorganisation, policy inertia and parsimony.[8] Instead, a more complex picture emerges, in which policy decisions shaped by a multitude of factors, including regional politics, attitudes of ratepayers and geography, determined hospital provision, often enhancing delivery for local populations. These findings add to some health historiography on Northern

Ireland, which points towards moderate progress in provision in the 1920s and 1930s, including the introduction of medical benefits under National Insurance legislation and the expansion of voluntary hospital provision.[9] These findings also help to address a lacuna in Irish poor law historical literature, which has mostly focused on the nineteenth and early twentieth centuries, with a lack of work on Northern Ireland in the interwar years.[10]

These insights have a significance beyond Northern Ireland. To date, studies of the new poor law in Britain have examined mainly ordinary relief, while medical relief remains an under-researched field.[11] Local authority healthcare has concentrated chiefly on English and Welsh examples of municipal care, with the post-1929 break-up of the poor law a key focus. Much of this wider work has challenged overly negative accounts of interwar municipal health. Instead, it has depicted a diverse, vibrant and expanding sector often shaped by perceived localised needs, local authority investment choices and traditions of healthcare.[12] Understandings of the multitiered system that emerged in Northern Ireland further add to these interpretations by showing that some local changes occurred under the poor law, like reforms in Britain. Yet, the failure of central government action and the persistence of permissive legislation meant that reform was highly localised, and many communities remained reliant on rudimentary poor law workhouses. Newly established, smaller political entities such as Northern Ireland shared some of the positive developments evident in larger countries. However, factors including weak central government and political divisions inherent to many new states established in this era stymied the capacity for reform.

Poor law reform prior to Irish partition

The Irish Poor Law Act of 1838, modelled on the new English law of 1834, introduced a countrywide system of relief based on the workhouse and financed by a local property tax. Synonymous with the horrors of the Great Irish Famine (1845–52), when workhouses were sites of disease and death, the poor law by the late nineteenth century provided ordinary and medical relief to much of Ireland's poor. Locally, it was administered by boards of guardians in each poor law union under the auspices of the central government authority, the Local Government Board (LGB). By the mid-nineteenth century, the system had 148 poor law unions, each with a workhouse. However, this number decreased with dissolutions and amalgamations, and, by 1900 it had reduced to about 130 unions in Ireland. Workhouses were the central institutional provision, while the dispensary system provided medical relief and rudimentary primary care.

By the early twentieth century, the Irish system had developed from its original objective of relieving the destitute poor. Irish workhouses increasingly became sites of medical care, which intensified after 1860. Medical provision was transformed under the 1862 Poor Law Act, which opened Irish workhouse infirmaries to the general sick poor, and eligibility was no longer confined to the destitute classes. The Act essentially established a hospital service for the poor law dispensary system that was set up initially in 1851 and provided outdoor medical relief.[13] Workhouse infirmaries provided medical and surgical care while also treating infectious disease patients, often in separate fever blocks. Many patients were older people with long-term, chronic medical needs, for which other sectors including the voluntary and county borough/council providers, by and large did not cater. By the turn of the century, the standard of care in workhouse infirmaries became increasingly professionalised. The controversial issue of untrained pauper and inmate nursing was forbidden in 1897 by the LGB. In Belfast, the workhouse became a site for nursing training and clinical instruction of medical students in Queen's Medical School. The increased association with medical training enhanced the sector's reputation.

Major deficiencies persisted with workhouse infirmaries despite these significant advances. The poor law was founded on principles of deterrence, and harsh conditions were intended to stave off only the truly destitute from applying. The more workhouse infirmaries were viewed as institutions for the sick, older people and infirm, the harder it was to justify principles of deterrence, but they remained associated with pauperism and poverty. Patients had to pass the workhouse gates and often underwent pauperising experiences such as being stigmatised by wearing pauper uniforms and living under disciplined regimes. A major problem was that workhouses were mixed institutions, serving a diverse range of 'inmates', including the able-bodied destitute, children, intellectually and physically disabled, and older people characterised as 'aged and infirm'. The separation of medical care from ordinary relief in mixed workhouses became a central demand of reformers. Both the 1906 Vice-Regal Commission on the Irish Poor Laws and the UK-wide Royal Commission on the Poor Law and Relief of Distress recommended such reforms. Direct poor law reform was not forthcoming, with the Liberal government instead focused on insurance-based measures including the 1908 Old Age Pension and 1911 National Insurance acts. While the medical benefits under the latter legislation were not introduced in Ireland due to opposition from the Catholic Church and Irish nationalism, which respectively feared increased state encroachment in medicine and higher taxation, these measures significantly altered the composition of workhouses in Ireland. Able-bodied and older people now had greater capacity to avoid the workhouse. By the time of Irish partition in 1921, the majority that turned to workhouses were the sick, as set out in Table 1.1. This was a significant change from 1910 when just over 35 per cent of inmates were classified as sick in workhouses throughout the island of Ireland, compared to 55 per cent in 1922 in Northern Ireland. After partition, workhouses' focus in Northern Ireland as sites of medical care for the sick expanded; they also continued to act as mixed institutions catering for multiple categories of people in need of treatment.

During the 1910s, some local boards of guardians implemented other aspects of poor law reform, primarily rationalisation and the closing of workhouses. The Poor Relief (Ireland) Act was introduced at the outbreak of the First World War, allowing boards of guardians to relieve inmates in other workhouses. This was originally only for workhouses that the military authorities had taken over for the accommodation of troops or war refugees, called 'interned aliens'. It was extended to all workhouses in 1916 and beyond the purview of war to relieve inmates in other workhouses.[14] This provision proved cheaper for poor law boards than meeting the full costs of their own institutions and was attractive to boards of guardians in the Ulster counties, soon to become Northern Ireland. Workhouses were viewed as too large, underutilised and costly in many rural areas. As early as 1916, the Irvinestown Board of Guardians in

Table 1.1 Categories of inmates/patients in Northern Ireland's workhouses on the last Saturday of March, 1922–38.

	1922	*1926*	*1930*	*1934*	*1938*
In workhouses					
Sick	2,693	3,085	3,027	3,337	3,399
Aged and infirm*	1,493	1,391	1,283	1,262	953
Children under 15, other than those sick in hospital	399	349	306	297	224
Lunatics, idiots and epileptics, other than those sick in hospital*	211	245	243	199	169
Mothers having infant children	71	88	72	80	61
All other classes	214	176	155	167	106
In extern institutions					
Extern Hospitals	24	42	51	73	54
Institutions for the blind, deaf and dumb*	181	208	95	76	75
Boarded out or nursing	340	339	325	379	363

Source: Ministry of Home Affairs, *Report on the Administration of Local Government Services in Northern Ireland, 1921/3–1937/8.*
* Infirm, lunatics, idiots, epileptics, blind, deaf and dumb were contemporary medical terms of the period.

County Fermanagh voted to close the workhouse and relieve the poor in neighbouring workhouses.[15] The Irvinestown Workhouse was small and, during 1913, received a mere 563 inmates (108,268 were relieved in Ulster's workhouses in this year) while costing ratepayers £672.[16] By 1920, ten Ulster boards of guardians either fully closed their institutions or boarded out healthy inmates. This locally driven measure was largely an Ulster development, and only ten boards of guardians introduced similar changes in the rest of Ireland.[17]

Boards of guardians' focus in Ulster on the reduction of poor law expenditure can be partly explained as a longer-term regional trend in poor relief. Late-nineteenth- and early-twentieth-century boards of guardians in Ulster were marked by fiscal parsimony, and expenditure on poor relief was lower than in the south and west of Ireland.[18] Ulster's lower poor relief expenditure was driven by numerous factors, including a greater ethos of Protestant 'self-help', often informed by sectarian tensions, and fears over fuelling inward migration from rural to urban regions. Furthermore, some Ulster poor law unions, especially those with a large Catholic population, were often poorer and could not afford to grant extensive relief.[19] The political composition of local boards of guardians was also important. In many areas with low expenditure, a residual socially conservative landlord class with little appetite for expanding provision remained in power into the early twentieth century.[20] The reduction of poor relief expenditure, often in sparsely populated regions with fully staffed workhouses that were scantly used, was a clear motivation for the full or partial closure of such facilities.[21]

The picture of boards of guardians controlled by socially conservative, largely Protestant, Ulster Unionists, who were driven by parsimony and aversion to investing in local healthcare, is, however, far from accurate. The historian Olwen Purdue has highlighted regional differences in poor law provision in pre-partition Ulster. Many boards of guardians in the east of Ulster, specifically in County Antrim, had come under the authority of middle-class political groupings before the similar transfer of power from the landed elite, albeit via nationalist politics, in Ireland's other provinces in the 1880s.[22] In contrast, the poor law in the west and south of the province continued to be run by the landlord class. This was due to a combination of economic and political factors. The west and south of Ulster were predominantly agricultural areas where the landlord class's power on boards of guardians persisted into the twentieth century. Unlike other parts of rural Ireland, where tenant farmers challenged the power of landlords on boards of guardians, unionist farmers' support for the landlord class solidified in the face of the emergence of nationalist politics.[23] While some areas in eastern Ulster, such as Ballymoney and Ballycastle, were also predominantly agricultural economies and, in the case of the latter, had a majority Catholic population, much of the region was industrialised where textile production was tied to a provincial linen industry and international market. Industrial and market towns such as Antrim, Ballymena, Lisburn and Portadown were the urban centres of this economic activity.[24] Much of eastern Ulster had a large unionist and Protestant majority with no substantial nationalist movement for landlords to rally opposition around locally. In turn, a mercantile and a middle class in towns and larger farmers in rural areas challenged the power of landlords on boards of guardians. The removal of the social elite from the running of boards of guardians at times led to a more liberal operation of the poor laws, evident in the election of female members after women were granted the right to sit on boards in 1896.[25] Liberal and female influence often led to more flexible, compassionate and progressive relief regimes in eastern areas compared to the harsher, socially conservative boards in the southern and western parts of Ulster.[26]

Traditions of more progressive poor law administrations in the east of Ulster were also evident in the development of poor law medical services, chiefly in the industrialised areas of County Antrim. In 1912, the Ballymena Board of Guardians agreed to build a new separate infirmary next to the workhouse. An extensive, populous and prosperous poor law union, the LGB sought the Ballymena Board to upgrade its existing medical services. The guardians agreed to build a new hospital at a cost of £6,000, provided through a loan from the LGB. During debates among the Ballymena Guardians, a clear commitment to delivering better hospital care for the sick poor was articulated. One guardian, Mr MacAuley, complained that conditions in the old infirmary made it a 'death trap'. Another guardian, Mr Kennedy, highlighted the mixing of ordinary and tuberculosis patients in the workhouse infirmary and stated that in the 'interests of Christianity' a new facility was needed. One of the strongest advocates for the new infirmary came from an LGB inspector named F. J. McCarthy. He reminded the guardians of their medical responsibilities and that 'in the interest of humanity alone it was necessary to see that the sick poor received every possible attention'. He maintained that a new hospital would be separate from the main workhouse building and that 'people could enter without feeling in any way that they were workhouse inmates, or they could be regarded as paupers'. McCarthy highlighted that the 'respectable poor' wished to receive non-stigmatising medical care which did not 'impair … their self-respect'.[27] The guardians agreed to build the new hospital, which opened in 1915. The newly named Waveney Hospital had eighty-eight beds and was modernised with electricity and x-ray machines. The guardians sought to enhance the interior, so much of the hospital, including the operating theatre, was covered with terrazzo paving and the wards with pitch pine wood.[28] Such an interior contrasted greatly with the harsh, austere mid-nineteenth-century workhouse. The new hospital was a positive step in poor law hospital services in Ballymena. It provided up-to-date and modern care, which separated the relief of poverty and medical provision while significantly weakening the stigma associated with poor law care. These local reforms were primarily justified by guardians and officials on the grounds of compassion and the wish to provide modern hospital care to the sick and poor.

Ballymena Workhouse, now free of all acute sick patients, developed as a centralised institution which received non-acute patients and inmates from neighbouring workhouses. In 1917, the Larne Board of Guardians decided to focus their institution solely on the sick poor while sending other, healthy inmates to Ballymena permanently. Thomas Nelson, clerk of the Larne Board of Guardians, believed this measure would remove the 'stigma of pauperism' and lead to an 'up-to-date and useful institution'. He argued that 'no institution for the treatment of the sick should be connected with the workhouse'.[29] Similar agreements were made for Ballymena Workhouse to receive inmates from Antrim, Ballymoney and Lisburn so that these workhouses could focus on solely providing medical care. These arrangements effectively brought about the local merging of poor law services, which allowed boards of guardians to concentrate on the sick poor while centralising other categories of inmates, especially the able-bodied poor, in a single institution in Ballymena.

The creation of Ballymena Workhouse as a centralised institution for the ordinary and non-acute sick inmates from four County Antrim poor law unions represented the local implementation of the policy recommendations of the Edwardian poor law commissions in Ireland and Britain. These not only sought the separation of medical care from ordinary relief but also the coming together of workhouses. While these policies were sought across the UK, they were not acted upon by the Westminster government during the 1910s. These changes also provided the basis for a multitiered poor law hospital system, which would become more pronounced during the interwar years. One tier of institutions solely focused on providing medical care, while other categories of inmates were either boarded out or centralised in institutions such as the Ballymena Workhouse. The second tier continued to provide mixed medical care in workhouses that offered inferior treatment for patients.

Poor law reform and the Irish Revolution

After the First World War, it was widely recognised that medical services in Ireland needed reform. The 1920 Irish Public Health Council recommended that the Westminster parliament introduce a bill to establish an Irish Ministry of Health like that created in England and Wales the previous year. It was envisaged that this central authority would bring about a coordinated health structure.[30] Before such legislation was introduced, major political transformations occurred. After the 1918 general election, Irish politics radically altered with the election of a majority of Sinn Féin members of parliament (MPs) committed to the establishment of an Irish republic, independent of the British Empire. Political violence soon engulfed much of the country, and the years between 1919 and 1923 have been termed the 'Irish Revolution' by historians. Irish republicans presumed that Ireland was a clear victim of English colonialism.[31] Through this prism, the poor law represented the harshness of British colonialism, and republicans vilified its administration as corrupt and immoral.[32] Reform of the poor law was a significant plank of the revolutionaries' social policies, and the 1919 Democratic Programme of the first meeting of the Irish revolutionary Dáil Éireann called for its replacement with a 'native, sympathetic scheme'. Reform was introduced initially by the revolutionary government and subsequently by the Irish Free State, which led to extensive administrative change, separation of medical care from ordinary relief in most institutions and a greater emphasis on the relief of the poor and sick in their own homes rather than institutional settings.[33]

The reforms were diluted by the deleterious finances of the newly independent Free State and the fiscal conservatism of the ruling Cumann na nGaedheal government. Yet the Free State's break-up of the poor law was significant. It preceded similar reforms in Britain, which did not come about until the 1929 Local Government Acts, which were separately enacted in Scotland, and England and Wales. Irish Free State reformers framed these as newly acquired benefits that were won through Irish independence. Such rhetoric was reflective of wider transnational trends in which increased citizenship rights for everyday people led to attempts to transform stigmatising relief systems to more substantial and progressive health and welfare regimes.[34] Yet the underpinning motivations for reform were complex and partly driven by the new state's economic challenges and need to reduce the cost of services and lingering concepts of the deserving and undeserving poor. Medical services for the acute and chronic sick were centralised in newly named county hospitals and homes, and more peripheral infirmaries focused solely on minor treatments. The closure of long-stay beds negatively impacted remote regions and often met with much local resistance. For example, in the early 1930s in the Atlantic seaboard County Kerry, there were calls to reopen wards in the Dingle District Hospital for long-stay patients instead of sending them to Killarney, located over forty miles away. Communication from the self-styled 'oppressed and infirm people of the western seaboard' complained to the local authorities: 'men and women, Irish speakers born and reared in the stronghold of the Gael have been forcibly ejected from the hospital at Dingle, compelled by brute force to leave their native heath and conveyed to the county home in Killarney'.[35] The anti-poor law rhetoric of reformers often did not correspond with the everyday and harsh realities associated with the closure of long-standing institutional provision.

Such central government reform was not forthcoming in the newly established Northern Ireland. The architects of the new northern state were primarily interested in quelling political and violent threats from Irish republicans. They had little interest or capacity to bring about significant social reform. Instead, reform was left in the hands of individual boards of guardians. As discussed later in this chapter, many of the areas of Northern Ireland with large Catholic populations, primarily in the west and south, were engulfed with political division, which dampened the potential for local government reform. This contrasted with the east of Northern Ireland, where the largely unionist and Protestant population ensured that nationalist–unionist divisions did not engulf boards of guardians.

The politically quiescent boards of guardians in the east had a far greater appetite to reform poor law medical services during the 1920s and 1930s. While the Northern Ireland government failed to introduce reform from above, boards of guardians turned to existing legislation under the 1898 Local Government (Ireland) Act. This allowed for the conversion of workhouses into district hospitals, the replacement of boards of guardians with boards of management/governors and the boarding-out of non-medical cases in other workhouses. Prior to partition, boards of guardians were largely insouciant towards the permissive legislation, and by 1919, only the Castlecomer Board of Guardians in County Kilkenny had introduced the measure.[36] In the vacuum of central government reform, it was adopted locally in Northern Ireland during the interwar years. From 1920 to 1940, twelve workhouses were transformed into district hospitals in the region.

Ten of the twelve poor law unions which implemented the reform had a Protestant majority population. As detailed in Table 1.2, boards of guardians in Antrim showed the greatest capacity for reform, and by 1929, six of the county's workhouses – Belfast was the exception – had become district hospitals. Two workhouses in County Down, one in Armagh and one in Banbridge also became district hospitals. The Limavady Guardians established a district hospital, also a unionist and Protestant majority region, in the northern part of County Derry/Londonderry. The only poor law unions with a Catholic majority that set up district hospitals were in Kilkeel in south County Down and Strabane, which bordered County Donegal in the Free State, in Tyrone in the west of Ulster. The establishment of district hospitals was, by and large, implemented by boards of guardians that were unionist in outlook, while areas with nationalist and Catholic majorities remained reliant on workhouses.

District hospitals had far better standards of care than workhouse infirmaries. As the interwar period progressed, boards of guardians invested significant amounts of money to upgrade their workhouse infirmaries into district hospitals. For example, the Larne Board of Guardians expended almost £45,000 to establish a district hospital, financed by £38,000 in loans to be repaid by the ratepayers and £7,000 in a labour grant from the government. Parts of the original workhouse were abolished or renovated, and a new wing was added, leading to a refurbished 100-bed hospital.[37] Another example was the renovated Newtownards Workhouse infirmary, renamed Ards District Hospital, which opened in 1932 at a cost of close to £50,000.[38] The hospital provided general medical and surgical treatment along with maternity and children's wards, and it was replete with an operating theatre and x-ray department. The refurbishment aesthetically transformed the former workhouse's

Table 1.2 Workhouses that were converted into district hospitals between 1920 and 1940, and religious breakdown of poor law unions.

County	*Poor law union*	*District hospital*	*Established*	*Religious breakdown**	
			(Year)	*Protestant*	*Catholic*
Antrim	Antrim	Massereene	1921	**25,149**	4,901
Antrim	Lisburn	Lisburn and Hillsborough	1920	**41,246**	8,100
Antrim	Larne	Larne	1929	**28,218**	6,196
Antrim	Ballycastle	Dalriada	1923	**6,476**	5,717
Antrim	Ballymoney	Route	1924	**22,130**	5,294
Antrim	Ballymena	Waveney	1921	**40,203**	10,115
Armagh	Lurgan	Lurgan and Portadown	1937	**36,568**	14,023
Derry	Limavady	Roe Valley	1930	**10,178**	8,923
Down	Newtownards	Ards	1932	**41,176**	3,164
Down	Kilkeel	Mourne	1927	8,076	**10,001**
Down/Armagh	Banbridge	Banbridge	1932	**30,016**	10,115
Tyrone	Strabane	Strabane	1922	10,303	**14,336**

Source: Ministry of Home Affairs, *Report on the Administration of Local Government Services in Northern Ireland, 1921/3–1937/8*.

interior. All windows had double sashes, and some were designed to give ventilation and glazed with vitaglass, which was a recently developed ultraviolet ray glass believed to have therapeutic qualities.[39] Walls were painted a 'sun colour' against 'natural teak doors', and floors were carpeted. This helped to address the phenomenological and environmental harshness of the interior of the former workhouse. It was fully modernised, with heat and electricity provided by a power plant on site.[40] Also, the Banbridge District Hospital was opened in 1932 at a cost of circa £70,000. The reconstructions were so extensive that inspectors from the Nuffield Trust commented in the early 1940s that 'little of the original workhouse [was] left'.[41] The large sums of money invested by boards of guardians ensured that the renovation of former workhouses significantly altered these institutions. No longer did they suffer from the stigma of the poor law. At the same time, the separation of ordinary relief and medical care was achieved, resulting in a fundamental reform of local poor law services.

Significant progress in diagnostics and staffing was also apparent in district hospitals. Many such hospitals outsourced laboratory and pathology diagnostic services. For example, the Ballymoney District Hospital sent specimens to Belfast for testing. Ballymena had some in-house facilities for routine bacteriological testing, while more complex specimens were sent to Queen's University in Belfast.[42] Such arrangements ensured that many district hospitals had access to the most advanced methods of diagnosing disease. The medical staffing in district hospitals also grew. Some hospitals employed visiting consultants and specialists to provide a level of expertise not previously associated with poor law provision. This was evident in the Ards District Hospital, which paid for visiting specialists from Belfast in medicine, ophthalmology, ear, nose and throat disease, dermatology, obstetrics and antenatal care. It also employed a senior medical officer, appointed when the institution opened in 1932. By the early 1940s, three house surgeons were also employed in the hospital.[43] The Lurgan and Portadown District Hospital was another facility that had access to much specialism, including a surgeon, a chief medical officer and two house doctors. More complicated cases were referred to voluntary hospitals in Belfast.[44] By 1942, a leading Northern Irish medic named Dr Frank P. Montgomery, a consultant radiologist in the Royal

Victoria Hospital, opined that district hospitals were 'fully modern and fully equipped for almost every type of general and specialised work'.[45] The enhanced standard of treatment in district hospitals ensured that they became popular with a broad proportion of the population. This was evident in the total numbers that turned to district hospitals, which grew almost fourfold from 3,545 in 1925–26 to over 12,300 by 1935–36 (see Table 1.3). The success of district hospitals was widely articulated. By the mid-1920s, the Ministry of Home Affairs reported that there was a 'steady increase' in the number of patients who turned to the former workhouses, and they were 'much appreciated by the residents in the several localities where they have been established'.[46] In 1930, the *Belfast News-Letter* proclaimed that the creation of district hospitals since the establishment of Northern Ireland was a 'great change for the better'.[47] The Nuffield inspectors commended district hospitals as a 'very great success'.[48] District hospitals emerged as well-equipped sites in which patients had access to modern medical technology, pathological and laboratory science, and increased medical staff including consultants and specialists.

Table 1.3 Number of patients in Northern Ireland's district hospitals, 1926/7–35/6.

District hospital	*1926–27*	*1929–30*	*1932–33*	*1935–36*
Massereene	654	733	755	954
Dalriada	329	361	389	476
Waveney	939	1,166	1,244	1,257
Route	303	337	474	709
Larne	–	–	765	1,202
Lisburn and Hillsborough	859	843	1,125	1,496
Roe Valley	–	–		632
Ards	–	–	1,764	2,803
Mourne	–	211	188	236
Banbridge	–	–	367	1,759
Strabane	461	230	563	840
Total	3,545	3,881	7,634	12,364

Source: Ministry of Home Affairs, *Report on the Administration of Local Government Services, 1921/3–1937/8.*

These improvements meant that district hospitals also appealed to not just the poorer classes but a broad social cohort, many of whom previously shunned poor law medical services. After the Lurgan and Portadown District Hospital was established, a poor law guardian named G. A. Locke believed that the hospital would treat 'rich and poor'.[49] Similarly, one letter writer to the local press in Ballymoney believed that Route District Hospital received patients from not just the poor but also 'the better class', including farmers, businesspeople and professionals.[50] Under the regulations, district hospitals had to relieve the sick poor first but, space permitting, could admit private patients who were to be treated in separate wards. Private doctors could treat and admit their patients, whereas previously, admission was done through a relieving officer who tested the patients' eligibility based on poverty.[51] Official policy encouraged the expansion of pay beds, and in 1927, the Local Government Commission recommended that district hospitals provide 'private' or 'semi-private' wards for better-off patients.[52] The trend of paying patients became more prominent as the district hospitals developed. As delineated in Table 1.4, in 1925, district hospitals generated £2,879 in charges, which grew to £19,541 by 1938. The admission of patients with greater means led government officials to report that district hospitals were 'meeting the needs of many persons who were reluctant to enter the old workhouse infirmaries'.[53] Many patients in district hospitals now paid or financially contributed to their care. For example, on 31 March 1935, the majority of patients – thirty-three of fifty-six patients – in Larne District Hospital made full or partial payment for their treatment.[54] Many of the private patients were not overly wealthy but often 'persons of small or moderate means'.[55]

An important motivation for boards of guardians to establish district hospitals was the greater capacity for private pay beds than in workhouses. This appealed to guardians who identified patient fees as an income generator. In 1920, the Strabane Board of Guardians believed that their planned district hospital would receive patients who were 'willing and able to pay thirty shillings per week'.[56] Such a growth in patient fee payment was also evident in interwar local authority healthcare in other jurisdictions. Poor law medical reform in the Irish Free State led to an increase in patient payment and broadened the social status of local authority patients.[57] During the interwar period, hospital provision became attractive to many who were not poor or destitute. District hospitals in Northern Ireland helped to provide acute hospital care for the respectable working and lower-middle classes who historically avoided the stigmatising poor law. The district hospital movement was as much about providing modern acute care to a wider social cohort as about enhancing provision for the poor.

In 1925, the Northern Irish government established the aforementioned Departmental Commission on Local Government Administration in Northern Ireland, which was tasked with examining all aspects of local government. The thirty-member Commission – chaired by Prof. R. J. Johnstone, who was MP for Queen's University, a gynaecologist and a leading member of the BMA, becoming its president in 1937 – convened for over two years and published its report in 1927. The Commission's recommendations were far-reaching and included the total abolition of workhouses, establishment of central homes for the relief of the able-bodied, separation of domiciliary medical care from the ordinary relief of destitution and creation of an efficient hospital scheme. The Commission's overriding recommendation was to remove the 'pauper taint' from welfare and healthcare provision.[58] Yet, the government failed to implement any of these reforms. Instead, local guardians set about reforming local provision, which one official from the Ministry of Home Affairs, D. L. Clarke, believed was 'in accordance with modern ideas and the general desire to separate the relief given under the poor law from hospital treatment'.[59] District hospitals represented the local implementation of policies articulated but not implemented by the central government. While the Northern Irish government faltered in developing hospital provision, some boards of guardians willingly stepped into the breach and established modernised and reformed local hospitals. In the face of ineffectual central government action, some boards proved innovative and dynamic.

A multitude of factors underpinned these locally driven reforms. Renovated district hospitals were expensive capital projects which were funded mainly by loans that were repaid by ratepayers, who were often more noted for keeping local taxation as low as possible. In turn, a degree of social and political collegiality in areas that were predominantly unionist and Protestant helped to secure support for these costly projects. Politically, local authorities were controlled mainly by unionists and had little challenge from nationalism. The Ulster Unionist Party faced disparate challenges from within the broad unionist political tradition along economic, religious, loyalist, liberal and labourist strands of opinion. Furthermore, independent unionists were elected to the Stormont parliament and local authorities.[60] Yet since the threat of home rule in early 1910s, unionists of different hues demonstrated considerable capacity to coalesce around the constitutional question which helped to quell divisions emanating from diverse interests.[61] Indeed, older traditions of radicalism and liberal unionism were often subsumed into the Ulster Unionist Party.[62] Divisions within unionism did not impede the creation of district hospitals. For example, the long-standing Newtownards poor law guardian, Thomas Bailie, was pivotal to the establishment of the Ards District Hospital, becoming vice-chairman of its first board of governors in 1932. He was also an independent unionist and successfully won a Stormont seat for North Down in 1941.[63] In this instance, political differences amongst unionists did not hamper the development of the district hospital. Also, guardians' decisions in unionist areas often reflected a high degree of collegiality and a desire to bring about more equitable health provision for local populations. Such sentiment was evident at the official opening of the Larne District Hospital in 1931 when the vice-chairman of the board of guardians, Mr C. M. Legg, described how the 'new hospital proved they were coming to see that the good of each was the good of all, that the health of the individual was the health of the community, that they loved not as individuals but as a corporate body'.[64] This rhetoric was reminiscent of a communitarian desire to unite and foster social bonds, albeit within predominantly unionist areas, through the provision of healthcare.

A pan-class movement of local hospital reform was evident, which drew support from not just locally elected guardians but also the upper classes. District hospitals now received philanthropy and charity redolent of the patrician and socially hierarchical voluntary sector. The Dalriada District Hospital received donations for its newly built facilities in 1922 and was gifted funds in 1925 to benefit 'the sick and suffering in the district'.[65] In 1933, the new Lurgan District Hospital received a gift of new x-ray equipment, valued at £1,000, from Ms Warring from a wealthy family associated with the linen industry.[66] Subsequently, the chairman of the Lurgan Board of Guardians, S. J. Wilson, described as a 'strong unionist and Orangeman', called on the 'merchant and linen lords' to contribute and provide charity for the district hospital.[67] District hospitals also received charitable bequests, such as in 1935 when the Larne District Hospital received £250 in the legacy of a deceased merchant named Alexander Holmes McMeekin.[68] This was a new departure from poor law medicine, which was reliant on funding from poor law rates. Such social collegiality was helped by the predominance of unionists and Protestants in these areas, ensuring that boards of guardians were not subject to the entrenched political and religious divisions evident in other parts of Northern Ireland. Similarly, labour politics were not overly influential in debates and motivations in reforming local hospital services. This contrasted with Belfast, where the labour movement was much more substantial and clear divisions existed among the Northern Ireland Labour Party and unionists in local health policies, which are discussed in Chapter 2. District hospitals drew support from across the social classes and combined upper-class philanthropic support with the efforts of elected local authorities.

Other motivating factors underpinning reform included civic pride combined with an intense localism. Local officials and politicians often boasted about their new hospitals. The Newtownards Guardians declared their aim was that the hospital 'should rank among the most up-to-date institutions'; a view endorsed by the Ministry of Home Affairs, Richard Dawson Bates, who specified it 'would stand second to none in the British Isles' at its official opening.[69] Local rivalries coloured much of the guardians' thinking, and many were propelled into action over fears that other areas would steal a march in hospital reform. The Lurgan Guardians started planning for a new hospital after cryptic claims that 'influences' orchestrated that a hospital was planned elsewhere to the detriment of the area.[70] When the hospital was completed, the chairman of the Lurgan Guardians believed the new institution 'would be the best in Ulster'.[71] Notions of civic pride, institutional loyalties and localism were very strong factors that brought about the reform of local poor law. Like developments in Britain, such reforms depicted a commitment on the part of the local authorities to a movement towards positive improvements in healthcare.[72]

District hospitals were significant attempts at local healthcare reforms, but they were not without major flaws. Firstly, there was a general lack of planning beyond the local which solidified fragmentation in the management of local authority hospitals. International health policy leanings had increasingly promulgated the regionalisation of care, in which interconnected hospital systems for large geographical areas, often organised around a teaching hospital, were viewed as the most efficient and effective method of organising provision. Such an approach was promoted in the UK's 1920 Dawson Report, although regionalisation of health services did not come about until the 1940s. In Northern Ireland, policies to merge local authority hospital services were aired by the 1927 Commission on Local Government Administration. Concerned with the multiplication of local authorities, lack of coordination and overlapping hospital administrations, the Commission's report recommended far-reaching administrative reforms. These included the abolition of boards of guardians, the joining up of all local authority health services under a single committee and medical officer of health at the county council level. This committee would have financial control, appoint officials and plan the hospital needs of each county in a 'uniform system of administration'.[73] This proposal was a radical restructuring of local government health provision, that had the potential to introduce an integrated hospital model, in which services were planned with the view of maximising the efficient use of beds and resources. However, legislation to bring about these reforms was not forthcoming. Instead, a highly localised regime, managed by individual local boards of management and governors, became entrenched. Boards of guardians also largely ignored other providers, including cottage hospitals and county infirmaries (focused on in Chapter 3). This often duplicated services available in towns, leading to competing interests and rivalries between institutions and localities. This was a missed opportunity and embedded traditions of localism and institutional loyalty in the management of hospital services, which would impede future attempts at greater coordination.

A second major problem facing the new district hospitals was how local authorities cared for longer-term or chronic patients, traditionally categorised as the 'aged and infirm' under the poor law. In Britain, the general concern was the achievement of a modern hospital service that provided short-term, acute and often successful medical interventions rather than low-level, long-term chronic care. As outlined by the historian Alysa Levene, the break-up of the poor law in 1929 in England and Wales led to better care for acute patients but not for the chronic and older poor. Levene noted that the 'residuum of the poor law' received second-class provision in low-quality and unmodernised buildings.[74] Authorities were less motivated to invest in costly and long-term treatment of illness associated with older persons, long-term physical impairments and mental health problems in need of complex social and medical support.[75] Similar trends were evident in Northern Ireland, where new district hospitals were primarily established to treat the acute and infectious sick. As already explained, many boards of guardians paid for their older and chronic inmates to be maintained in other workhouses. This was the case in County Antrim, where Ballymena Workhouse had become a centralised institution of sorts, which, since the 1910s, received ordinary 'inmates' from neighbouring boards of guardians.[76] Institutions that remained workhouses were inevitably lower quality buildings, lacked investment and had minimal staff, ensuring that many older and chronic patients received inferior care in direct contrast to treatment in the modernised district hospitals.

The separate treatment and management of chronic and acute illness proved challenging to maintain. The reality was that many chronic long-term patients suffered acute episodes and needed access to district hospitals, while others developed ongoing care needs as inpatients. In turn, many chronic patients continued to be treated in district hospitals. This drew criticism from many medics who saw chronic, incurable patients as blocking beds that would be better utilised for younger, acute patients.[77] GPs in Ballymoney complained to the Route Hospital's Board of Management that the prevalence of 'chronic' patients attenuated the facility's intended focus on acute care and that it was in danger of 'reverting back to the status of a workhouse infirmary'.[78] The Nuffield Trust identified the 'old and infirm' as making up many district hospital patients who were only 'in hospital because no other proper accommodation [was] available'. It called for the establishment of separate homes for such cases to 'relieve the more expensive hospital beds'.[79] The prevalence of chronic patients in district facilities portrayed the difficulty local authorities had in transforming institutions which had traditions of chronic care into fully acute hospitals. Despite the protestations of some medics, many patients with longer-term needs continued to be treated in the newly reformed district hospitals.

The district hospital ideal of acute care was further undermined by the failure to develop long-stay alternatives. The 1927 Commission into Local Government Administration sought the relief of long-term patients in county homes, like those developed in the Irish Free State, that would act as a mixed institution, freeing up district hospitals to focus on acute care.[80] However, the failure to act on the 1927 Commission meant that county homes were never introduced in Northern Ireland, leaving the outdated and inadequate unreformed workhouses to serve, unsuitably, as mixed institutions. By the 1940s, the Nuffield inspectors argued that the voluntary sector should offer such provision and highlighted the religious-run Bethany Home in Northampton, England, as an example. Such institutional long-stay provision was hampered by only 650 voluntary beds available in Northern Ireland.[81] Patients with congenital intellectual disabilities were housed in some district hospitals. This was exacerbated by Northern Ireland's lack of separate institutional provision for the intellectually disabled, which existed in Britain under mental deficiency legislation.[82] Medics and hospital administrators' capacity to remove longer-term patients was curbed by the lack of specialised institutional care outside of the stigmatising workhouses. The specialised medical field of gerontology and treatment of illness associated with old age had yet to gain traction, and the health outcomes of chronic patients were modest, increasing their reliance on institutional care. It was not until the post-war years that policymakers focused on deinstitutionalisation and the creation of alternative domiciliary provision. The obstinance of long-term patients in hospitals designed for the acute sick was not confined to Northern Ireland. It was also evident in the Irish Free State where 'mixed' provision persisted in some areas.[83] Similarly, the 1929 reforms in Britain were weakened by the ongoing need to care for older persons and chronic patients in former workhouses in trends which continued into the latter twentieth century.[84] Northern Irish boards of guardians that sought to reshape institutions into modern acute hospitals were not alone in finding the separate treatment and management of acute and chronic patients elusive. However, central government's lack of action hindered them more.

Workhouse infirmaries

In many areas, workhouse infirmaries remained unreformed, leading to inferior care and conditions compared to the upgraded district hospitals. Thirteen workhouses remained in Northern Ireland by the late 1930s. Four workhouses were in areas with unionist and Protestant majorities. Outside Belfast, these three workhouses – Coleraine, Ballymena and Armagh – all acted as centralised facilities that took inmates and long-term chronic patients from other institutions that had been transformed into district hospitals. While district hospitals provided modernised acute care, workhouse infirmaries represented local authority failure to reform and invest in services for local populations. The inferiority of workhouse infirmaries was based on multiple factors. Firstly, many workhouses continued to act as mixed institutions. As outlined in Table 1.1, workhouses increasingly catered for the sick. Still, other categories, including older people, children (often born out of wedlock), intellectually disabled and able-bodied continued to be relieved, albeit in reduced numbers as the period progressed. The mixing of these categories of inmates with the sick under one roof ensured that medical treatment remained associated with the relief of poverty and was inherently stigmatising. Secondly, conditions were exacerbated by many boards of guardians' failure to invest in austere and dated workhouses. In 1938, Dr Leonard Kidd deprecated workhouse infirmaries for being 'unfit in structure and equipment for modern medical and surgical work'. He highlighted that some were lit by oil lamps and lacked telephones.[85] Kidd was a leading medical

Table 1.4 Breakdown of income sources for district hospitals in 1925, 1932 and 1938.

	1925	*1932*	*1938*
	£	£	£
From guardians	19,972	25,361	70,212
Hospital charges	2,879	5,293	19,541
Other receipts	1,818	2,965	1,999
Total	24,669	33,619	91,752

Source: Ministry of Home Affairs, *Report on the Administration of Local Government Services, in Northern Ireland 1921/3–1937/8*.

Table 1.5 Unreformed workhouse infirmaries and religious breakdown of poor law unions in Northern Ireland, 1921–40.

County	*Poor law union*	*Religious breakdown**	
		Catholic	*Protestant and other*
Antrim	Ballymena**	10,115	**40,203**
Antrim	Belfast	97,096	**311,457**
Armagh	Armagh	19,249	**24,860**
Derry	Magherafelt	**19,139**	16,968
Derry	Coleraine	6,486	**23,269**
Derry	Londonderry	**29,838**	25,355
Down	Downpatrick	19,229	**19,967**
Down	Newry	**32,969**	16,425
Fermanagh	Enniskillen	**12,501**	11,256
Fermanagh	Lisnaskea	**14,162**	9,078
Tyrone	Omagh	**24,672**	15,683
Tyrone	Dungannon	**15,868**	14,382
Tyrone	Castlederg	**5,717**	5,493
Tyrone	Clogher	**6,982**	6,762

Source: Ministry of Home Affairs, *Report on the Administration of Local Government Services in Northern Ireland, 1921/3–1937/8.*

* These figures are based on the 1911 census and published in the North-Eastern Boundary Bureau, *Handbook of the Ulster Question* (Dublin: Stationery Office, 1923), p. 51.

** The Ballymena workhouse was a separate institution to the Waveney District Hospital.

professional and BMA member who had been a prominent figure in the poor law 'strike' of 1902–4, when doctors throughout Ireland sought increased remuneration.[86] The Nuffield Trust was even more scathing of workhouse infirmaries and stated: 'the interior, to modern eyes, is frankly repellent ... [with] primitive types of sanitary appliances coupled with the all-pervading odour of carbolic acid combine to make these workhouse barracks repulsive to those of us who live in happier circumstances'.[87] Unrenovated mid-nineteenth-century workhouses were far from appropriate surroundings for the treatment of the sick. These harsh environments contrasted greatly with the upgraded district hospitals, in which a greater emphasis on patients' phenomenology led to far superior interiors. Desultory underinvestment and neglect of workhouses ensured that the stigmatising taint of poverty remained associated with such provision.

Furthermore, medical care in workhouse infirmaries was even more greatly diminished by the lack of medical staff, which contrasted with the growth in general, specialist and consultancy medical services in district hospitals. Kidd complained that many workhouse infirmaries were without a resident medical official.[88] The lack of medical staff was evident in larger city workhouses as well as smaller institutions. For example, there was only one full-time medical officer in the 107-bed Derry/Londonderry city workhouse infirmary, named 'Waterside', which was reliant on visiting medics.[89] Rudimentary medical expertise was compounded by reliance on outdated equipment. For example, the Nuffield Trust described how the 'cold and dark' 195-bed Dungannon Workhouse did not establish an x-ray facility until the 1940s and had a 'primitive' and rarely used operating theatre.[90] The lack of medical expertise and equipment restricted the capacity of workhouse infirmaries to provide acute care, ensuring that many patients in these institutions were invariably the chronically sick poor. The prominence of chronic, often older patients contributed to these institutions' high mortality rates. In 1938, workhouses had 2,317 deaths, which made up 13 per cent of all deaths in Northern Ireland and was nearly three times greater than the 832 deaths in the twelve district hospitals.[91] Many workhouse infirmaries were rudimentary with insufficient medical expertise, equipment and harsh interiors, which meant that this tier of provision was inferior to the better-developed district hospitals.

Some boards of guardians made investments in their infirmaries, resulting in modest improvements in the standard of care provided. The Newry Guardians received a loan of £25,000 in 1934 to invest in the infirmary and build a nurses' home.[92] The Nuffield inspectors recognised that reconstructed poor law infirmaries were 'some of the most comfortable and attractive hospitals' that they viewed.[93] While the Belfast Board of Guardians had an infamously parsimonious poor relief regime, it was more willing to invest in developing the infirmary, spending £198,192 on 'improvements and extensions' between 1925 and 1932.[94] Yet the continued association with the poor law ensured that workhouse provision, even in more modernised infirmaries, remained stigmatising.

A key factor in boards of guardians' failure to reform workhouse infirmaries was the political and religious divisions that enveloped

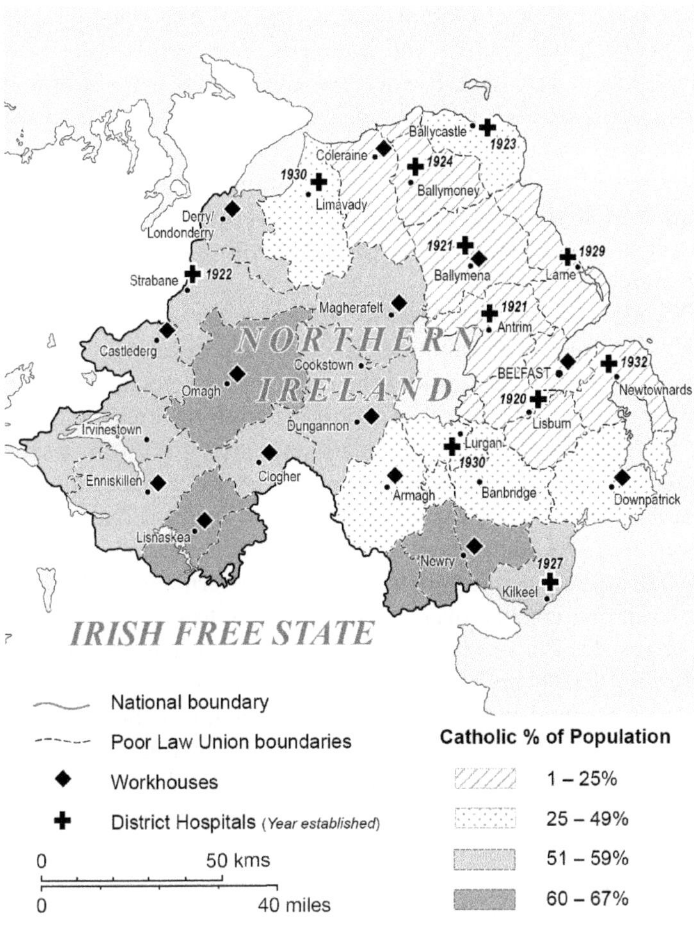

Map 1.1 Workhouses and district hospitals and religious composition of poor law unions, 1939. *Source:* See source in Table 1.5.

much of Northern Ireland. Firstly, most workhouses were in counties in the south and west of Northern Ireland, which had a large Catholic and nationalist population. As outlined in Table 1.5, nine out of thirteen (excluding the Belfast workhouse, which was an exception due to its size) workhouse infirmaries were in poor law unions with majority Catholic populations. Many of these areas were marked by much upheaval during the years of the Irish

Revolution, followed by entrenched political and religious bitterness between nationalists and unionists. The former were on the losing side of the Irish Revolution and partition for whom the creation of Northern Ireland was catastrophic, and which was to be challenged and discredited. These political circumstances contrasted greatly with most regions that established district hospitals, which were characterised by more collegial political and social relations cushioned by unionist majorities that supported the Northern Irish state.

During the Irish Revolution, nationalist areas witnessed much political tumult and militarisation, which negatively impacted poor law medical services and the capacity for reform. The British military took over some workhouses, mainly in areas with large Catholic and nationalist populations where the war between Britain and Irish republicans was intense. A 1922 inspection of the Lisnaskea Workhouse, partially occupied by the British army, in the border area of County Fermanagh, revealed egregious conditions. Officials in the nascent Northern Ireland government's Ministry of Home Affairs reported overcrowding in the infirmary, including the use of a bathroom as a schoolroom and the fact that the nurses' sitting room was in the master's office. Precariously, the laundry for the fever hospital was undertaken in the main hospital's kitchen, risking cross infection.[95] The workhouse in Newry in County Down was close to the border and was taken over by the army after the dissolution of the board of guardians by the Northern Irish government. It was the scene of attempted bomb attacks by republicans, including a mine attack in 1922.[96] The use of workhouses by the military also obstructed attempts to introduce reforms. In Strabane in County Tyrone, the military's occupation of the workhouse in 1921 impacted the guardians' plans to transform the building into a district hospital.[97] Efforts at developing the district hospital were further undermined by another military takeover of the institution in February 1922.[98] The Strabane Guardians were determined to reform their infirmary and 'get the taint of the workhouse from the hospital'. In early 1922, they succeeded in establishing a district hospital, one of the few workhouse infirmaries that were reformed in nationalist areas.[99] While the Strabane Guardians forced through reforms, the militarisation of the era undercut the capacity of workhouse infirmaries to enhance provision and care. This contrasted with regions of the new Northern Irish state which experienced little, if any, disruption, such as County Antrim, where boards of guardians were busily planning and implementing reforms.

Disorder surrounding partition impacted local authority medical services most severely in parts of the new Northern Irish state where local government became a focal point for political and sectarian tensions. Prior to Irish partition, republicans won power on many local authority bodies, which subsequently declared allegiance to the revolutionary Dáil Éireann parliament in Dublin. After partition, the Free State and Northern Ireland governments targeted political dissent at a local government level. In the Free State, the power of local authorities was attenuated through temporary dissolutions in areas that sided against the government in the Irish Civil War.[100] By the late 1920s, the Irish Free State further eroded local government power, centralised appointments of senior local government officials and introduced full-time managers into local administration.[101] These helped to centralise power and dispel potential political dissent from the local state.[102] In Northern Ireland, many nationalist local authorities, primarily in the counties in the west including Tyrone, Fermanagh and Derry/Londonderry, refused to recognise the Northern Irish state and pledged allegiance to the Irish Free State. In turn, politically dissenting local authorities were temporarily dissolved and placed in the hands of full-time officials called administrative commissioners. For example, the Strabane Board of Guardians was disbanded in April 1922 for declaring allegiance to the Free State. Armed police and soldiers prevented an attempt to convene a meeting, and the defenestrated guardians subsequently condemned the 'tyrannical brutal methods of the Belfast Parliament'.[103] Similarly, the mid-Ulster Cookstown Board of Guardians was dissolved in March 1922 after it was reported the 'Sinn Féin-cum-Nationalist majority' refused to 'recognise Northern Ireland'.[104] The Newry Board of Guardians was also temporarily dissolved.[105] In these exceptional circumstances, local poor law reform was extremely unlikely.

In the early years of Northern Ireland, many nationalists became ever more isolated from local government. In September 1922, the Northern Irish government enacted the Local Government Act, which imposed a declaration of allegiance to 'King George and the Northern Government' upon members and officials of local authorities, further alienating many nationalists.[106] Discrimination against the nationalist and Catholic population was evident in the devolved government's interference with local government. During the early 1920s, the Ministry of Home Affairs redrew electoral boundaries under the Leech Commission, which brought about unionist command of some local authorities that previously had nationalist majorities. In some cases, these changes blatantly consolidated unionist power, while in other areas, discrepancies in boundaries that were originally drawn up in the 1840s were addressed. Nationalists widely boycotted the Leech Commission, which further strengthened the influence of local unionists in reshaping boundaries. In 1922, electoral proportional representation, introduced across the island in 1920 by the British government to protect political minorities, was abandoned in Northern Ireland, which was inimical to nationalist interests in local government. These measures were introduced to secure Northern Ireland's place within the United Kingdom and prevent republican and nationalist political dissent from local government. Nationalist repudiation of the machinery and legitimacy of Northern Ireland, which included the boycotting of local government elections, further dampened their input into the government's early administrative reforms. Nationalist loss of control of local authority bodies was apparent in the 1920s. The most spectacular losses were in the west – Fermanagh and Tyrone County Councils and Londonderry Corporation.[107] These factors coalesced to cement nationalism's implacable opposition to local government, which was now effectively dominated by unionism.[108]

Any interpretation, however, that the lack of local poor law reform resulted from unionist domination and discrimination must be tempered. Many nationalists were socially conservative and not overly associated with more progressive poor law policies. In the Free State, poor law reform was marked by financial prudence, parsimony and harsh attitudes to some of the poor.[109] Northern Irish boards of guardians that returned to nationalist hands in 1924, such as Newry and Clogher, failed to develop district hospitals. Cookstown in County Tyrone provides an indicative example of the complexities that undermined reform. In 1919, the guardians voted to close the workhouse, temporarily relieve the poor in a neighbouring union and develop a district hospital. Long-standing ratepayer fears of rising costs led to the suspension of the hospital's plans, which were further derailed by the turmoil of the early 1920s.[110] The nationalist-run board was dissolved in March 1922 after it passed a resolution that refused to recognise the Northern Irish government.[111] The board was placed under the command of Commissioner Watkins, who administered the poor laws for over two years. Watkins had little interest in poor law reform and focused on reducing the rates in the union, although he was considered amenable to representations from Catholic interests.[112] The turbulent political and administrative disruption caused by the Irish Revolution and its aftermath led to the Cookstown inertia in poor law reform.

Dealings with central government complicated attempts at further reform. Following the 1924 local government elections, the Cookstown Board was reconstituted, but by this stage, it was in unionist hands after nationalists boycotted local government to protest gerrymandering.[113] In 1927, the unionist-run Cookstown Guardians attempted to resurrect plans for a district hospital, which soon became entangled in complex legal wrangling with the Ministry of Home Affairs over the guardians' wish to purchase a new building and not renovate the existing workhouse. Central government also sought more ambitious proposals for the hospital, although guardians' concern with the potential burden on the ratepayers ensured their plans were constricted by fiscal conservativism.[114] While the disruption of the early 1920s undermined the potential for local government reform, parsimony and bureaucracy proved to be more long-term factors which prevented the Cookstown Board of Guardians from establishing a district hospital.

The neighbouring Dungannon Poor Law Union was another example of poor law reform being hampered by political imbroglio between nationalists and unionists. Although located in County Tyrone, which had a predominantly nationalist and Catholic population, the religious and political demography of the Dungannon Poor Law Union was more evenly divided, with a slim Catholic majority.[115] In January 1920, discussions on the board of guardians commenced regarding reforming the workhouse infirmary.[116] Soon after, in the May 1920 local government elections, nationalists narrowly defeated the unionists in the contest for the Dungannon Rural District Council by nine councillors to eight. Its membership overlapped with the board of guardians. At the first meeting of the newly elected board, the unionist members were accompanied by the Ulster Volunteers and police. At the same time, the military was held in reserve in case of disorder. In extraordinary scenes, the unionist councillors insisted that the outgoing unionist chairman, W. S. Bennett, who was no longer an elected guardian, would have the first and casting vote, ensuring that unionists remained in charge of the board. The meeting descended into chaos, and both the nationalists and unionists elected their own officers. This was a blatant attempt by the unionists to maintain authority or, as the *Irish Independent* reported, to 'convert a unionist body [from] what the electors made a Sinn Féin-Nationalist council'.[117] In the ensuing legal battle, the King's Bench in Dublin ruled that Bennett acted illegally and a new vote of officers should be undertaken.[118] Soon after, three nationalists were elected to the governing positions of the board of guardians. In February 1921, the new chairman of the Dungannon Board of Guardians, John Doris J. P., proudly expressed that he was the 'first of his faith [Catholic] and nationality [Irish nationalist] to preside at that board'.[119] Doris was a long-standing nationalist in the area, representative of the socially conservative version exposed by Joe Devlin (as opposed to the more radical Sinn Féin), and a member of the Catholic and nationalist fraternity Ancient Order of Hibernians.[120]

Against the backdrop of the Irish Revolution and partition, the board again became engulfed in political division. During a meeting in early 1923, the nationalist-controlled board refused to pass an address to the Duke of Abercorn, the Governor of Northern Ireland, leading to the unionist guardians leaving the gathering in protest.[121] The nationalist chairman, Doris, asserted that the board sought a 'United Ireland' while another guardian, Cush, highlighted how the electorate in County Tyrone 'declared their determination' for Irish independence in the 1918 general election.[122] The impending hearing of the Leech Commission further aggravated nationalists who believed they would be disadvantaged in any redrawing of electoral divisions. Doris complained, in reference to the 1922 Local Government Act, that the 'very first act passed by the Belfast Parliament was to take away any power the minority possessed, and Judge Leech was coming to Dungannon ... to complete the preparation of that infamy'.[123] Nationalists in Dungannon, like many across much of Northern Ireland, boycotted the hearings on the redrawing of local government boundaries, subsequent local elections and involvement in local government, ensuring that the board of guardians passed back to unionist power, further embittering relations.

Politicisation and division on the Dungannon Board of Guardians left little capacity to bring about the poor law reform evident in other parts of Northern Ireland. Instead, the standard of provision suffered. In August 1923, the Ministry wrote to the Dungannon Guardians complaining that conditions in the workhouse infirmary were 'far from satisfactory', highlighting the lack of accommodation for both patients and nurses and that patients were treated in the able-bodied men's wards of the main body of the facility. The Ministry called on the guardians to devise a scheme to transform the workhouse into a district hospital.[124] District hospitals required much investment on the part of local ratepayers and social and political collegiality among guardians and wider society, as evidenced in the more homogenous parts of Northern Ireland. Such consensus and communitarianism seemed impossible amid the deep political division that enveloped the Dungannon Guardians.

Nationalist and unionist relations in Northern Ireland became more stable after 1925. The former was increasingly despondent after the failure of the Boundary Commission to bring about any alteration in territory, and predominantly Catholic and nationalist areas remained in Northern Ireland. Nationalists partly re-engaged with the institutions of the Northern Irish state, including participation in the Northern Ireland parliament and local government bodies. This was evident on the Dungannon Board of Guardians, where nationalists retook their seats, although the body remained under the authority of unionists. Proceedings often degenerated into political acrimony on the town's local authorities. For example, during a meeting of the Dungannon Rural District Council, whose members were also guardians, nationalists claimed that they suffered 'bigotry' and decisions on the unionist-controlled council were made in the 'Orange Hall'. This was in reference to long-held nationalist suspicions of the Protestant Orange Order's shadow over Northern Irish public life.[125] The Orange Order, or Loyal Orange Institution, in Northern Ireland, is a fraternity dedicated to Protestantism and maintaining the British connection. Against such a charged political and sectarian backdrop, attempts at local poor law reform did emerge but were ultimately unsuccessful. Proposals to develop a new

£30,000 district hospital were discussed throughout the late 1920s and 1930s in Dungannon. This ultimately failed to garner enough support from local guardians or ratepayers, and the new hospital was not built. Opposition was mostly from ratepayers who balked at the prospect of increased local taxation. While such resistance was not necessarily demarcated along nationalist–unionist lines – for example, the Nationalist MP for the Tyrone East Constituency in the Northern Irish House of Commons, Joseph F. Stewart, supported the scheme while other nationalist ratepayers opposed it – the general political division in the region made consensus-based decisions on costly local social reforms difficult.

The continuance of the workhouse infirmary in Dungannon was reflective of the failure of local authority policymaking in interwar Northern Ireland. The dominance of the political and sectarian divisions, especially during the early 1920s, and the discontent and mutual suspicion that these spawned throughout the 1920s and 1930s dwarfed social concerns. While it is not within the capacity of this study to examine local policymaking on every board in Northern Ireland, similar dissension was evident in many other areas which failed to develop district hospitals.

The persistence of poor law medicine embedded a multitiered local authority hospital framework in Northern Ireland. Northern Ireland's eleven district hospitals provided modernised acute care to an ever-increasing number of patients. Many of these had the capacity and willingness to pay for semi- or fully-private treatment. The thirteen workhouse infirmaries remained underfunded, unreformed and often for longer-term, chronic patients considered the 'residuum' of the poor law. This ensured inequality of provision along multiple levels. Firstly, this was evident between acute and chronic patients; the latter received second-class treatment compared to the former, who were invariably younger, more economically active and had greater survival rates. Secondly, access to the better district hospitals was also based on locality and the willingness of local boards of guardians to upgrade their infirmaries. The general trend observed in this analysis, with some exceptions, was that unionist areas were more willing to bring about reform. Poor law unions with substantial Catholic and nationalist populations, however, were hampered by political upheaval surrounding partition and ineluctable political and religious divisions. In turn, a local health divide became intertwined with political and religious fissures, which deepened the disillusionment of many Catholics and nationalists with the Northern Irish state.

Why did Northern Ireland fail to reform the poor law?

A key question that emerges is why Northern Ireland's government failed to bring about reform centrally and instead relied on the initiative of local authorities. The poor law's continuation is viewed as one of Northern Ireland's most significant failures in the field of health and welfare, and evidence suggests that it lagged behind the rest of the United Kingdom in social policy. Historians have largely viewed this as reflecting the Northern Irish government's social conservatism, fiscal parsimony and policy inertia.[126] Yet, poor law reform was a policy concern of the new devolved government. As already highlighted, the 1927 Commission promised to centralise the administration of health and hospital services. Instead, the report was bypassed, and a highly localised hospital structure became even more entrenched.

The failure to bring about these reforms was based on multiple central government failings. Local government reform was a complex proposition which the Ministry of Home Affairs seemed ill-equipped to perform. This was recognised in 1928 by the Prime Minister, James Craig, when he dampened expectations for the introduction of legislation and stated 'no time will be lost ... [but] no one who understands local government and all its intricacies can expect a bill to be introduced so soon after the issue of the Report'.[127] In 1931, Dawson Bates argued that the slow progress of reform was partly due to the proposals' 'complicated and comprehensive nature'.[128] Administrative capacity was further hindered by the lack of a dedicated central government bureaucracy, such as the Ministry of Health in England and Wales, the Board of Health in Scotland or the Department of Local Government and Public Health in the Free State. Northern Irish health services and local government remained under the Ministry of Home Affairs, which was also responsible for internal security in a country where a large minority challenged the legitimacy of the state. The Northern Irish Ministry of Home Affairs lacked the capacity and experience to bring about complex reform of hospital and health administration.

Other areas of health reform took precedence. The most significant medical policy initiative in interwar Northern Ireland was the introduction of national health insurance. As previously noted, medical benefits were not introduced in the original 1911 National Insurance Act. Still, unionists favoured the legislation, and in 1930 the Northern Irish National Health Insurance Act was passed, whereby most subscribers became entitled to general practitioner care. The Northern Irish government was also under pressure from London to introduce the benefit. The British government was looking to adopt conventions proposed at the International Labour Conference – this is one of the few instances when London pressed Northern Ireland on any health policy during the interwar years.[129] The introduction of medical benefits altered the poor law and removed large numbers from the dispensary system, which was a form of outdoor medical relief. The measure did not impact hospital provision, and, as in Britain, insured workers were not covered for such treatment.[130]

Northern Irish preference for national health insurance over poor law reform also demonstrated other important dynamics shaping policy. Medical benefits were confined to the insured and primarily benefited the employed classes and their dependents, particularly in Northern Ireland's industrialised economic base in the north-east. It excluded many of the long-term sick, poor and older people. Some in unionism, including the labourist strands, were committed to keeping Northern Ireland apace, or step-by-step, with social legislation and expenditure in Britain, helping to maintain political support from the Protestant working classes.[131] Such influences were evident in the government's commitment to maintaining unemployment benefits at wider British levels despite edging Northern Ireland close to bankruptcy during the economic depression.[132] Medical benefit had far more political capital for unionism than poor law reform. By the 1930s, centralised poor law reform would have had the greatest impact in the provincial towns and rural areas of Northern Ireland. Here the workhouses largely persisted and had the highest proportion of nationalists, negating the political capital of reform for the unionist government.

The government's indifference toward reform was equalled by many within the higher echelons of the medical profession. Long recognised as key actors in shaping health systems and policies, medics were a powerful interest group in Northern Ireland. Their position was strengthened by a weak, socially conservative unionist government which had scant interest in challenging their power. The profession was well-organised with a provincial body, the Ulster Medical Society, while numerous branches of the BMA existed in Northern Ireland. It was also intertwined with the government, and many MPs in the Ulster Unionist Party were doctors. The medical reaction to the reforms proposed in the Commission's 1927 report was muted. The Tyrone branch of the BMA emphasised that the Commission's report largely repeated the Edwardian poor law inquiries and perceptively predicted that the 'same fate was likely to attend the present report, since there seemed little enthusiasm for it on the part either of the general public or the government'. The branch contended that the profession remained 'lukewarm' towards the proposals.[133] Johnstone did criticise the government's inertia in parliament and, in 1931, lamented that many 'respectable working people' were forced to rely on the poor law, and that it was a 'great mistake that ... the taint of the poor law should hang over this very important medical service'.[134] However, the indifferent and disinterested response from the medical profession ensured little medical agitation to force the reforms emerged.

The medical profession's lacklustre interest in poor law reform stemmed from multiple factors. Local authority medical officials were slower to organise than other branches of medicine. They often lacked influence within the profession compared to the medical consultant and specialist elite in voluntary hospitals. The prevalence of poor and largely chronic, long-term patients with the meagre likelihood of cure further undermined the sector's status. The medical profession's lack of interest in local government reforms contrasted with its response to the introduction of the panel system under the national health insurance schemes. This impacted all of Northern Ireland's GPs, who were now ensured a basic income. Similar interest was demonstrated when the panel system was initially introduced in Britain, where the potential to negotiate generous remuneration for GPs weakened any initial opposition from the BMA.[135] Northern Ireland's medical representative bodies were often preoccupied with the scheme's introduction and terms and with shaping its subsequent workings.[136] Doctors' focus on national health insurance drained any impetus for campaigning for poor law reform. The medical profession's interest in poor law reform was also diluted by the strong position of medical voluntarism in Northern Ireland (see Chapter 3). Local government encroachment on fields of medicine that voluntary hospitals provided – mostly acute and specialist care – was often met with medical opposition. Medical voluntarism had little interest in supporting a new layer of district hospitals that provided acute care.

The medical profession's failure to substantially support the proposed reforms reveals much about health policy formulation in interwar Northern Ireland. Health system histories have explored the varying degrees of influence that interest groups, social classes and organised labour or structural biases of institutions such as government departments have had in shaping care.[137] In Northern Ireland, class and labour politics were often of secondary importance in a political culture shaped by constitutional and religious divisions inherent to the nationalist and unionist nexus.[138] Labour politics may have influenced government action on national health insurance, but it did not extend to poor law reform. Shortcomings of the labour movement allowed for the medical profession to shape health policy in Northern Ireland to a larger extent than in Britain or other countries with stronger labour movements. The lack of a dedicated health department in central government further strengthened the medical profession's influence over policy.

Conclusion

This analysis of interwar poor law health reform highlights multiple themes relating to Northern Irish health policy and politics. At one level, Northern Ireland's interwar health services depicted a capacity to bring about genuine reform. In turn, the overly simplistic interpretations that Northern Ireland trailed the rest of the United Kingdom in bringing about local health reform have been challenged. District hospitals represented a significant reform, which provided modernised healthcare to not just the poor but also attracted those of somewhat greater, if still modest, means. In this sense, the district hospital movement represented a policy commitment by local boards of guardians and ratepayers to develop healthcare for the benefit of the wider community. Northern Ireland was capable of real and positive changes in health, often predicated on social collegiality and communitarianism.

Yet, such an optimistic scenario is problematised by the multitiered model that emerged. District hospitals relied on the continuation of numerous workhouses, which housed non-acute patients and other inmates in second-class care. This imbalance was further complicated by the fact that district hospitals were mostly restricted to areas with unionist majorities. At the same time, predominantly nationalist places, by and large, failed to benefit, further alienating an already embittered and despondent minority, who also suffered from multiple other disadvantages and much discrimination in Northern Ireland. This points to the importance of the role of politics in shaping local health policies. Nationalist–unionist divisions on local boards of guardians often undermined reforms, indicating that politics, albeit sometimes inadvertently, subdued the health policy capacity of many local bodies.

At a wider level, Northern Ireland's picture of a multitiered poor law hospital framework, weak central government, intense localism and sectional interest groups is illustrative of the challenges faced by many new and small countries that emerged in the interwar period. Although some of the more positive historiographical understandings of interwar health, identified in larger countries, are applicable to Northern Ireland, the intractable political and religious tensions diminished the capacity to build a health service which benefited the whole of the population. These barriers were more common to newer countries that emerged after post-First World War nationalist challenges to larger imperial entities, often characterised by political, sectarian and communal violence. The ensuing divisions fragmented communities and societies, such as in Northern Ireland, which impeded health reform, leading to benefits and services that were unevenly distributed. In this sense, Northern Ireland's experience of poor law reform further complicates wider understandings of interwar health, which have mostly focused on larger political entities.

Another key theme that emerges is the strength of sectional interests and stakeholders in health policymaking to the detriment of a planned health system. District hospitals represented a medical localism which filled the vacuum of central government inaction and weakness. Such localism became an entrenched force and powerful stakeholder in the Northern Irish medical landscape. Fragmentation of hospital services became further embedded, which diminished the potential for greater integration, coordination and more efficient administration. District hospitals largely operated independently of each other, leading to duplication as local and institutional loyalties took precedence over the planning of services. The lack of centralised power not only fostered disjointed localism but also allowed sectional interest groups to hold much sway over policymaking. The power of the medical profession, another major stakeholder, was also evident in its lack of concern for poor law reform. This contrasted with the profession's greater focus on medical benefit and the growth of Northern Ireland's prestigious voluntary hospital sector, as evidenced in Chapter 3. In place of central government action, localism, the medical profession and medical voluntarism emerged as the key actors in health. The interplay between these stakeholders and a slowly reforming and centralising state are further explored throughout this book. As detailed and analysed in later chapters, tensions and conflict between these forces would come to the fore in the 1940s and post-war years as health planners attempted to unravel the power structures that became embedded in the interwar years.

Notes

1 D. Harkness, *Northern Ireland since 1920* (Dublin: Helicon Limited, 1983), p. 4.

2 D. M. Fox, *Health Policies, Health Politics: The British and American Experience, 1911–65* (Princeton, NJ: Princeton University Press, 1985); E. P. Hennock, *The Origin of the Welfare State in England and Germany, 1850–1914: Social Policies Compared* (Cambridge: Cambridge University Press, 2007); M. Gorsky, 'Hospitals, finance and health system reform in Britain and the United States', *Journal of Health Politics, Policy and Law*, 37:3 (2012), 365–404.

3 H. L. Clark and B. M. Doyle, 'Imperial and post-imperial health care before welfare states', *European History Review*, 28:5–6 (2021), 617–35.

4 J. Darwin, 'A third British Empire? The dominion idea in imperial politics', in J. Brown and W. R. Louis (eds), *The Oxford History of the British Empire: Volume IV: The Twentieth Century* (Oxford: Oxford University Press, 1999), pp. 64–87.

5 County infirmaries were separate from the poor law and funded by a combination of county councils/city corporations and charitable sources.

6 Public Record Office of Northern Ireland, Belfast [hereafter PRONI], CAB/4/267, Poor law and medical services reform, 21 August 1930.

7 *Poor Law Reform Commission (Ireland). Report of the Vice-Regal Commission on Poor Law Reform in Ireland. Volume I*, HC [Cd 3202], 1906; *Report of the Royal Commission on the Poor Laws and the Relief of Distress*, HC [Cd 4499], 1909.

8 Jackson, 'Local government in Northern Ireland, 1920–73', pp. 57, 60.

9 D. S. Lucey and G. C. Gosling, 'Paying for health: Comparative perspectives on patient payment and contributions for hospital provision in Ireland', in Lucey and Crossman (eds), *Healthcare in Ireland and Britain*, pp. 81–100; P. Martin, 'Ending the pauper taint: Medical benefit and welfare reform in Northern Ireland, 1921–39', in V. Crossman and P. Gray (eds), *Poverty and Welfare in Ireland, 1838–1948* (Dublin: Irish Academic Press, 2011), pp. 223–36.

10 V. Crossman, *Poverty and the Poor Law in Ireland, 1850–1914* (Liverpool: Liverpool University Press, 2013); V. Crossman, *Politics, Pauperism and Power in Late Nineteenth-Century Ireland* (Manchester: Manchester University Press, 2006); P. Gray, *The Making of the Irish Poor Law, 1815–43* (Manchester: Manchester University Press, 2009); O. Purdue and G. Laragy, *Poverty, Children and the Poor Law in Industrial Belfast, 1880–1918* (Liverpool: Liverpool University Press, 2024).

11 M. A. Crowther, *The Workhouse System, 1834–1929: The History of an English Social Institution* (London: Batsford Academic and Educational, 1981); F. Driver, *Power and Pauperism: The Workhouse System, 1834–1884* (Cambridge: Cambridge University Press, 1993); L. Hollen Lees, *The Solidarities of Strangers: The English Poor Laws and the People, 1700–1948* (Cambridge: Cambridge University Press, 1998).

12 Levene *et al.*, *Cradle to Grave.*

13 Crossman, *Poverty and the Poor Law in Ireland, 1850–1914*; Barrington, *Health, Medicine and Politics in Ireland.*

14 *Local Government Board Report for Ireland for 1917*, HC [Cd 8765], 1917–18, p. xxx.

15 *Ulster Herald*, 28 October 1916.
16 *Local Government Board Report for Ireland for 1914*, HC [Cd 7561], 1914, pp. 269–71.
17 *Local Government Board Report for Ireland for 1920*, HC [Cmd 1432], 1920, pp. xxvii–viii.
18 For a regional analysis of poor relief in late nineteenth- and early twentieth-century Ireland, see M. Cousins, *Poor Relief in Ireland, 1851–1914* (Bern: Peter Lang, 2011), 31–80; Crossman, *Poverty and the Poor Law in Ireland 1850–1914*, 52–62.
19 Cousins, *Poor Relief in Ireland*, p. 59.
20 O. Purdue, 'Poor relief in the north of Ireland, 1850–1921', in Crossman and Gray (eds), *Poverty and Welfare in Ireland*, pp. 23–36.
21 *Local Government Board Report for Ireland for 1917*, p. xxx.
22 O. Purdue, 'Poverty and power: the Irish Poor Law in a north Antrim town, 1861–1921', *Irish Historical Studies*, 37:148 (November 2011), 567–83.
23 Purdue, 'Poverty and power', 573.
24 A. Bielenberg, *Ireland and the Industrial Revolution: The Impact of the Industrial Revolution on Irish Industry, 1801–1922* (London: Routledge, 2009), especially Chapter 3.
25 D. Urquhart, *Women in Ulster Politics, 1890–1940: A History Not Yet Told* (Dublin: Irish Academic Press, 2000), p. 112.
26 Purdue, 'Poverty and power', 583; for an analysis of regional differences internal to Ulster in poor relief expenditure, see Purdue, 'Poor relief in the north of Ireland', pp. 23–36.
27 *Ballymena Observer* [hereafter *BO*], 24 May 1912.
28 *Ballymena Weekly Telegraph* [hereafter *BWT*], 17 February 1915.
29 *Larne Times* [hereafter *LT*], 7 July 1917.
30 *Report of the Irish Public Health Council on the Public Health and Medical Services in Ireland*, HC [Cmd 761], 1920; I. Milne, *Stacking the Coffins: Influenza, War and Revolution in Ireland, 1918–19* (Manchester: Manchester University Press), p. 232.
31 J. K. Knirck, 'The Dominion of Ireland: The Anglo-Irish Treaty in an imperial context', *Éire-Ireland*, 42:1 (2007), 230.
32 Lucey, *End of the Irish Poor Law?*, pp. 2, 18.
33 Lucey, '"These schemes will win for themselves the confidence of the people": Irish independence, poor law reform and hospital provision', *Medical History*, 58:1 (2014), 46–66.
34 Frohman, 'The break-up of the poor laws', 982; G. Finlayson, *Citizen, State, and Social Welfare in Britain 1830–1990* (Oxford: Oxford University Press, 1990), pp. 165–6.
35 Quoted in Lucey, *End of the Irish Poor Law?*, p. 160.

36 Lucey, 'These schemes will win for themselves the confidence of the people', 50.
37 *LT*, 28 March 1931.
38 *North Down Herald and County Down Independent* [hereafter *NDHCDI*], 2 April 1932.
39 J. Sadar, 'The healthful ambience of vitaglass: light, glass and the curative environment', *Architectural Research Quarterly*, 12:3–4 (2008), 269–81.
40 *NDHCDI*, 2 April 1932.
41 NPHT, *Survey of the Hospital Services*, p. 78.
42 NPHT, *Survey of the Hospital Services*, pp. 77, 78.
43 NPHT, *Survey of the Hospital Services*, p. 76; *NDHCDI*, 2 April 1932.
44 NPHT, *Survey of the Hospital Services*, p. 86.
45 F. P. Montgomery, 'The future of the hospitals', *UMJ*, 11:2 (1942), 116.
46 Ministry of Home Affairs [hereafter MHA], *Report on the Administration of Local Government Services in Northern Ireland, 1926* (Belfast: HMSO, 1927), p. 47.
47 *Belfast News-Letter* [hereafter *BN*], 15 December 1930.
48 NPHT, *Survey of the Hospital Services*, p. 26.
49 *Portadown Times* [hereafter *PT*], 5 February 1937.
50 *Ballymoney Free Press and Northern Counties Advertiser*, 5 July 1928.
51 *LT*, 28 March 1931.
52 Departmental Commission on Local Government Administration in Northern Ireland, *Report of Departmental Commission on Local Government Administration in Northern Ireland: presented to Parliament by His Grace the Governor of Northern Ireland* (Belfast: HMSO, 1927), p. 106.
53 MHA, *Report on the Administration of Local Government Services... 1926*, p. 47.
54 PRONI, HOS/5/1/9/B/1, Moyle District Hospital, Larne, Register of Insured Patients, 1934–48.
55 MHA, *Report on the Administration of Local Government Services in Northern Ireland, 1927* (Belfast: HMSO, 1927), p. 54.
56 *SC*, 27 December 1920.
57 Lucey, 'These schemes will win for themselves the confidence of the people'.
58 PRONI, CAB/4/267, Poor Law and medical services reform, 21 August 1930.
59 *Larne Times*, 28 March 1931.

60 For the various strands of independent unionism, see C. Reid, 'Protestant challenges to the "Protestant State": Ulster unionism and independent Unionism in Northern Ireland, 1921–39', *Twentieth Century British History*, 19:4 (2008), 419–45.
61 A. Grant, *Derry: The Irish Revolution, 1912–23* (Dublin: Four Courts Press, 2018), p. 21.
62 For example, Robert Gordan Sharman-Crawford disavowed his family's reformist political agenda to firmly become a member of the unionist establishment in the new devolved Northern Ireland, see P. Gray, *William Sharman Crawford and Ulster Radicalism* (Dublin: University College Dublin Press, 2023), p. 356.
63 *NDHCDI*, 30 January 1932.
64 *LT*, 28 March 1931.
65 *BN*, 11 December 1922; *BN*, 28 December 1925.
66 *Witness*, 28 April 1933.
67 *PT*, 27 March 1936. For Wilson's career, see *PT*, 29 July 1955.
68 *BN*, 12 March 1935.
69 *NDHCDI*, 2 April 1932.
70 *PT*, 5 September 1930.
71 *PT*, 27 March 1936.
72 A. Levene, 'Between less eligibility and the NHS: The changing place of poor law hospitals in England and Wales, 1929–39', *Twentieth Century British History*, 20:3 (2009), 325.
73 MHA, *Report on the Administration of Local Government Services in Northern Ireland, 1931* (Belfast: HMSO, 1931), pp. 195–7.
74 A. Levene, 'Between less eligibility and the NHS', 325.
75 G. Weisz, *Chronic Disease in the Twentieth Century: A History* (Baltimore, MD: Johns Hopkins University Press, 2014), p. 178.
76 *NDHCDI*, 15 December 1928.
77 M. D. Moore, *Managing Diabetes, Managing Medicine: Chronic Disease and Clinical Bureaucracy in Post-War Britain* (Manchester: Manchester University Press, 2019), p. 56.
78 PRONI, HOS/9/1/1/4, Minutes of Route Hospital Committee, Ballymoney, 30 November 1944.
79 NPHT, *Survey of the Hospital Services*, p. 14.
80 *Report of Departmental Commission on Local Government Administration in Northern Ireland*, p. 79.
81 E. M. Hickey, 'The problem of the Aged in Northern Ireland', *UMJ*, 15:2 (November 1946), 151.
82 NPHT, *Survey of the Hospital Services*, pp. 13–14.
83 Lucey, 'These schemes will win for themselves the confidence of the people'.

84 Levene, 'Between less eligibility and the NHS', 337; M. Gorsky, '"To regulate and confirm inequality"? A regional history of geriatric hospitals under the English National Health Service, *c.*1948–*c.*1975', *Ageing and Society*, 33:4 (2013), 615.
85 L. Kidd, 'A Ministry of Health for Northern Ireland', *UMJ*, 7:4 (October 1938), 235.
86 Privilege and Jones, 'Crisis and scandal', 39.
87 NPHT, *Survey of the Hospital Services*, p. 26.
88 Kidd, 'A Ministry of Health for Northern Ireland', 235.
89 NPHT, *Survey of the Hospital Services*, p. 86.
90 *Ibid.*, p. 81.
91 R. J. Lawrence, 'The health services in Northern Ireland', *Public Administration* 34:3 (Autumn 1956), 294.
92 *Northern Whig* [hereafter *NW*], 11 May 1934.
93 NPHT, *Survey of the Hospital Services*, p. 26.
94 PRONI, BG/7/A/128, Belfast Board of Guardians minute book: Abstract of account and clerk's half-yearly statements, 30 September 1932.
95 PRONI, BG/20/BC/5, Lisnaskea Board of Guardians letter book, Medical Officer Dr McCloy report of Lisnaskea Workhouse, 9 November 1922.
96 *Larne Times*, 6 May 1922.
97 *Strabane Chronicle* [hereafter *SC*], 1 January 1921.
98 *SC*, 25 February 1922.
99 *SC*, 11 February 1922.
100 Lucey, *End of the Irish Poor Law?*, pp. 58, 62.
101 M. E. Daly, *The Buffer State: The Historical Roots of the Department of Environment* (Dublin: Institute of Public Administration, 1997).
102 M. Potter, *Municipal Revolution in Ireland: Local Government in Cities and Towns since 1800* (Dublin: Irish Academic Press, 2011), pp. 289–301.
103 *SC*, 8 April 1922.
104 *BN*, 18 March 1922.
105 *BN*, 21 April 1922.
106 *SC*, 16 September 1922.
107 P. Buckland, *The Factory of Grievances. Devolved Government in Northern Ireland, 1921–39* (Dublin: Gill and Macmillan, 1979), p. 226.
108 Harkness, *Northern Ireland*, pp. 25–8.
109 Lucey, *End of the Irish Poor Law?*
110 *Mid-Ulster Mail*, 19 September 1936.
111 *BN*, 18 March 1922.
112 *Mid-Ulster Mail*, 31 May 1924.
113 *Mid-Ulster Mail*, 4 June 1924; *Derry Journal*, 4 June 1924.

114 *Mid-Ulster Mail*, 13 July 1929, 8 March 1920, 19 September 1936.
115 For a study of Tyrone's politics during the Irish Revolution, see F. McCluskey, *The Irish Revolution, 1912–23: Tyrone* (Dublin: Four Courts Press, 2014).
116 *BN*, 24 January 1920.
117 *Irish Independent*, 14 June 1920.
118 *Irish Weekly and Ulster Examiner*, 4 December 1940.
119 *NW*, 26 February 1921.
120 *Mid-Ulster Mail*, 20 October 1934.
121 *Londonderry Sentinel* [hereafter *LDS*], 10 February 1923.
122 *Irish Weekly and Ulster Examiner*, 17 February 1923.
123 *LDS*, 10 February 1923.
124 *Mid-Ulster Mail*, 11 August 1923.
125 *LDS*, 12 June 1930.
126 Buckland, *Factory of Grievances*, pp. 160–3.
127 Northern Ireland Parliament, *Northern Ireland House of Commons Debates* [hereafter *NIHoCD*], 9, 6 March 1928 (Belfast: HMSO, 1928), pp. 29–30.
128 PRONI, CAB/4/293, Cabinet Secretariat, Cabinet Conclusions, Reform of Poor Law, medical, public health and local government services, 11 November 1931.
129 PRONI, CAB4/206, Cabinet Secretariat, Cabinet Conclusions, Note by the Minister of Labour on Draft International Conventions on Health Benefits, 26 March 1928.
130 Martin, 'Ending the pauper taint', p. 230.
131 P. Bew, P. Gibbons and H. Patterson, *Northern Ireland, 1921–2001: Political Forces and Social Classes* (London: Serif, 3rd ed., 2002).
132 C. Nolan, 'Creating jobs, manufacturing unity: Ulster unionism and mass unemployment 1922–34', *Contemporary British History*, 15:2 (2001), 7.
133 'Ireland', *BMJ*, 2:3492 (10 December 1927), 1113.
134 *NIHoCD*, 13, 19 May 1931, pp. 1903–4.
135 M. Gorsky, 'Hospitals, finance, and health system reform in Britain and the United Kingdom, c.1910–50: Historical revisions and cross-national comparison', *Journal of Health Politics, Policy and Law*, 37:3 (June 2012), 371.
136 For example, S. McComb and J. S. Peatt, 'National Health Insurance Notes – Belfast & County Areas', *UMJ*, 1:1 (January 1932), 65–6.
137 Gorsky, 'Hospitals, finance and health system reform', 367.
138 A. Edwards, *A History of the Northern Ireland Labour Party: Democratic Socialism and Sectarianism* (Manchester: Manchester University Press, 2009), pp. 8–12.

2

Municipal healthcare and maternity and child welfare and the limits of labour: a case study of Belfast Corporation

The focus now turns to municipal healthcare, another facet of the mixed economy of healthcare during the interwar era. While the previous chapter depicted the importance of nationalist–unionist politics in determining local poor law reform in provincial Northern Ireland, the politics of the labour movement in interwar healthcare is now explored. This monograph's overall focus is on Northern Ireland, but this chapter provides a case study of Belfast's failure to implement local authority maternity and child welfare policies. This case study approach is justified by Belfast's potential for labour politics and its high infant mortality rate in these years. Furthermore, this case illuminates wider patterns in interwar healthcare across Northern Ireland. The constraints of progressive and feminist health policies in the region are revealed, indicating that the politically dominant Ulster unionism, which favoured minimal central or local state action, remained key to shaping Northern Ireland's healthcare. While poor law reform was often impeded by nationalist–unionist divisions, maternity and child welfare were restricted by unionism's opposition to labour politics. This indicates the limitations of broader historiographical understandings of the unionist step-by-step policy, which sought to keep welfare measures in line with wider UK levels. This was to show the benefits of the union while also solidifying unionist political unity through high public spending. Like the Northern Ireland government's failure to reform poor law healthcare, as outlined in Chapter 1, intransigence to maternity and child welfare illustrates that unionism's parity with Britain policy did not extend to certain groups. The failure to develop maternity and child welfare also underscores the power of the medical profession as a key stakeholder in health provision, another key finding from Chapter 1. Powerful medical figures were antithetical to the growth of municipal health to protect the interests of the medical voluntary sector and their autonomy from the local state; the power of medical voluntarism is further explored in Chapter 3.

Politics and the potential of labour

As set forth in the previous chapter, politics played a key role in shaping local authority healthcare. In provincial Northern Ireland, policy inertia was often a result of intractable political and religious divisions and had less to do with ideological differences about health strategy. In Belfast, the political landscape differed, with the Northern Ireland Labour Party being stronger and having a greater focus on agitating for progressive local authority social policies. The city was Northern Ireland's largest urban and industrialised centre where labour politics inherently appealed to much of its nearly 400,000 population, many of whom were working class. Labour politics could transcend the sectarian and nationalist–unionist divide and had the potential to threaten the dominance of the Ulster Unionist Party among the Protestant working classes.

Experiences in Britain showed that the Labour Party had a significant impact on local authority health provision. Labour's policies were shaped by, firstly, the Socialist Medical Service Association (SMSA) and, secondly, the Socialist Medical Association (SMA), which subsumed the former after its establishment in 1930. Made up of left-wing medics committed to creating a socialised medical service free and open to all, both the SMSA and SMA were affiliated to the Labour Party and informed the movement's increased concern with social conditions and not just economic matters. At the core of the SMA and Labour Party's plans was a remodelled health service under direct democratic governance, in which local government would play a key role. Central to these plans was the creation of health centres, which were to provide a comprehensive and merged service of both curative and preventive care. Radically, consultants and general practitioners were to be grouped together, ensuring that patients could receive primary and secondary care.

Centres were to be deeply connected with hospitals, including voluntary institutions whose autonomy and lack of state oversight the SMA viewed critically.[1] This was an early version of socialised medicine, which envisaged the radical expansion of local authority responsibilities and a weaker voluntary system.

The growth of the labour movement throughout interwar Britain led to local authority successes and opportunities to implement socialised visions of municipal health. By 1939, the Labour Party held an average of 35 per cent of seats on county boroughs, with majorities on eighteen.[2] Increased Labour Party involvement in municipal politics influenced healthcare and hospital policies. In the Yorkshire cities of Leeds, Sheffield and Middlesbrough, the character of local Labour Party activity and the influence of socialism all shaped healthcare policies, albeit this varied from city to city.[3] A strong, adversarial and combative Labour presence could lead to the rapid development of municipal services. This was evident in the high-spending Barnsley Borough where local Labour Party political activity prioritised maternity and child welfare. Labour councillors viewed such services as vital to raising the bar for disadvantaged families.[4] In the Labour bastion of Glasgow, strong support for extended municipal healthcare by leading Labour advocates helped to enhance services despite the persistence of shortcomings.[5] In that city during the interwar years, Mary Barbour – a motivated Labour councillor – was instrumental in the extension of women's services such as maternity and child welfare provision.[6] In London the advance of an SMA-inspired model of municipal healthcare came to the fore after Labour won elections for many boroughs and London County Council in 1934.[7] Many Labour boroughs in London developed 'cradle-to-grave' healthcare. Central to this local authority approach were the aforementioned 'all-in' health centres, which sought to provide a comprehensive array of primary and preventive health services delivered by multidisciplinary teams to working people.[8] Across Britain, particularly in London, Labour politics promoted a socialised version of municipal healthcare.

The likelihood of Belfast Corporation becoming a bastion of socialist healthcare was limited. The 1920 municipal elections witnessed significant success for the recently established Belfast Labour Party (morphed into the Northern Ireland Labour Party in 1924), which won thirteen of the sixty seats, drawing non-sectarian support from the Catholic and Protestant working classes, often to the cost of unionist candidates.[9] However, the resurgence of the constitutional question during the Irish Revolution and partition, combined with the subsequent abolition of proportional representation, weakened the labour movement in the 1923 election to Belfast Corporation. In turn, Labour won a mere two seats while the Unionist Party's number increased from thirty-seven to fifty, and nationalists decreased from ten to eight. The NILP's support fluctuated throughout the interwar years but never seriously threatened unionist power on Belfast Corporation. The nationalist percentage of seats remained stable in the 13-to-17 per cent bracket.[10] Furthermore, municipal electoral politics in Belfast was marked by increased apathy in the interwar years. Between 1920 and 1939, 85 per cent of municipal seats went unopposed, the majority going to unionists. Represented mainly by businessmen, the unionist-run Corporation was invariably concerned with keeping rates low and the administration run on business lines.[11] Many of these unionists were marked by social conservatism and opposition to the labour movement, undermining the potential for municipal growth in health services.

The Corporation's frequent mismanagement also thwarted the prospect for progressive social policies. The Megaw Inquiry into Belfast Corporation's Housing Committee reported in 1926. It identified corruption, neglect by officials and failure of leading unionist councillors, which brought about the resignation and prosecution of senior officials and halting of the Corporation's housing programme.[12] While the Corporation was reformed in the 1920s, its social and health services continued to be plagued by maladministration. The 1941 Whiteabbey Inquiry led to the suspension of the Belfast Corporation Tuberculosis Committee after prolonged allegations of malpractice in tendering, nepotism and a breakdown of trust between the medical staff and councillors.[13] The social conservatism of Ulster Unionism and the maladministration of municipal business weakened much of the Corporation's activity.

The circumstances for progressive and socialist policies were weak, but the NILP's pursuit of economic and social policies was at times influential despite its small presence on the Corporation. The election of Harry Midgely as a councillor in 1925 ensured a strong and persistent labour voice on the Corporation. Midgely was a leading Belfast trade unionist and labour politician who remained a councillor until 1949. After he was elected NILP chairman in 1932, he dominated the party and continued to adopt militantly leftist positions.[14] He was very active on Belfast Corporation and agitated for improvement in educational and social services, often in conflict with the socially conservative strands of unionist councillors. He frequently criticised the government and the Corporation's record in areas such as housing, free school books and meals for necessitous children.[15] Midgley also campaigned on health services, including the elimination of fees for patients in rate-aided hospitals run by the Corporation, claiming that 'charging for a patient was wrong'.[16] Midgley succeeded in raising the threshold for free treatment in the city's Purdysburn Fever Hospital from ten to twenty shillings after rent deductions. The town clerk highlighted that the 'great majority' of patients were, as a result, exempt from payment.[17] Midgley later complained about any charges for patients in infectious diseases hospitals, maintaining that similar treatment was free in British municipal facilities. He lamented during one meeting that if he 'had enough people' on the Corporation, the measure would be implemented.[18] Such comments indicated the limitations of Midgley and the NILP on the Corporation. Many other policies failed to be implemented, such as an unsuccessful attempt to introduce free school books in 1931.[19] Nevertheless, the labour movement was a persistent voice that agitated for growth in municipal healthcare. This was most evident in Belfast, where the labour movement had its strongest base, while there was less of a focus in other parts of Northern Ireland where the NILP was much weaker.

Other strands of the socialist movement also sought the expansion of municipal healthcare. Belfast had a high proportion of females in the industrial workforce, above all in the city's large textile industry. By the late nineteenth century, over 70 per cent of the city's 24,245 textile labour force were female.[20] The labour movement adopted a more gendered platform with the establishment of the Central Women's Section of the Northern Ireland Labour Party in 1924. Women who had been prominent suffragists such as Margaret McCoubrey, the former leader of the Belfast-based Irish Women's Suffragist Society, backboned this body.[21] The Central Women's Section agitated for a range of issues, including greater protection for marginalised women who had children out of wedlock, raising the age of marriage and employment rights of married female teachers, as well as health matters, including maternity and child welfare and school meals for poor children.[22] McCoubrey was elected as the NILP's first female councillor on Belfast Corporation for the Ormeau Ward in 1929. This was a significant victory for the labour and feminist movements in Belfast, indicating that female participation in progressive politics was not as muted as often assumed in interwar Belfast and Northern Ireland.[23] By the late 1920s, Belfast Corporation was increasingly politicised along class and gender lines. The NILP and feminist activists agitated for more progressive social and health policies which challenged the Corporation's deep-rooted parsimony and social conservatism.

Medical officer of health and plans for growth

The labour movement may have been important to the agitation for the growth in municipal health services, but it was far from the only factor that could bring about reform and expansion. In England and Wales, county boroughs controlled by traditional elites with modest labour influence often experienced municipal healthcare growth. Notions of civic pride, influential medical professionals and a general commitment to community public health were factors in municipal expansion in non-Labour English and Welsh boroughs.[24] Medical officers of health were often crucial to the success of municipal health provision and could play the role of an active lobbyist for local growth. Belfast Corporation appeared willing to recognise the potential benefits of having an active and energetic medical officer of health (MOH) when it appointed Dr Charles Thomson to the position in 1929. Thomson was previously the MOH of the Deptford Borough in London and published in public health journals and the *British Medical Journal*.[25] He had a reputation for expertise in health education, maternity and child welfare and diphtheria immunisation schemes.[26] His appointment over local candidates was viewed as a break from the Corporation's 'system of patronage' which the municipal administrative reforms, emanating from the housing corruption scandal of the late 1920s, sought to eradicate.[27] As an outsider, Thomson's experience in

London ensured he was exposed to a very different municipal culture than in Belfast, where health services had rapidly grown, often with the backing of the labour movement and influenced by the SMA. Thomson's appointment had the potential to challenge Belfast Corporation's stubborn unwillingness to grow many municipal health services.

The record of medical officers of health, generally in Britain during the interwar years, is mixed. An active, energetic and determined MOH could positively impact the health of local populations. This was most famously evident in the English Borough of Rochdale, where the MOH Andrew Topping's reform of maternity services led to an immediate drop in the town's high maternal mortality rates in 1932.[28] MOsH however, have also been the source of controversy within the broader historiography for their failure to address the health impacts of the economic depression of the early 1930s. The historian Charles Webster has criticised local MOsH for underplaying the effects of unemployment on ill health due to officialdom's politically motivated attempts to present an overly optimistic picture of standards during the economic and political crisis of the depression.[29] They were culpable for failing to publicise the extent of the poor nutritional status of schoolchildren and mothers during an era when public health debates had become engulfed in the wider politics of the economic depression. Many leading health officials in Britain often played a valuable propaganda function in convincing people that welfare services contained the medical problems associated with the depression.[30] In this sense, many MOsH failed to put the concerns of their communities to the fore and instead capitulated to political pressure. Public health officials also often resorted to blaming the victims, such as 'bad motherhood' for infant mortality, rather than the social causes that gave rise to illness.[31]

For much of the interwar years, Belfast's poor record in infant health was a major concern. Belfast's infant mortality rate (IMR) was persistently high, and it had one of the worst records of any city in Britain or Ireland. Figure 2.1 provides a quinquennial comparison of IMR in Belfast, Dublin, Liverpool and Sheffield. For the 1925–29 and 1930–34 periods, Belfast had the highest IMR of the four cities, while during 1935–39, it was second only to the infamously unhealthy city of Dublin. In 1929, Belfast's record of

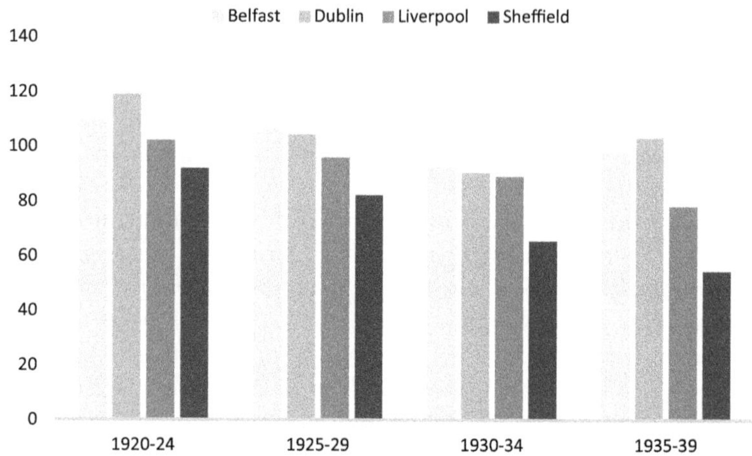

Figure 2.1 Quinquennial IMR in Belfast, Dublin, Liverpool and Sheffield, 1920–39

Table 2.1 County borough expenditure on maternity and child welfare per 1,000 of population in Belfast, Dublin, Liverpool and Cardiff and the English and Welsh mean in 1936.

	Belfast	*Dublin*	*Liverpool*	*Cardiff*	*English and Welsh mean*
Maternity and child	34.62	31.08	166.57	116.18	99.55

Sources: MHA, *Local Taxation Returns, 1935/6* (Belfast: HMSO, 1936); Levene *et al.*, *Cradle to Grave*, 68–71.

infant deaths reached its nadir and was the highest recorded of any British or Irish borough. Belfast's poor record in infant health was compounded by the failure of the city's corporation to develop maternity and child welfare (MCW) provision substantially. In contrast to many British boroughs, where purpose-built local MCW clinics, municipal maternity hospitals and extensive free milk schemes were all features of an expanding municipal service, Belfast Corporation's provision was extremely circumscribed. As outlined in Table 2.1, Belfast's expenditure on maternity and child welfare was substantially lower than in comparable cities, such as Cardiff and Liverpool, and the wider English and Welsh mean.

The failure to substantially develop services in Belfast and Northern Ireland was at odds with wider UK and transnational trends. By the early twentieth century, an international maternity and infant movement emerged in direct response to high infant and maternal mortality rates and falling fertility.[32] Westminster's Notification of Births Acts 1905 and 1915 and the Midwives (Ireland) Act 1918 legislated for the development of maternity and child welfare and the regulation of maternity services.[33] The 1918 Maternity and Child Welfare Act confirmed the importance of maternal and child welfare in the sphere of public health policy. It empowered local authorities to provide services for infants and expectant and nursing women, including antenatal and postnatal services along with free and subsidised milk and food depots; dental care was also included.[34] Furthermore, it provided central government grants of up to 50 per cent of local government expenditure, ensuring that funding was not solely reliant on local authority rates but also general taxation.[35] In response to this legislation, Belfast Corporation established a Maternity and Child Welfare Committee in 1918. The Committee initially progressed well, and by 1922, five clinics were established, in which 1,225 babies were medically examined, and women made 24,387 attendances. Milk was distributed to 'necessitous cases', and grants were made to voluntary maternity homes and hospitals in the city.[36] Clinics often held baby clubs in co-operation with voluntary women's groups. For example, the Charlotte Street Clinic was run by the Women's United Service, and Lady Aberdeen's Women's National Health Association set up its first baby club in Belfast in 1908.[37] The Corporation's MCW scheme funded these clinics and provided medical staff, and by 1927, three municipal part-time medical officers were employed to run the service.[38] Despite these early successes, provision failed to grow substantially, and Belfast fell far short of what was provided in many British municipalities. Belfast's persistently high infant mortality rate compounded what was viewed as the Corporation's failure to grow municipal maternity and child welfare.

After he was appointed medical officer of health, Charles Thomson was keen to bring about change in Belfast Corporation. He reportedly had 'strong convictions regarding reform of the whole [Public Health] department'.[39] Thomson promised to be the proactive type of medical officer of health who could provide local health leadership and shape policymaking, as identified in the historiography of municipal health in interwar Britain.[40] He quickly flagged Belfast's high infant mortality rate as a significant health concern. His assertion that infant deaths from diarrhoea were due to maternal ignorance about unsanitary food preparation and lack of breastfeeding was reflective of victim blaming evident in many health ideas around motherhood during this era.[41] Such an emphasis was largely directed at poorer working-class women and often failed to offer improvised women lifestyle alternatives.[42] However, unlike many of his counterparts in Britain who were diffident about associating ill health with poverty, Thomson also blamed Belfast's high rate of infant deaths on poverty, unemployment and malnutrition. He connected malnutrition to ill health and reported that infant deaths from prematurity, atrophy, debility, pneumonia and bronchitis were 'due to poverty [and] insufficient food', believing that 'a thin and badly nourished mother tend[ed] to produce a thin baby below weight'.[43] While Thomson partly resorted to blaming women for infant deaths, his willingness to link mortality to social conditions represented a more radical and progressive approach to municipal health.

Thomson soon devised an ambitious plan to reshape municipal maternity and child welfare. In early 1930, he recommended that two new centres be built to offer multidisciplinary health services to women and children. Each centre was to provide primary and consultancy care along with personal health services, including venereal disease treatment; dental, ophthalmic and ear, nose and throat surgeries were also to be established. Services were to include antenatal and postnatal classes, laboratory analysis and sunlight therapy; distribution of dried milk and dining halls for expectant and nursing mothers were also included.[44] Thomson also proposed a new municipal hospital for children on the disused site of the Townsend Street Maternity Hospital, an orthopaedic clinic for children with disabilities and the consolidation of health visitations.[45] These proposals dwarfed the city's existing municipal MCW care or anything that any other local authority provided in Northern Ireland.

Attempts to provide interdisciplinary care and harmonised primary, consultancy and public health provision under one roof represented a radical overhaul of medical practice and the role of local government authorities in Northern Ireland. This model of health proposed by Thomson in Belfast echoed leftist and socialist medical policies and was akin to the SMA's plans for municipal health in London.[46] Along with such an unprecedented amalgamation of health services, the local government model promised healthcare that was democratically run, funding that was locally controlled, and eligibility that was to be based on medical need. This contrasted with the cultures and structures inherent to the older providers of healthcare in Northern Ireland. The voluntary sector, which is examined in greater detail in Chapter 3, was predicated on the paternalism of the social elite and charitable concepts of deservingness and shaped by the interests of leading medical professions and hospitals. The poor law sector remained stigmatising for many, in which entitlement was often predicated on poverty and the standard of care lagged other sectors. District hospitals did represent progress, but patients were increasingly expected to financially contribute to their care in that tier. Instead, Thomson offered an early version of socialised healthcare that challenged the predominance of the poor law and voluntary sectors as providers.

Thomson's proposals were fraught with political and professional tensions. Belfast Corporation was marked by a traditional unwillingness to overburden ratepayers, while Thomson's plans were inevitably costly and would lead to an increase in rates. Politically, socialised municipal healthcare was closer to the labour movement than the dominant Ulster unionism. This was further complicated by the powerful voluntary hospital sector, which was politically and socially interconnected with the higher echelons of unionism.[47] These hospitals often viewed local government healthcare with suspicion and resisted state encroachment on their independence and power. In turn, the labour movement and SMA had long reservations about the system and sought voluntary consolidation with the public authorities.[48] Resistance to the plans was inevitable.

The scheme was initially met with support despite the potential for opposition. The Corporation's Maternity and Child Welfare Committee approved the scheme. However, it cost an estimated £33,000, which represented a major increase in the annual cost of £6,000 that Belfast spent on MCW.[49] The measure garnered support from not just the labour movement but also some within unionism, including the chair of the committee and the Unionist Party councillor Samuel McLoughlin. The unionist *Belfast Telegraph* newspaper noted that Thomson's proposals were costly but maintained: 'lives are precious, and it is time something was done to supplement our efforts'.[50] Many Ulster Unionists were anxious not to lose ground among the Protestant working class to the NILP and independent unionists on socio-economic issues.[51] Potential unionist unease about an overly socialist measure was diluted by approval from the socially conservative Protestant faiths including the Church of Ireland, Presbyterian and Methodist churches.[52] Unsurprisingly, NILP members of the corporation backed the measure. The NILP leader and councillor Samuel Kyle welcomed the scheme and emphasised that the high infant mortality rate in Belfast was not one of which they 'were particularly proud'.[53]

Political and medical opposition

Despite support from some within unionism, Protestant churches and the labour movement, the plans were quickly undone. The Corporation voted for Thomson's plan but on the condition that the central government funded 50 per cent of the estimated cost. Predicating the scheme on central government backing was precarious. Since partition, the Northern Ireland administration was disinclined to increase funding to local authority health services, notably maternity and child welfare. In 1924, the Ministry of Finance set the maximum budget for maternity and child welfare from central coffers at a mere £4,300 for the whole of Northern Ireland, although the 1918 legislation provided for government funding of up to 50 per cent of local authority expenditure.[54] In lieu of increased central funding, the government promoted the role of charity and voluntarism. In 1926, James Craig informed the Belfast Women's Advisory Council, a non-sectarian and feminist body formed as part of the Women's Section of the NILP, that there would be no increased government funding for MCW until 'it [was] clearly established that voluntary effort [had] failed'.[55] For much of the 1920s, the government was unwilling to fund MCW, which was unlikely to change for Thomson's plans, revealing the insincerity of the Corporation's support for extended MCW in Belfast.

The likelihood of success was further lessened by opposition from leading unionists who articulated traditional ratepayer concerns.

During a Windsor Women's Unionist Association meeting, the Ulster Unionist Lord Mayor of Belfast Corporation, Sir William Coates, commented that the proposed scheme's increase on the rates had to be considered. He contended that the 'maternity and child welfare scheme would be a tax on the rates – pure and simple'.[56] Coates was circumspect about the scheme on financial grounds. The attendance of the Minister for Finance, Hugh Pollock, who had ultimate approval for the request for increased central government spending, at the meeting did not bode well for the proposals. Unsurprisingly, the government was unwilling to commit to the increased funding immediately and informed the Corporation in March 1930 that it was considering the measure. The timing of this communication was crucial as the Corporation's estimates for the forthcoming financial year had to be confirmed by the start of March, ensuring that the government's procrastination would delay the scheme for at least twelve months. Coates refused to agree to the full costs being paid by the Corporation and highlighted the importance of 'rigid economy' and the adoption of a 'cautious view' towards increasing welfare costs.[57] Thomson's MCW proposals were duly shelved.

Opposition was also evident from some sections of the medical profession. Dr Williamson, a medical doctor and Unionist Party elected alderman to the Corporation, opposed the extension of maternity and child welfare. Williamson was a senior member of the Corporation and chaired its Public Health Committee. He contradicted Thomson and claimed that the infant mortality figures in Belfast were inflated by women coming from outside the city to give birth in the city's institutions. Williamson criticised Thomson for 'decry[ing] Belfast on every occasion and ma[king] the city a laughingstock', maintaining that the poor law and voluntary sectors already provided provision for mothers and their infants. He also resorted to victim blaming and opined that many infant deaths were avoidable with more 'intelligent and efficient instruction in the care of children'.[58] Despite his prominence in Belfast public health, Williamson ignored the wider social causes of ill health and emphasised the role of the voluntary and poor law sectors but demoted municipal responsibility. Much of Williamson's criticism was echoed in the local unionist press. The *Belfast News-Letter* focused on the reputational harm created by the spotlight on the city's high infant mortality rate. In an editorial, it asked if 'our reformers could manage to air their grievances and carry on their propagandist work without damaging unnecessarily the reputation of Belfast in cross-Channel quarters'.[59] During a debate to support the plans at the General Assembly of the Presbyterian Church, a medic named Dr Acheson also questioned the infant mortality rates, claiming that the medical profession 'would refuse to endorse Dr Thomson's figures'.[60] Some doctors traduced Thomson with claims that he did not understand Belfast's medical landscape and sought to discredit the veracity of the infant mortality figures that he highlighted.

Influential figures in Northern Ireland's medical establishment were also antithetical to the scheme. Northern Ireland's powerful medical voluntarism was deeply interconnected with the unionist and Protestant social and political elite and was key to shaping health and hospital policies. Representatives of the powerful medical voluntary sector opposed the expansion of municipal MCW. The leading medical and political figure, Prof. R. J. Johnstone (Unionist Party MP and senior BMA member, who also headed up the Northern Ireland Departmental Commission on Local Government Administration), opposed the measure. He informed the Northern Ireland House of Commons that many in the medical profession believed Thomson's proposed municipal scheme was inimical to Belfast's interests and that 'the money [would] be very badly spent'. Instead, Johnstone praised the voluntary and poor law sectors for undertaking 'very good work' in maternity and child welfare.[61] Opposition from the medical establishment can be explained by fear of the expansion of local authority care in fields and specialities that were traditionally in the voluntary sector. Moreover, medical voluntarism in Belfast simultaneously developed the Royal Maternity Hospital, as will be further explored in Chapter 3. Opened in 1933 it was spearheaded by Johnstone and the Royal Victoria Hospital. Thomson's scheme threatened to municipalise services that the voluntary sector was committed to and potentially weakened philanthropic funding via increased local taxation. Thomson's socialistic and municipal scheme offered a very different vision of healthcare than that of elite, hierarchical and paternal medical voluntarism.

In the face of opposition from the political and medical establishment, the labour and feminist movements continued to agitate for the measure. During a Belfast Corporation meeting, McCoubrey heavily criticised the central government's failure to increase the state grant and made a thinly veiled accusation against councillors who opposed the measure: she stated '[I] ... hoped that no member of the Council by hint, word, or look had insinuated to the government that the Council would be content with a modified scheme'.[62] A deputation of Belfast's Women's Advisory Council lobbied the Minister for Home Affairs to increase maternity and child welfare grants.[63] Similarly, the trade union movement also sought the adoption of the proposals. The Textile Operatives' Society of Ireland, which represented 'a large body of women, call[ed] upon the Ulster government to immediately give effect to the scheme for maternity and child welfare as suggested by Dr Thomson'.[64]

A renewed attempt to bring about increased funding was made in early 1931 when the Corporation's estimate for the forthcoming financial year had to be finalised. Some 150 members of the Belfast Women's Advisory Council attended a meeting of Belfast Corporation seeking the proposed increase in maternity and child welfare. McCoubrey led the deputation and contextualised the issue within a gender framework. She said: 'whilst the Council, as city fathers, were arguing and debating in regard to necessary financial adjustments, the deputation [was] there as city mothers to impress upon them that the most important aspect was the care of the infant life of the city'. The gendered nature of the issue was further highlighted by McCoubrey when she challenged the councillors' apparent commitment to financial parsimony and the protection of the ratepayers as an overly male concern by declaring 'the women ratepayers were willing to face that expenditure'.[65] The Belfast feminists also viewed their efforts as part of a wider, transnational movement to agitate for women's rights. The international feminist press reported the protest in a piece written by Dora Mellone, the former suffragist and leading Belfast member of the Irish Women's Suffrage Federation.[66] Although largely ineffective in the face of entrenched unionist social and political conservatism, the agitation portrayed the political and gendered character of healthcare debates.

Central government intransigence

The Northern Irish government was divided over whether to support maternity and child welfare. For much of the interwar years,

Northern Irish officials attempted to maintain parity with British social welfare levels, which historians have identified as a step-by-step policy.[67] In 1922, the Northern Irish cabinet pledged that welfare legislation passed in Westminster would be replicated in Northern Ireland, regardless of the strain on public finances.[68] This policy focused on contributory insurance welfare, evidenced in Northern Ireland's introduction of medical benefits and contributory pensions for widows, orphans and older people, along with the maintenance of unemployment and old-age pension payments at UK-wide rates.[69] Yet, the unionist government and cabinet were divided between what historians have termed 'populists' and 'anti-populists'. Populists sought to stave off the appeal of socialism by addressing the concerns of working-class Protestants through high social spending and sectarian arguments and rhetoric. In contrast, anti-populists eschewed using extravagant public expenditure to appeal to working-class Protestants and offered a more conciliatory approach to Catholics.[70] Populists are viewed as emerging as the dominant view within government, evidenced through the failure to bring about non-sectarian education reform and increased expenditure on social security measures, such as unemployment and medical benefit.[71]

Tensions over maternity and child welfare surfaced in the male-dominated Northern Irish cabinet (all twelve members in the inter-war years were male) between the populist and anti-populist wings of government. The populist and step-by-step Minister of Home Affairs, Dawson Bates, supported increased government grants to fund local authorities.[72] Bates's support for maternity and child welfare was deeply political and motivated by a fear of the increased popularity of the labour movement. In April 1929, Bates wrote to the Minister of Finance, Hugh Pollock, claiming that the NILP 'had found a weak spot in our armour' and would make 'very strong capital out of our neglect' of maternity and child welfare.[73] In early 1930, the issue came to a head in cabinet after Belfast Corporation sought part funding for Thomson's plan. Bates again strongly supported government funding and informed the cabinet that the lack of financial support led to MCW being in 'a state of arrested development' and that Belfast's infant mortality rate should be 'comparable with England'.[74] The populist Bates was explicitly sensitive to Belfast's unfavourable comparison to cross-channel services and population health, which threatened the step-by-step policy viewed as key to unionist unity. It was also inimical to the unionist commitment that devolution would not negatively impact standards of care. While the feminist and labour movement's commitment to maternity and child welfare was based on women's rights and progressive health policies, Bates, in contrast, was principally motivated by the maintenance of unionist political unity.

The Minister of Finance, Hugh Pollock, fiscally conservative and noted anti-populist, was vehemently opposed to Bates and the Corporation's request to partially fund the services. Pollock criticised Belfast Corporation for basing the scheme on state support and 'throwing' on the government the 'whole moral responsibility for its adoption or rejection'.[75] Pollock deprecated claims that the government lagged Britain in funding local authorities. He argued that Belfast Corporation greatly benefited from state financing of education and police, unlike local authorities across Britain. The Corporation was, according to Pollock, in 'complete ignorance of the present advantages which they enjoy'. He claimed:

> There can be no comparison between the financial relations of government *vis-à-vis* British as against Northern Irish local authorities. If Belfast claims a fifty per cent Child Welfare Grant because such grants are made to British towns, it follows that they must be prepared to undertake comparable liabilities, because parity in benefits postulates parity in responsibilities.[76]

Pollock determinedly proclaimed: 'the time has come when we must stand firm against these flank attacks by the Corporation'.[77] He succeeded: the cabinet denied the Corporation's request, and the government remained quiescent in the field of maternity and child welfare. This demonstrated the limits of the government's step-by-step policy, in which parity in social welfare was only achieved for contributory insurances and pensions, which invariably favoured the predominantly Protestant employed and industrialised classes. The government was less willing to fund services that it viewed as the remit of local government or the voluntary sector, which often supported the poor, sick, women and children. The government's intransigence, combined with the Corporation's unwillingness to meet the full costs, ensured the arrested development of municipal maternity and child welfare and a lower standard of care than offered by local authorities in Britain.

Tensions between the Northern Irish government and Belfast Corporation had existed since the creation of Northern Ireland. Central government frustrations with Belfast Corporation also emanated from the local authority's maladministration, unearthed in the 1920s by the Megaw Inquiry.[78] Central–municipal government tensions were apparent throughout interwar Europe as both sides sought to take powers from each other, pass on costs and establish final authority for action or inaction.[79] The devolved context of Northern Ireland exacerbated matters. Belfast Corporation's power dwarfed all other local authorities and rivalled the central state.[80] The proposed MCW scheme became entangled in the wider financial quagmire between central and local government.

Further crisis

While Thomson's ambitious proposals were in abeyance, the politics of welfare once again came to the fore in 1932 when Belfast felt the full impact of the economic depression. High levels of unemployment severely impacted social conditions, and Belfast's population health was at a low ebb. High infant mortality rates again hit the city, and in July 1932, the number reached 119, the highest level since 1920 and a clear indication that the economic depression had significantly impacted health.[81] Welfare provision for the unemployed had become highly politicised. In Britain, proposed cuts to unemployment benefits led to much political division within the Labour government. The controversy was ultimately a key factor in its demise, the subsequent split in the Labour Party and the election of a National Government in 1931.[82] In Belfast, the relief of the unemployed generated much political and social unrest. The Belfast Board of Guardians were notoriously slow to grant relief to the able-bodied uninsured and those whose unemployment insurance had expired after two years and were no longer entitled to benefits.[83] Similar to the Corporation's stance on maternity and child welfare, the guardians sought to shift the financial and moral responsibility for increased relief payments to central government, which the latter bitterly resisted.[84] This came to a head in 1932, during the height of the economic depression, when the guardians, oblivious to the effect of chronic unemployment, curbed relief payments because they considered many applicants were undeserving; attitudes which were combined with anti-Catholic sectarianism. Prolonged street violence erupted in protest at Belfast Board of Guardians' low relief payments, popularly known as the 'Outdoor Relief Riots', in October 1932. A rare occurrence of cross-religious Catholic and Protestant working-class agitation marked this unrest.[85] The politics, distress and violent protest of the economic depression that engulfed much of Britain were widely evident in Belfast.

In the context of the economic depression and the city's ill health and high infant mortality rates, Thomson renewed attempts to expand municipal maternity and child welfare in 1932. In contrast to his original 1930 plans for fully reformed and expanded services, this time, he solely focused on emergency measures to address malnutrition. This was reflective of highly politicised public health debates in Britain during the interwar years. Officialdom, according to the historian Charles Webster, sought to downplay the link between unemployment and malnutrition due to political pressure to ignore the failures of public health and socio-economic policies of the coalition governments, which faced voluminous social commentary on the plight of working people scourged by unemployment and poverty.[86] Malnutrition was key to debates about the role of public health and the state in the politically charged years of the economic depression.

Thomson did not shy away from the issue of malnutrition and highlighted the connection between unemployment and poor health. He reported that many parents were in 'such poverty' that they could not afford to buy milk or food for their infants, that the Corporation's provision of free milk was exhausted and did not meet 'the needs of necessitous, expectant and nursing mothers and infants'. Many women had to be removed from the recipient lists prematurely to provide for new cases.[87] After completing a survey of one hundred mothers who attended maternity and child welfare clinics, Thomson identified 'a state of malnutrition and debility in the expectant mothers', seventy-four of whom were in unemployed households.[88] To combat infant deaths, Thomson sought the introduction of temporary free meal services for women and infants.[89] The scheme proposed to provide 1,250 meals on a weekly basis for which he sought six thousand pounds. Thomson's focus on poverty and nutrition was reflective of his progressiveness. In this regard, he was representative of some public health officials who pursued policies to address ill health, malnutrition and the effects of unemployment.[90]

Opposition to the measure emerged. Alderman Duff claimed that the provision of meals was the responsibility of the poor law. He criticised Thomson for following English local government, where the poor law had been abolished in 1929 and subsumed by municipal authorities. Councillor Lowe, a doctor, similarly attacked the scheme, asking: 'how many churches have we got in Belfast? All these are feeding the people. Free breakfasts, free dinners, free teas, free beds. My God, the whole thing's free'. Lowe's comments echoed notions about welfare creating dependency, which were also evident on the Belfast Board of Guardians concerning outdoor relief.[91] The NILP councillor Midgley retorted that some doctors such as Lowe were motivated by professional self-interest and opposed the expansion of services that 'cut across their private practice'.[92] The Corporation narrowly voted for the scheme, but the plans collapsed after the failure to get a tenderer. Belfast Corporation's response to the distressed economic and social conditions of 1932 was largely a failure. Recalcitrance to Thomson's plans was based on traditional opposition from some in the medical profession to municipal expansion in services. This was combined with resistance from many councillors to accept that the municipality had a role in tackling malnutrition, which they viewed as the remit of the poor law and voluntary sectors.

Conclusion

This focus on maternity and child welfare has provided multiple insights into health politics and policies in Northern Ireland, which are key themes with which this work is concerned. Utilising the case study of Belfast Corporation's approach to maternity and child welfare, the arrested potential for socialistic healthcare policies in Northern Ireland is identified. The policies unsuccessfully pursued by the medical officer of health, Thomson, were inspired by the London-orientated SMA and sought to replicate services provided in many Labour-run local authorities in Britain. Thomson also did not shrink from the realities of unemployment and attempted to expand provision to meet the health consequences of the economic depression. The Northern Ireland and Belfast labour and feminist movements, often inspired by wider international campaigns for women's rights, recognised Thomson's progressive policies and threw their full support behind them. The plans to expand such provision offered a version of healthcare largely unavailable in Northern Ireland, especially concerning maternity and child welfare, that was democratically managed, free from the pauperising poor law and paternalistic charity, and staffed by medical local authority employees. Maternity and child welfare also became deeply politicised as unionism inevitably rejected what was viewed as a NILP measure.

At one level, Belfast seemed to have the most propitious conditions – fledgling labour success in local and general elections, urbanisation, industrialisation and a large workforce, many of whom were women – in Northern Ireland for the implementation of such progressive, leftist health policies. The city's high infant mortality rate depicted the need for increased provision. Yet the appetite for such progressive policies in Belfast and Northern Ireland was dampened by the dominance of the Ulster Unionist Party, which ensured social conservatism, commitment to ratepayer savings and acquiescence to the socially hierarchical voluntary sector. The power brokers at central and local government, predominantly male and unionist, rejected the proposals, which was a clear indication of the constraints of progressive health policies and politics in the region.

Ostensibly, the unwillingness of the central government to increase the grant for expanded services or the Corporation to meet the full cost of services prevented growth in maternity and child welfare. This painfully illustrates the restrictions to unionism's step-by-step welfare policy, which sought to maintain support from the working classes by keeping social services at wider UK levels. This pledge, however, was largely for insurance-based schemes and did not extend to supporting local authority services. The government was willing to fund insurance-based welfare such as unemployment benefits, national health insurance and state pensions, which helped to maintain and reward a productive, largely unionist workforce. It was far less willing to support local authority provision, which often provided for the most needy and vulnerable but least politically significant groups in society.

Deeper systemic factors also lay behind central and local government's inactivity in this field. The debate around maternity and child welfare was highly gendered. Some of the most vocal campaigners for maternity and child welfare were female activists, while the government cabinet was all male, and the Belfast Corporation was predominantly of that gender. The gendered nature of the issue was not lost on feminist campaigners, such as McCoubrey, who wily highlighted that the mostly male cohort of councillors were unwilling to invest in female-oriented provision. The male unionist decision-makers in both central and local government were unperturbed and easily batted away a measure that feminists agitated for.

Other factors were also inimical to growth in municipal care. Many in the medical profession opposed the measure, chiefly private practitioners and the powerful voluntary sector, whose independence was threatened by the increased municipalisation of healthcare. Voluntary healthcare, as outlined in Chapter 3, was far more successful in developing maternity provision in Northern Ireland. Socially hierarchical, medically controlled and politically conservative, medical voluntarism differed from the more democratically focused, labour and feminist-orientated municipal healthcare envisaged in Thomson's plans. These represented two contrasting and, at times, competing visions and cultures of healthcare and welfare. Northern Ireland's labour and feminist movements, however, were ultimately too weak to bring about substantial municipal provision.

Notes

1 J. Stewart, *The Battle for Health: A Political History of the Socialist Medical Association, 1930–51* (Brookfield: Ashgate Publishing Company, 1999), pp. 23–5, 43–53.

2 Levene *et al.*, *Cradle to Grave*, p. 90.

3 B. M. Doyle, 'Labour and Hospitals in urban Yorkshire: Middlesbrough, Leeds, and Sheffield, 1919–38', *Social History of Medicine*, 23:2 (2010), 374–92.

4 Levene *et al.*, *Cradle to Grave*, p. 123.

5 C. Williamson, 'To remove the stigma of the Poor Law': The 'Comprehensive' ideal and patient access to the municipal hospital service in the city of Glasgow, 1918–39', *History*, 99:1 (2014), 78.

6 A. M. Hughes, *Gender and Political Identities in Scotland, 1919–39* (Edinburgh: Edinburgh University Press, 2010), p. 123.
7 Stewart, *Battle for Health*, p. 89.
8 E. Jones, 'Nothing too good for the people: local Labour and London's interwar health centre movement', *Social History of Medicine*, 25:1 (2012), 84–102.
9 G. Walker, 'The Northern Ireland Labour Party in the 1920s', *Saothar*, 10 (1984), 19.
10 S. O'Connell, 'An age of conservative modernity, 1914–68', in S. J. Connolly (ed.), *Belfast 400: People, Place and History* (Liverpool: Liverpool University Press, 2012), p. 281; I. Budge and C. O'Leary, *Belfast: Approach to Crisis. A Study of Belfast Politics, 1613–1970* (London: The Macmillan Press, 1973), pp. 186–7.
11 C. V. Loughlin, *Labour and the Politics of Disloyalty in Belfast, 1921–39: The Moral Economy of Loyalty* (Basingstoke: Palgrave Macmillan, 2018), pp. 73–5.
12 Budge and O'Leary, *Belfast: Approach to Crisis*, pp. 147–8; C. E. B. Brett, *Housing A Divided Community* (Dublin: Institute of Public Administration, 1986), pp. 16–22.
13 Privilege and Jones, 'Crisis and scandal', 39–43.
14 L. M. White, 'Midgley, Henry Cassidy ("Harry")', in J. McGuire and J. Quinn, *Dictionary of Irish Biography* (hereafter *DIB*), Vol. 6, McGuire-Nutt (Dublin: Cambridge University Press, 2009) pp. 503–5.
15 *BN*, 13 January 1934; G. Walker, *The Politics of Frustration: Harry Midgley and the Failure of Labour in Northern Ireland* (Manchester: Manchester University Press, 1985), p. 41.
16 *BN*, 3 July 1928.
17 PRONI, LA7/2EB/119, County Borough of Belfast Council minutes, Public Health Committee meeting, 4 November 1930, p. 613; Public Health Committee meeting, 2 December 1930, p. 960.
18 *BN*, 4 April 1934.
19 *Belfast Telegraph* [hereafter *BT*], 2 January 1931.
20 O. Purdue, 'Surviving the industrial city: the female poor and the workhouse in late nineteenth-century Belfast', *Urban History*, 44:1 (2017), 72.
21 T. Clavin, 'McCoubrey (Morrison), Margaret', in *DIB*, https://www.dib.ie/biography/mccoubrey-morrison-margaret-a10131 (accessed 20 November 2024); M. Hill 'Women, War and Welfare: The co-operative crusades of Margaret Taylor McCoubrey, 1880–1956', *Familia: Ulster Genealogical Review*, 32 (2016), 38–59.
22 PRONI, D3311, Central Women's Section of the Northern Ireland Labour Party minute book, 11 June 1928, 7 January 1929, 2 January

1930; *BN*, 28 February 1930; *BN*, 23 October 1930; *NW*, 5 March 1932.

23 M. Hill and M. Ward, 'Conflicting rights: The struggle for female citizenship in Northern Ireland', in E. Breitenbach and P. Thane (eds), *Women and Citizenship in Britain and Ireland in the Twentieth Century: What Difference Did the Vote Make?* (London: Bloomsbury Publishing, 2012), pp. 117–8.

24 Levene *et al.*, *Cradle to Grave*; J. Neville, 'Explaining local authority choices on public hospital provision in the 1930s: A public policy hypothesis', *Medical History*, 56:1 (2012), 56.

25 C. S. Thomson, 'Small-pox and vaccination', *BMJ*, 1:43 (6 January 1923), 43; *ibid.*, 'Administrative problems connected with puerperal fever and puerperal pyrexia', *Journal of the Royal Society of Promotion of Health*, 48:5 (1 January 1927), 236–44.

26 *BT*, 30 January 1929.

27 *BT*, 2 March 1928.

28 Levene *et al.*, *Cradle to Grave*, p. 82; Gorsky 'Did public health fail?', 181.

29 Webster, 'Healthy or hungry thirties?', 110–29.

30 J. Welshman, 'School meals and milk in England and Wales, 1906–45', *Medical History*, 41:1 (January 1997), 18.

31 A. Mold, P. Clark, G. Millward and D. Payling, *Placing the Public in Public Health in Post-War Britain, 1948–2012* (London: Palgrave Macmillan, 2019), p. 2.

32 V. Fildes, L. Marks and H. Marland, 'Introduction', in *ibid.*, *Women and Children First: International Maternal and Infant Welfare, 1870–1945* (Abingdon: Routledge, 1992), p. 1.

33 L. Earner-Byrne, *Mother and Child: Maternity and Child Welfare in Dublin, 1922–60* (Manchester: Manchester University Press, 2007), pp. 10–11.

34 H. Hendrick, *Child Welfare: Historical Dimensions, Contemporary Debates* (Bristol: Policy Press, 2003), p. 65.

35 PRONI, LA7/9AD/1, Belfast County Borough MCW Committee minutes, 6 November 1918.

36 PRONI, LA7/9DA/24, Belfast County Borough Medical Officer of Health Report, 1922, p. 47.

37 PRONI, LA7/9AD/1, Belfast County Borough MCW Committee minutes, 24 April 1919; A. Evans, 'Health in Belfast: The vital statistics of poverty', in F. W. Boal and S. A. Royle (eds), *Enduring City: Belfast in the Twentieth Century* (Belfast: Blackstaff Press, 2006), p. 248; for the role of babies' clubs in public health in Ireland, see Earner-Byrne, *Mother and Child*, p. 10; M. Ó hÓgartaigh, 'Flower power

and "mental grooviness": Nurses and midwives in Ireland in the early twentieth century', in B. Whelan (ed.), *Women and Paid Work in Ireland, 1500–1930* (Dublin: Four Courts Press, 2000), pp. 133–47; I. Finn, 'Women in the medical profession in Ireland, 1876–1919', in Whelan (ed.), *Women and Paid Work in Ireland*, pp. 102–99.

38 PRONI, LA/79/DA/25, Belfast County Borough Medical Officer of Health Report, 1927, p. 40.

39 *NW*, 4 March 1929.

40 Levene *et al.*, *Cradle to Grave*, p. 82; J. Welshman, 'The Medical Officer of Health in England and Wales, 1900–1974: watchdog or lapdog?', *Journal of Public Health Medicine*, 19:4 (1997), 443–50; M. Gorsky, 'Local leadership in public health: the role of the medical officer of health in Britain, 1872–1974', *Journal of Epidemiological Community Medicine*, 61:6 (2007), 468–72.

41 PRONI, LA/7/9/DA/25, Belfast County Borough Medical Officer of Health Report, 1929, p. 54.

42 J. Jenkinson, *Scotland's Health, 1919–48* (Oxford, Peter Lang, 2001), p.147.

43 PRONI, LA/7/9/DA/25, Belfast County Borough Medical Officer of Health Report, 1929, p. 54.

44 PRONI, LA7/9/AD/1, Belfast County Borough MCW Committee minutes, 27 January 1930.

45 *BT*, 28 January 1930.

46 E. Jones, 'Nothing too good for the people: Local Labour and London's interwar health centre movement', *Social History of Medicine*, 25:1 (2012), 84–102.

47 The interconnectedness of Ulster unionism and voluntary hospitals is explored in Chapter 3.

48 Stewart, *Battle for Health*, pp. 25, 50.

49 *Witness*, 07 February 1930.

50 *BT*, 28 January 1930.

51 For example, Thomas Henderson was an independent unionist councillor, elected to Stormont in 1929, who had a socio-economic platform, see Reid, 'Protestant challenges to the "Protestant State"', 430.

52 PRONI, LA/7/9/AD/1, Belfast County Borough MCW Committee minutes, 12 February 1930.

53 *Witness*, 7 February 1930.

54 MoF, *Financial Relations*, p. 6.

55 PRONI, CAB/9/B/53/3, Cabinet Secretariat, Ministry of Home Affairs B files, Prime Minister meeting notes: deputation from the Belfast Women's Council, 21 March 1926.

56 *BN*, 14 February 1930.

57 *BN*, 25 February 1930.
58 *BN*, 4 March 1930.
59 *BN*, 4 March 1930.
60 *BT*, 7 June 1930.
61 *NIHoCD*, 13, 10 March 1931, p. 236.
62 *BN*, 25 February 1930.
63 *BN*, 20 March 1930.
64 *BN*, 30 May 1930.
65 *BN*, 3 February 1931.
66 *The International Women's News*, March 1931, p. 87; M. Ward, 'Conflicting interests: The British and Irish Suffrage movements', *Feminist Review*, 50 (summer 1995), 142.
67 Buckland, *Factory of Grievances*, pp. 150–2; G. Walker, 'The Northern Ireland Labour Party', in F. Lane and D. Ó Drisceoil (eds), *Politics and the Irish Working Class, 1830–1945* (Basingstoke: Palgrave Macmillan, 2005), p. 235.
68 Reid, 'Protestant challenges to the "Protestant State"', 426.
69 R. J. Lawrence, *The Government of Northern Ireland: Public Finances and Public Services, 1921–64* (Oxford: Oxford University Press, 1965), pp. 45–50; Martin, 'Ending the pauper taint'.
70 For an exploration of such tensions within unionism, see P. Bew, P. Gibbons and H. Patterson, *Northern Ireland, 1921–2001: Political Forces and Social Classes* (London: Serif, 3rd ed., 2002), pp. 48–64.
71 N. C. Fleming, 'The first government of Northern Ireland, education reform and the failure of anti-populist Unionism, 1921–25', *Twentieth Century British History*, 18:2 (2007), 146–69.
72 Other prominent 'populists' included the Northern Irish Prime Minister James Craig and the Minister for Labour, J. M. Millar; see Buckland, *Factory of Grievances*, p. 160; for an outline of Bates political career, see R. Hawkins, 'Bates, Sir (Richard) Dawson', in *DIB*, https://www.dib.ie/biography/bates-sir-richard-dawson-a0491 (accessed 20 November 2024).
73 PRONI, CAB/9/B/53, Cabinet Secretariat, Ministry of Home Affairs B files, MCW schemes, Bates to Pollock, 23 April 1929.
74 *Ibid.*, Memorandum to Cabinet on MCW schemes from Ministry of Home Affairs, 11 March 1930.
75 *Ibid.*
76 *Ibid.*
77 *Ibid.*
78 Budge and O'Leary, *Belfast: Approach to Crisis*, pp. 147–8.

79 B. M. Doyle and A. McElligott, 'The rise and fall of European municipal power since 1800', *International Journal of Regional and Local Studies*, 7:1/2 (2011), 17.

80 In 1930 the Corporation's annual expenditure was £3,086,568 compared to the Northern Irish state's £11,830,748; see MHA, *Local Taxation Returns, 1929/30* (Belfast: HMSO, 1930); MoF, *Financial Relations*, p. 20.

81 PRONI, LA/7/2/EB/129, Belfast County Borough MCW Committee minutes, 24 August 1932, p. 511.

82 D. Howell, *MacDonald's Party: Labour Identities and Crisis, 1922–31* (Oxford: Oxford University Press, 2002), p. 4.

83 S. Riordan, 'Politics, economy, society: Northern Ireland, 1920–39', in T. Bartlett (ed.), *The Cambridge History of Ireland: Vol. 4, 1880 to the Present* (Cambridge: Cambridge University Press, 2018), pp. 319–20.

84 Buckland, *Factory of Grievances*, pp. 157–9.

85 For an overview of the extensive literature on the Outdoor Relief Riots, see McLoughlin, *Labour and the Politics of Disloyalty in Belfast*, pp. 26–7. Also see P. Devlin, *Yes We Have No Bananas: Outdoor Relief in Belfast, 1920–39* (Belfast: Blackstaff, 1981).

86 Webster, 'Hunger or Healthy', 114–15; see also J. Lawrence, 'Class, "affluence" and the study of everyday life in Britain, c. 1930–64', *Cultural and Social History*, 10:2 (2013), 276; I. Gazeley, A. Newell, K. Reynolds and H. Rufrancos, 'How hungry were the poor in late 1930s Britain?', *Economic Historical Review*, 75:1 (2022), 81.

87 PRONI, LA/2EB/129, Belfast County Borough MCW Committee minutes, 24 August 1932, p. 511.

88 PRONI, LA/2EB/129, Belfast County Borough MCW Committee minutes, 15 November 1933; *ibid.*, Report on the scheme for feeding expectant and nursing mothers for sixteen weeks ending 31 March 1933, p. 6.

89 PRONI, LA/2EB/129, County Borough of Belfast Council and Committee minutes October–December 1932, Finance Committee meeting, p. 57.

90 Welshman, 'The Medical Officer of Health in England and Wales, 1900–1974'.

91 Buckland, *Factory of Grievances*, p. 158.

92 *BT*, 2 December 1932.

3

Voluntarism and hospitals in interwar Northern Ireland

Introduction

After examining poor law and municipal provision in Chapters 1 and 2, the book's focus now turns to charitable and voluntary hospital provision. Before the nationalisation of voluntary hospitals in the United Kingdom in 1948, these were central to the mixed economy of healthcare of the early twentieth century in an era when they emerged as the most advanced and sophisticated medical institutions. It is argued in this chapter that some voluntary hospitals in Northern Ireland brought about a degree of collaboration and organisation that was not overly evident in poor law and local authority provision. This resembled some cities in interwar Britain, which witnessed coordination between providers, leading to localised health systems.[1] Such integration was evident on Grosvenor Road in Belfast, where a medical site revolved around three hospitals – Royal Victoria, Royal Maternity and Royal Hospital for Sick Children. It was brought about by an influential nexus and coalition of leading medical consultants, academic medicine and the social elite; these groupings coalesced politically under Ulster unionism. This powerful force was mirrored outside Belfast where a medical voluntarism, comprised of the local social and economic elite, leading provincial medics and unionist politicians, supported and managed county infirmaries and cottage hospitals. This chapter posits that this unionist medical voluntarism emerged as the most powerful interest group in interwar Northern Irish healthcare.

The extent to which medical voluntarism represented a coherent hospital structure is also examined. It is argued that while the Grosvenor Road medical site reflected a nascent hospital model, the overall inability to include other voluntary facilities, mainly the Mater Hospital, and local authority institutions stymied the potential for a more joined-up interwar service. Institutional loyalties and competition between hospitals are highlighted as another barrier to greater coordination in provincial Northern Ireland, where the development of local authority district hospitals threatened county infirmaries. Overall, a disaggregated system of voluntary hospitals, independent of local authority provision, is depicted.

Also, the changing financial base of voluntary hospital funding and the increased importance of working-class contribution schemes are explored. The chapter explains how increased demand for access to healthcare in many voluntary hospitals challenged the entitlement of the poor to medical charity. It argues that medical voluntarism failed to provide for patients beyond the poor and working classes. The sector was weakened by its inability to extend entitlement to white-collar, middle-class and fee-paying patients, who increasingly turned to hospitals for treatment. Restrictions on entitlement diminished the popularity and success of medical voluntarism.

Historians have largely not explored medical voluntarism on the island of Ireland. Some work has highlighted the potential for historical research into voluntary healthcare.[2] While studies on philanthropy in Ulster have included the exploration of early-nineteenth-century Presbyterian evangelicalism, general surveys of charity in the nineteenth and early twentieth century and the Belfast Charitable Society, focus on medical voluntarism has largely concentrated on county infirmaries in the late eighteenth century and traditional institutional histories.[3] This is the first study to examine medical voluntarism and voluntary hospitals in Northern Ireland after partition.

What were voluntary hospitals?

Voluntary hospitals were first and foremost charitable institutions that were independent from central and local government. General infirmaries originated in the eighteenth and early nineteenth centuries in response to the medical needs of urban populations during industrialisation. By the mid to late nineteenth century, specialist voluntary hospitals emerged. Voluntary hospitals were more advanced and prestigious than local authority and poor law institutions. They focused on acute medicine, and many voluntary hospitals did not treat the long-term chronic, infirm and infectious sick. They were also deeply connected to the medical profession and associated training. Medical consultants and specialists provided their services *gratis*, often relying on hospitals' wealthy subscribers for private practice. Voluntary hospitals were funded mainly by charity and received little support from local rates or general taxation. Boards of management and governors, drawn from subscribers, ran voluntary hospitals. The poor were entitled to access voluntary hospitals, while governors and subscribers could also give access through subscribers' notes. The working classes who paid into hospital contribution schemes also had an entitlement.

General and specialist voluntary hospitals were, by and large, an urban phenomenon. As depicted in Table 3.1, many voluntary beds (1,637 or 70.2 per cent of the total in 1940) in Northern Ireland were in this category, and most were in Belfast. Northern Ireland's leading medical institution was the Royal Victoria Hospital, which originated in the Belfast Fever Hospital and General Hospital, dating back to 1791 and received its royal charter in 1875. The other major general voluntary hospital in Northern Ireland was the Mater Infirmorum, a Catholic facility established by the Sisters of Mercy nursing religious order in 1883. Belfast also witnessed the expansion in specialisations common to the mid- to late nineteenth century, spurred on by the growth of medical knowledge and professional rivalries.[4] Voluntary hospitals were prominent across cities on the island of Ireland. Irish cities – both north and south – generally had more voluntary beds than British cities of similar sizes (see Table 3.2). This was most evident in Dublin, where Catholic voluntary hospitals grew from the mid-nineteenth century alongside the older Protestant-orientated voluntary hospitals, which dated from the late eighteenth and early nineteenth century. This led to one of the most extensive voluntary systems in Britain or Ireland. Voluntary provision in Belfast was greater than in many British cities but smaller than in Dublin. In British cities, Catholic general voluntary hospitals were uncommon, even in places with large Catholic populations such as Glasgow and Liverpool. The Catholic

Table 3.1 Voluntary hospital beds in Northern Ireland, circa 1921–40.

	Est.	*circa 1921*	*circa 1940*
General hospitals			
Royal Victoria Hospital	1791	323	538
Mater Infirmorum	1883	270	318
Specialist hospitals			
Belfast			
Benn Ulster Eye, Ear and Throat Hospital	1871	30	32
Foster Green Hospital for Consumption and Chest Disease	1879	76	199
Nervous Diseases Hospital and Epileptic Colony	1896	16	30
Hospital for Sick Children	1873	45	86
Incorporated Maternity Hospital/Royal Maternity Hospital	1794	32	85
Ophthalmic Hospital	1848	25	28
Samaritan Hospital for Diseases of Women	1873	30	50
Ulster Hospital for Children and Women	1872	46	106
Our Lady's Hospital and Oratory, Beechmount	1934		140
Derry/Londonderry			
Eye, Ear and Throat Hospital	1896	19	25
Total		**912**	**1637**
City/county infirmaries and fever hospitals			
Armagh County Infirmary, Armagh	1797	50	70
City and County Infirmary, Derry/Londonderry	1789	65	100
Fermanagh County Hospital, Enniskillen	1820	59	64
Tyrone County Hospital, Omagh	1825	66	97
County Antrim Infirmary, Lisburn	1780	55	60
County Down Infirmary, Downpatrick	1797	60	70
Newry Fever and General Hospital, Newry	1825	24	32
Total		**379**	**493**
Cottage Hospitals			
Ballymena Cottage Hospital, County Antrim	1881	23	23
Cushendall Cottage Hospital, County Antrim	1885	11	15
Smiley Cottage Hospital, Larne, County Antrim	1903	26	21
Bangor Cottage Hospital, Bangor, County Down	1869	24	32
Coleraine Cottage Hospital, County Derry/Londonderry	1885	17	45
Cowen Heron Cottage Hospital, Dromore, County Down	1900	15	16

(*Continued*)

Table 3.1 (Continued)

	Est.	*circa 1921*	*circa 1940*
Hopefield Cottage Hospital, Portrush, County Derry/Londonderry	N/A	N/A	N/A
The Robinson Memorial Hospital, Ballymoney, County Antrim	1933		29
Total		**116**	**181**
Total voluntary beds in Northern Ireland		**1,407**	**2,331**

Source: This data was collated from numerous sources including *Burdett's Hospitals and Charities: Being the Yearbook of Philanthropy and the Hospital Annual* (London: Scientific Press, 1919); *Burdett's Hospitals...* (London: Scientific Press, 1930); NPHT, *Survey of the Hospital Services of Northern Ireland* (Belfast: Privately Printed for the Northern Ireland Regional Hospital Committee, 1944), pp. 64–88.

Table 3.2 Voluntary hospital beds per 1,000 of the population in Irish and British cities, 1911 and 1940.

	1911	*1940*
Belfast	2.31	3.27
Dublin	5.85	4.56
Glasgow	2.01	3.2
Liverpool	1.54	2.49
Sheffield	1.36	2.31

Source: Voluntary Hospital Database: http://www.hospitalsdatabase.lshtm.ac.uk/ (accessed 1 September 2020); B. R. Mitchell, *British Historical Statistics* (Cambridge: Cambridge University Press, 1988).

Mater Infirmorum increased Belfast's bed count. Belfast's voluntary hospital structure witnessed much growth during the interwar years with a significant increase in beds, as evidenced in Table 3.1, and the building of new hospitals.

Outside Belfast, county and city infirmaries formed another layer of medical voluntarism and provided general acute and surgical care. These hospitals witnessed little growth during the 1920s and 1930s. Staffed by the county surgeon, they were the main source of specialist and consultant provision in provincial Ulster and dated back to the County Infirmaries Act of 1765.[5] Two county fever infirmaries offered infectious disease provision under the 1818 Hospitals (Ireland) Act. The patients were mostly the poor and working classes, although more middle-class individuals increasingly turned to these hospitals during the interwar years. Local authorities, such as county councils, had an important role in funding and managing the institutions. Predominantly funded by voluntary and patient contributions, they also received grants from county councils. The boards of management were made up of subscribers and county councillors. Despite such local government involvement, the hospitals were considered voluntary institutions and differed in prestige and prominence from workhouse infirmaries.[6] This facet of the management of county infirmaries differed from the Belfast voluntary hospitals, which had little input from the local or central state. At the same time, there was no similar type of voluntary hospital in Britain.

Eight cottage voluntary hospitals also existed in provincial Northern Ireland. Established in the late nineteenth and early twentieth century, they were confined to more prosperous, largely unionist rural areas and towns in counties Antrim, Down and Derry/Londonderry. The local gentry were often central to their establishment. For example, in Larne, the landed Smiley family funded the building of the eponymous Smiley Cottage Hospital, which opened in 1903.[7] The failure of philanthropic efforts in the west and south of Northern Ireland spoke of the inadequacies of voluntarism in areas where the social elite, traditional benefactors of cottage hospitals, was predominantly unionist in outlook but much of the population was Catholic and nationalist. This echoed trends in local authority care, where similar geographical demarcations along political and religious lines were evident in the poor law reform of workhouses into district hospitals, as described in Chapter 1. The underdevelopment of cottage hospitals was evident in that they provided a mere 181 (8 per cent) of 2,331 voluntary beds in Northern Ireland by 1940. This was proportionally smaller than cottage hospitals in Britain, where one study identified that they provided as many as 17 per cent of all voluntary hospital beds.[8] This category did not represent a major aspect of voluntary care in Northern Ireland and was not as important as in Britain.

In the vein of medical voluntarism, cottage hospitals mostly provided general acute care. They did not cater to patients found in poor law institutions, such as chronic and infectious disease cases. They allowed GPs, often restricted from treating their patients in the large urban voluntary hospitals, to admit and treat them in

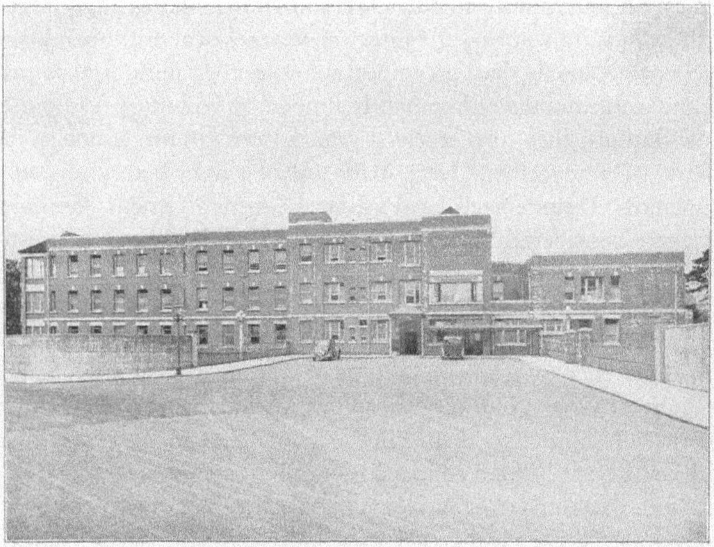

(v) The Royal Maternity Hospital, Belfast. (opened October, 1933.)
Architects - Messrs Young and MacKenzie, Belfast.

Figure 3.1 Royal Maternity Hospital, Belfast, circa 1933. *Source: NIHA Annual Report for the Year Ending 31 Dec. 1951* (Belfast: NIHA, 1952), n.p.

hospitals, ensuring that they retained patients and fees.[9] Cottage hospitals had a reputation for providing homely care in pleasant surroundings but not the more advanced or specialist treatment provided in Belfast's voluntary hospitals. Socially, these hospitals predominantly catered for patients with some means who looked to avoid poor law institutions.

Ulster unionism and medical voluntarism

Medical voluntarism was politically tied to the unionist and Protestant establishment and was key to policymaking in Northern Ireland. Voluntary hospitals and the medical profession have received scant attention as an interest group in Northern Irish politics compared to other organisations such as the Orange Order, churches, and business and farmer lobbies.[10] The medical profession, closely connected with voluntary hospitals, represented in the main by the BMA, has long been identified as an influential pressure group in medical policymaking in Britain.[11] In Northern Ireland, a powerful cohort intersected between the medical profession, voluntary hospitals and Ulster unionism. Many senior medical leaders in voluntary hospitals were also Ulster Unionist Party MPs. In total, fourteen Ulster Unionist MPs were medics during the lifespan of the Northern Irish parliament.[12] Many were elected for the Queen's University constituency and had leading positions in voluntary hospitals. For example, R. J. Johnstone, a professor of gynaecology, sat in the Northern Ireland House of Commons from 1921 until he died in 1938. Johnstone was a central figure in medical voluntarism and led the establishment of the Royal Maternity Hospital in 1933, acting as the first chairman of the hospital's board of management.[13] Johnstone's seniority in the medical profession throughout the UK was evident when he became president of the BMA in 1937.[14] In particular, the Royal Victoria's medical leadership was deeply connected with unionist politics. The chair of the board in the 1930s was Lieutenant-Colonel Mitchell, a surgeon and Unionist Party MP for Queen's. Another Royal Victoria consultant, Howard Stevenson, was elected to Stormont in 1938 as an Ulster Unionist MP for Queen's.[15] Unionism, the medical profession and voluntary hospitals were intertwined.

The interconnections between unionism and medical voluntarism in Northern Ireland were not confined to medics but were also immanent to the non-medical leadership of voluntary hospitals. Many lay members of boards of management of voluntary hospitals were prominent unionist politicians. This was evident in Belfast where Herbert Quin, the one-time Unionist Party MP (1944–49) for Queen's University and later member of the Northern Ireland Senate (1950–68), Stormont's upper chamber, was the chair of the Royal Victoria. Quin was a barrister and Orange Order member.[16] Outside Belfast, much of the voluntary hospital leadership was drawn from prominent figures in provincial unionism. For example, John Milne Barbour, an industrialist and unionist who sat in the Northern Irish parliament as an MP for Antrim constituencies from 1921 to 1959, chaired the Antrim County Infirmary.[17] Lord Bangor, a Unionist Party member of the Northern Ireland Senate, chaired the Down County Infirmary's Board of Management.[18] The Bangor Cottage Hospital's annual meetings were often chaired by the Unionist Party MP and one-time speaker of the Northern Ireland House of Commons, Sir Harry Mulholland.[19] Similarly, H. B. W. Armstrong was the chair of the Armagh County Infirmary. He was a unionist member of the Senate, the Vice Lieutenant of County Armagh, and was briefly elected to the Westminster House of Commons in the early 1920s.[20] Such figures were influential in government and often calibrated health policy towards the mutual needs of elite medics and medical voluntarism. Leading voluntary hospitals and the medical profession represented a powerful interest group at the heart of Ulster unionism and the Northern Irish government.

Medical voluntarism sat easily with the social elite that populated much of the upper echelons of unionism. Firmly rooted patrician unionism had much influence in Northern Irish politics and society. Often referred to as 'Big House Unionism' or the 'Ulster Squirearchy', these elites dominated much of unionist political, social and civic life until the post-war years when they increasingly faced criticism for being out of touch.[21] Medical voluntarism drew on elite charity, which its critics viewed as a preserve of the wealthy and upper-class condescension.[22] Medical voluntarism enveloped social hierarchy, philanthropy, limited state intervention and diluted bureaucracy. Such concepts were synonymous with the socially conservative inchoate Northern Irish unionist state and its elite. In Northern Ireland, voluntary hospitals were embraced by a unionist aristocracy, whose place among the localised political and social elite was strengthened after partition and the establishment of the new country.[23] Although much of the aristocracy's economic power, primarily landed families, had waned, their social status and commitment to Ulster unionism provided many with civic and leadership roles. The Royal Victoria Hospital received support from the aristocracy, and in 1926, the Marquess of Dufferin and Ava became its chairman. The hospital also had much patronage from Belfast's industrial elite. In the early 1920s, William Pirrie – chairman of Harland and Wolff Shipbuilders and the First Viscount Pirrie – was its patron before he died in 1924.[24] The hospital's annual meetings were civic events and frequently addressed by Northern Ireland's leading figures, including the Prime Minister, James Craig and the Lord Chief Justice, Sir Denis S. Henry.[25]

Outside Belfast, the provincial landed elite was integral to voluntary hospitals, often providing financial support, acting as patrons and heading up appeals for funding. Aristocratic women regularly took a prominent role through ladies' committees by fundraising and organising social occasions, flag days and gala events. For example, in 1929, the Countess of Clanwilliam led an appeal fund for the County Down Infirmary, which involved hosting a *fête* on the family's Montalto Estate.[26] This philanthropy allowed the aristocratic elite to continue to be relevant in Northern Irish society. Medical voluntarism drew on the support and patronage of Northern Ireland's elite, who also pervaded the paternalistic leadership of the Ulster Unionist Party and Northern Irish government. This nexus between the political, social and medical elite ensured that medical voluntarism was a powerful pressure group in Northern Ireland's healthcare system, society and government.

In many instances, the aristocracy's role was titular, and they did not participate in the day-to-day management of voluntary hospitals, which, instead, was often in the hands of a middle- to upper-class business, industrial and professional elite. For example, by 1940, the Royal Victoria's board comprised fifteen life governors, fifteen annual subscribers and five members of the medical and surgical staff. Three members – Sir Dixon, Lady Dixon and Lady Byres – had aristocratic titles, but they rarely attended management meetings. Instead, a cohort representative of prominent businessmen and professionals were the most active members.[27] James Blessington was a governor who regularly attended management meetings of the Royal Victoria. He was a senior partner in the leading Belfast estate agency, Blessington Fair & Co, treasurer of the Winder Presbyterian Church, and member of the Ulster Reform Club and Masonic Order.[28] Other active members of the board included Archibald Scott, chairman and managing director of the New Northern Spinning & Weaving Limited Company, and John Higginson, managing director of an eponymous cotton converters company.[29] For such individuals, sitting on the hospital's board of management was part of their broader philanthropic activity, which was apposite to their assumed station in life and confirmed their social status.[30] At another level, these people had much professional experience relevant to the management and governance of hospitals. The involvement of these elites further strengthened medical voluntarism.

Voluntary hospitals, integration and academisation of medicine

At the time of partition, Northern Ireland's voluntary hospitals were marked by a lack of alignment. Management of voluntary hospitals was highly autonomous and disconnected from each other, local authority provision and poor law infirmaries. This was in keeping with wider British developments in which the management of pre-NHS voluntary hospitals has been criticised by contemporaries and historians alike for the lack of integration, overlap of provision and competition between hospitals. Contemporary bodies such as the Political and Economic Planning advocacy group, which was formed in 1931 and undertook a survey of social services across Britain, claimed that voluntary hospitals were self-governing institutions, jealous of their independence and only loosely associated with each other.[31] Many viewed medical voluntarism as failing to offer a coherent systems approach to healthcare organisation.

These negative interpretations of medical voluntarism have been challenged. Scholarship has stressed that health services in some pre-NHS British cities and regions were marked by spatial organisation around a central urban and voluntary teaching hospital, which acted as a focus for medical specialism and scientific expertise.[32] The historian D. M. Fox terms this as 'hierarchical regionalism', which he views as the key organising principle in British and American health services for much of the twentieth century.[33] Promoted by many medical experts, such ideas promulgated the organisation of health services around regional structures to ensure that an area's services worked together to establish referral mechanisms and rationalise patient flows to appropriate institutions. Britain's 1920 Dawson Report adumbrated the first blueprint for a regional hierarchy of tertiary (specialist hospitals), secondary (general hospitals) and primary care. The Dawson Report was quickly shelved due to the difficulties of creating such a model. It, however, was credited with the popularisation of regional health policies, especially among leading civil servants (more recent work, however, points towards earlier regional policies in the development of late-nineteenth-century isolation hospitals).[34]

Case studies of some interwar British cities and regions have described highly sophisticated, coordinated and regionalised health services.[35] One of the most systematic approaches emerged in Aberdeen under the direction of a 'Joint Hospital Scheme', where the city's voluntary hospitals, municipal clinics and the university's new medical school relocated to a singular green-field site. Effectively, a medical-government-academic 'complex' emerged which represented new structural changes in medicine and the merger of the branches and providers of healthcare.[36] Such collaboration was undoubtedly exceptional, and voluntary hospitals, after all, emerged from a tradition of individual initiative and little government involvement.[37] These examples show that amalgamation policies were evident in some, but not all, interwar British cities.

Before partition, some collaboration between medicine, education and hospital care emerged. The historian J. V. Pickstone described the emergence in the early twentieth century of new networks, or 'technoscientific communities', in which elite medicine, academia and industry coalesced to transform the organisation of health.[38] Such networks were nurtured in Belfast through medical education, initially evident in the city's main hospitals' role as teaching units for Queen's Medical School. This was facilitated in 1908 when Queen's University left the Royal University of Ireland collegiate, leading to the establishment of the Faculty of Medicine. Queen's Medical School now had greater independence from the Dublin-dominated Irish medical establishment. Academic, medical and industrial networks were brought about at an individual level. For example, during the 1910s, William Crawford, a leading industrialist and chairman of the Flax Spinning company, was also the chairman of the Royal Victoria's Board of Management and sat on the university's governing body, the Senate.[39] Such networks were influential and powerful and helped to bring together voluntary hospitals and medical education.

After partition, Northern Ireland's academic leadership sought the development of new scientific networks. Sir Richard Livingstone, the Vice-Chancellor of Queen's University between 1924 and 1933, was committed to developing the institution's education and research capacities. Livingstone believed that political devolution offered Queen's many opportunities. In 1924, he maintained that the university may have been financially 'poorer' than its English contemporaries, but that 'self-government' could act as a stimulus to intellectual life. Queen's position as the sole university in Northern Ireland offered many advantages.[40] In 1925, he commented that 'industry or public health or public life' would greatly benefit from collaboration with the 'chief body of scientific experts in Ulster' located in the university.[41] He further committed to engaging with wider society when he stated '*de jure* we are the University of Ulster. But if we are to be so in fact, the more interests of the community we touch, the more classes we serve, the more roots we strike in the soil, the stronger we shall be'.[42] Agriculture was one field in which extensive government, industry and academic collaboration emerged. Central to the Northern Irish economy and employment, by 1924, the government's newly established Ministry of Agriculture provided funding for Queen's to undertake teaching and research.[43] Collaboration between Queen's, central government and farmers' representatives helped to merge the various branches of agriculture.[44]

Livingstone also promoted similar coalition-building in medicine. In the early years of Northern Ireland, medical education in Queen's was of a relatively high standard. In 1925, Dr Alan Gregg, head of the Rockefeller Foundation's European health programme, considered Queen's as the leading school on the island. However, he noted its lack of research or major contributions to medicine.[45] The university recognised the importance of deepening the connection between Queen's Medical School and its teaching hospitals, primarily the Royal Victoria. Yet the relationship between the medical school and teaching hospitals was highly fragmented and marked by logistical, administrative and operational complexities. This was worsened by the distance of over one mile between the Royal Victoria and Queen's.[46] In 1927, Livingstone believed medical education and research were largely detached by the distance between the pathological and bacteriological laboratories in Queen's campus and the teaching hospitals. Drawing on his experience of visiting medical schools in Toronto, McGill, Harvard and Columbia, he averred that university laboratories and hospitals should be closely connected.[47] In turn, Livingstone planned to locate the university's laboratories closer to voluntary hospitals. This represented a reorientation of medical knowledge and management. Laboratory science was already in public health services but resisted by medics in the voluntary sector, whose autonomy was threatened by new modes of organisation and fear of subjection to medical specialities supported by salaries rather than private medicine.[48] These fears were overcome, and bench science became an integral part of the diagnosis and treatment of disease in hospital medicine.[49] Pathology could also prove a valuable source of income for medical schools by conducting routine investigations for local authorities and practitioners.[50]

Greater co-operation between hospitals and universities was also in line with reforms in medical education. Medical reformers in the US and Britain promoted closer relations and the establishment of full-time university professional clinical chairs and units housed adjacent to, or even in, general teaching hospitals.[51] This was epitomised by Abraham Flexner's report for the Carnegie Foundation in the United States, which sought greater synergy between medical schools and hospitals.[52] Flexner was influential in Britain and gave evidence in 1911 to the Royal Commission on University Education in London, which recommended that the medical schools of three London hospitals be incorporated into the University of London. After the First World War, the new Chief Medical Officer of Health in Britain, George Newman, promoted this academicisation of medicine and new management of hospitals.[53]

Greater collaboration between Queen's University and the Royal Victoria strengthened both institutions and was, unsurprisingly, widely supported. In 1928, the university's Senate resolved to transfer the department of pathology and bacteriology to the vicinity of the Royal Victoria.[54] The Senate highlighted two advantages to the move: the replacement of the existing inadequate pathology facilities and the proximity of the university's teaching and research to a 'great hospital'.[55] Medics in the Royal Victoria were equally enthusiastic. They recognised it benefited the diagnosis and treatment of disease, training of medical students and advancement of scientific knowledge, which modelled the 'modern tendency' in America and England where scientific departments were adjacent to teaching hospitals.[56] The new pathology institute was a joint venture between the university and the hospital. The Royal Victoria provided the site at a 'fair rent', and Queen's erected the building, which was to be shared between the two institutions.[57] The Institute of Pathology was formally opened by the Prime Minister in 1933 on a site next to the Royal Victoria (an overhead bridge physically connected the two buildings) on the Grosvenor Road in west Belfast. It provided laboratories and educational facilities for eighty students.[58] Significantly, this enhanced the greater academicisation of hospital medicine.

This coalition building was not confined to the Royal Victoria and Queen's University. The Grosvenor Road site developed into an even greater harmonised complex for medical services when the Royal Maternity Hospital and Royal Hospital for Sick Children were built in the 1930s. Plans had been in place since 1928 to amalgamate the Royal Victoria and Belfast Incorporated Maternity Hospital, and legislation was passed in 1931, which dissolved the latter.[59] Combined with the construction of a new hospital building, this merger illustrated the power of medical voluntarism in shaping the evolution of Northern Irish healthcare during the interwar years.

The medical, political and social elite of Northern Ireland spearheaded the establishment of the new maternity hospital. Drawing on traditional philanthropy, the aristocracy headed the fundraising campaign to build the new hospital, which included public appeals by the Duchess of Abercorn, and Lord Dufferin and Ava were important supporters of the cause.[60] Long-standing figures in the medical elite, many of whom were deeply connected with the Ulster Unionist Party, such as Professor Johnstone, were also key to the creation of the Royal Maternity. These figures were representative of the political, social and medical establishment that backboned the Northern Irish government, Ulster unionism and medical voluntarism. They also had much influence. Impressively, £150,000 was raised from the selling of assets, donations, the Duchess's public appeal and a labour grant from the Ministry of Labour under the Unemployment Relief Acts.[61] The ability to raise such finance was significant, although it was not without difficulties and repeated appeals were made to the public for donations.[62] The Royal Maternity opened in 1933 with sixty-four beds, which increased to one hundred by 1939. The Royal Hospital for Sick Children relocated from its Queen's Street premises to a new building near the Royal Victoria in 1932, funded primarily by philanthropy – £90,000 of the approximate total cost of £108,000 was raised by charity. Some central and local government funding was forthcoming, and the Ministry of Labour provided a £18,000 grant for labour costs and Belfast Corporation supplied the land.[63] The opening of these two new hospitals in the 1930s showed the strength of medical voluntarism in Belfast and Northern Ireland.

The development of the Grosvenor Road medical complex was mutually beneficial to the three hospitals and the university. As early as 1929, the *Belfast Telegraph* highlighted that the 'coordination of the Royal Victoria, Children's Hospital and Maternity Hospital in the future will make for economy and secure the best service for all'.[64] The shared interests of the three hospitals and the university were widely acknowledged. Livingstone was enthusiastic about the benefits accrued by the medical school from the 'hospital centre' and having a 'General, Maternity and Children's Hospital in close conjunction with the University Institute'.[65] Co-operation between the hospitals and the pathology institute led to the sharing of auxiliary services such as clinical pathology, bacteriology, pathology and biochemistry.[66] Royal Victoria further embedded its status as the leading hospital in Northern Ireland with far greater access than other general hospitals to the most up-to-date methods of diagnosis and treatment.

By the late 1930s, the Grosvenor Road medical complex had emerged as the most well-developed medical site in Northern Ireland. The three hospitals had almost 40 per cent of all voluntary beds in Northern Ireland. Deeply connected to Queen's Medical School, the hospitals could draw on unparalleled knowledge, expertise and research. In the context of this study, it represented the first major attempt at the synchronisation of medical services in Northern Ireland and developed as a voluntary hospital system modelled on wider trends in hospital organisation and management in Britain and the United States. Although based in Belfast, the architects of this new system saw this site as serving the whole of Northern Ireland. The devolved context of Northern Ireland further necessitated a self-sustaining medical system and acted as an impetus for the development of this medical centre. Much rhetoric framed the development within the context of meeting the needs of the new devolved country. The Grosvenor Road medical complex illustrates locally driven health system building. It mirrored developments identified by historians in some interwar British cities. The nascent medical site also revealed the power brokers of medicine in the newly established Northern Ireland. It was underpinned by a nexus of powerful medical, academic, social and political elites. These were the driving forces behind a medical voluntarism, which developed an increasingly sophisticated, joined-up and modernised hospital structure.

A divided health system

The extent to which the development of the Grosvenor Road medical complex represented a value-neutral expression of technocratic advance, identified in Fox's work on American and British national health policy, is questionable. Local health systems were often shaped by different interest groups seeking to advance their positions.[67] The Grosvenor Road complex primarily benefited the university and three voluntary hospitals at the cost of other medical institutions, including the Catholic Mater Infirmorum Hospital and Belfast Workhouse, by this stage renamed City Hospital. This coalition was deeply rooted in the Northern Irish establishment and intertwined with the upper echelons of Ulster unionism and the Northern Irish government. Other groups who were excluded from this elite, such as Catholics and nationalists or progressive and labour-orientated health movements, had little, if any, involvement in this new medical power base in Northern Ireland.

Religious differences, entangled with political division, often fragmented health systems and health education in Irish cities. The medical historian Greta Jones has described attempts in the Irish Free State in the 1920s, promoted by the Rockefeller Foundation, to enhance co-operation between the two major institutions of medicine in Dublin (Trinity College and University College) with the aim of one united first-rate school. These efforts failed because of religious and political tensions. Middle-class demand for medical professional opportunities also dampened calls for a reduction in medical schools.[68] In Dublin, religious rivalries marked medical education and students' choice of medical school for much of the twentieth century.[69]

In some ways, medical developments in Belfast were intertwined with political and religious divisions which pervaded Northern Irish society. While many voluntary hospitals did not have a specific religious purpose, the boundaries between religion and philanthropy were less marked and originated in Victorian charity and Christianity.[70] Although largely under lay management, many of Northern Ireland's hospitals were viewed as being associated with Protestants. For example, the management of hospitals such as the Royal Victoria and Royal Maternity was largely dominated by Protestants. Similarly, Queen's Medical School faculty was mostly made up of Protestants, even if students came from across the religious divide. Furthermore, the development of Grosvenor Road into Northern Ireland's hospital power base was brought about by a medical, political and philanthropic elite reflective of the largely unionist establishment, with minimal involvement from Catholics, nationalists or the labour movement. The voluntary hospitals on the Grosvenor Road medical site were not under religious control. Still, they were inherently tied to a medical, political and social establishment that had no incentive to accommodate nationalist and Catholic concerns.

The exception to the largely lay Protestant-run voluntary hospitals was the Catholic Mater Infirmorum Hospital in Belfast. Catholic religious nursing sisters had developed hospitals in many countries where they became important providers of hospital services.[71] Similarly, in Northern Ireland, the Mater was a significant hospital. As a teaching hospital, professors of medicine and surgery, along with groups of students, visited the Mater for consultation and teaching. Students could, in their final year, live in the Mater as resident clerks and dressers, which counted as part of their clinical course.[72] By 1940, the Mater's 318 beds made it the second largest general voluntary hospital in Northern Ireland.

While the Mater was a leading hospital in Belfast and Northern Ireland, it had little involvement in the evolving organisation of voluntary hospital services. Located on the Crumlin Road in north Belfast, the Mater was geographically isolated from the Grosvenor Road medical complex and disconnected from the newly built Queen's Pathology Institute. The location of the pathology institute compounded the Royal Victoria's status as the major general hospital in Northern Ireland but disadvantaged the Mater. Some Catholic interests opposed the measure. Two Catholic members of Queen's Senate, including a former medical consultant in the Mater named Mr J. B. Moore, unsuccessfully opposed the original proposal to relocate the university's pathology department next to the Royal Victoria.[73]

The Mater's reticence towards the Grosvenor Road medical complex stemmed from the complicated relationship Catholics and nationalists had with Northern Irish officialdom. For many within unionism, Catholicism was synonymous with disloyalty and the new Northern Irish state was highly suspicious of the Catholic population.[74] Little effort was made to distinguish constitutional and revolutionary methods of opposition to partition, evidenced in the Northern Irish government's dealings with the Mater Hospital. In 1925, the Ministry of Home Affairs rejected an application from the hospital to expand its facilities by acquiring land from the nearby Crumlin Road prison. The authorities feared that many of the students and staff in the Mater would have political sympathies with republican prisoners in the jail.[75] Such official suspicion of the Mater contrasted with the support that the Grosvenor Road development received. Equally, the Mater authorities were suspicious of any encroachment from an officialdom that allowed discrimination against Catholics. This mutual distrust further exacerbated divisions along religious and political lines in Northern Irish hospital medicine. The Catholic Church also undertook the building of a proto-welfare state, which not only included the Mater Hospital but also a network of schools, orphanages, magdalene asylums and relief organisations such as the St Vincent de Paul in Northern Ireland. This network acted as a state within a state, which many Catholics believed protected their religious identity in a hostile and discriminatory Northern Ireland. The maintenance of the Mater's independence from the unionist and Protestant establishment was key to the Catholic community's identity.

The isolation of the Mater from advances in Northern Ireland's voluntary hospitals, however, cannot solely be attributed to a chauvinistic Ulster unionism unwilling to accommodate Catholic interests. Experiences south of the Irish border demonstrated that opposition from the Catholic religious hierarchy to scientific developments, medical collaboration and state involvement in voluntary care was inimical to medical progress. Irish voluntary hospitals run by religious orders undercut doctors' authority and research.[76] Religious hierarchical influence also impeded health reform in the Irish Free State. For example, in the early 1920s, attempts to reform nursing provided by religious orders in local authority hospitals in County Kerry were undermined by the local Catholic bishop.[77] Other countries with large Catholic populations witnessed resistance to increased lay power in hospitals run by religious authorities in the early twentieth century. In some hospitals in Barcelona, tensions between Catholic religious authorities and lay and clinical management stymied the professionalisation of training of medical students and nursing.[78] Religious authorities resisted increased secular control of Catholic voluntary hospitals. The Mater's greater co-operation with the Grosvenor Road medical complex would have required some dilution of religious power. This would have been resisted regardless of the wider political and religious divisions in Northern Irish society. While Catholics were justified in their distrust of the unionist establishment and fear of discrimination, Catholic religious authorities were also resistant to scientific progress and the professionalisation of health services. Overall, the religious and political makeup of Northern Ireland led to divisions in medical voluntarism. This embedded fragmentation in the voluntary hospital sector and ensured that coordination of services was restricted to the Grosvenor Road complex and excluded the Mater Hospital. This was reflective of the intractable fissures in Northern Irish society, where mutual suspicion led to entrenched divisions. A mixture of well-founded Catholic suspicion of the state intermingled with ecclesiastical resistance to increased lay management were insuperable obstacles to greater alignment of medical voluntarism in Northern Ireland.

Voluntarism and government

While the development of the Grosvenor Road medical site was important for Northern Ireland's healthcare, direct financial support from the Stormont government was unforthcoming. The Northern Irish government officially supported it, and leading unionist politicians provided important backing that was helpful in charitable fundraising efforts. Both the Royal Maternity and the Institute of Pathology received grants for labour costs from the Ministry of Labour. Yet the Irish Public Health Council's call for greater central government funding for voluntary hospitals in 1920 was not forthcoming, and backing for hospitals or scientific research failed to emerge.[79] This differed from the Irish Free State, where the government-run Irish Sweepstakes generated large non-exchequer funding for Irish hospitals, which gave central government some leverage over voluntary hospital policies. The socially conservative Northern Irish government viewed medical voluntarism as separate from the state, ensuring there was no policy or financial intervention in most voluntary hospitals in the interwar years (county infirmaries were the exception, which are addressed in a later section of this chapter).

Central government's hesitancy or inability – it was hampered by severe financial difficulties for much of the 1920s and 1930s – to invest in medical facilities was demonstrated in 1931. After the Rockefeller Foundation agreed to fund the Irish Free State to develop a centralised state laboratory (this grant was subsequently withdrawn in 1933 after objections from Dublin's competing medical schools in Trinity College and University College), Livingstone sought support from the government for similar funding from Rockefeller to develop a proposed 'Ulster Institute of Public Health' as a state laboratory.[80] The economically conservative Minister of Finance, Hugh Pollock, advised the Prime Minister not to create a state laboratory. Pollock maintained that it would be 'difficult to make a good case' in 'a small area' such as Northern Ireland for a state laboratory, commenting that it was 'outside our financial capabilities'.[81] The laboratory never progressed, depicting the unionist government's unwillingness to support medical initiatives, even when the possibility of substantial funding from bodies such as the Rockefeller Foundation existed.

There was potential for the harmonisation of local government healthcare and medical voluntarism. One of the best examples of consolidation, already highlighted in this chapter, occurred in Aberdeen. Here, the assertiveness and ideas of successive local authority MOsH were central to bringing together the city's medical school, voluntary hospitals and local authority health services.[82] More common was the joint activity between local government and voluntary hospitals in developing specialist work such as contracting laboratory services and venereal disease and infant welfare clinics.[83] Indeed, the growth of local authorities' public health responsibilities often acted as a bridge between the two sectors.[84] This was also evident in some parts of Northern Ireland. By the 1930s, some voluntary cottage hospitals in provincial Ulster were contracted by local authorities to provide health services. For example, Ballymena Cottage Hospital received funding from the County Antrim Tuberculosis Committee to treat such patients.[85] The same local authority partly funded the building of a sun parlour in the Hopefield Cottage Hospital in Portrush for local authority tuberculosis patients.[86] After the Venereal Disease Act in 1917, local authorities were obligated to care for venereal disease sufferers, and the Belfast Corporation funded clinics in the Royal Victoria and the Mater hospitals.[87] It also funded medical attendance, laboratory testing and diagnosis of venereal disease in the Royal Victoria.[88] Within a Northern Irish context, this took on added significance, as the health officials had to be sensitive to religious sensibilities. The Northern Irish government was at pains to uphold the moral values of the churches in the treatment of venereal disease.[89] Furthermore, the Corporation's Maternity and Child Welfare Committee also part-funded an antenatal clinic in the Royal Maternity.[90] The convergence of local authority and voluntary hospital activity was evident in the provision of some public health responsibilities such as maternity and child welfare, tuberculosis and venereal disease.

Yet the role of local government in medical voluntarism in Belfast was confined to such public health functions. It did not extend to acute or specialist medicine, the well-established preserve of voluntary hospitals. Local authority officials, such as the MOH, had little influence on the Grosvenor Road medical site, which was dominated by medical voluntarism. At times, key representatives of medical voluntarism resisted local government attempts at expansion. This was evident in Belfast Corporation's plans to expand maternity and child welfare services, which, as highlighted in Chapter 2, were successfully resisted by leading medical figures such as Prof. R. J. Johnstone, who instead spearheaded the establishment of the voluntary Royal Maternity Hospital. Similarly, the Belfast workhouse had little engagement with the more prestigious voluntary sector. The workhouse infirmary was modernised during the 1920s and 1930s and was a teaching hospital for Queen's Medical School. However, it was still the poor relation to the more prestigious voluntary hospital sector and isolated from the increased combination of provision and expertise in the Grosvenor Road complex. Medical voluntarism had little interest in supporting local government expansion in areas that threatened its pre-eminence, such as acute medicine and specialist services. Professional self-interest also motivated medics' resistance to local government expansion. They feared the advent of a local government-salaried service and the loss of private practice.

The emergence of the Grosvenor Road medical complex was the result of collaboration between the university and medical voluntarism. The site undoubtedly emerged as the most prominent, advanced and sophisticated medical facility in Northern Ireland. While it was the beginning of a harmonised hospital system, this coalition failed to include local authority healthcare. It proved incapable or reticent to reach out to the Mater Hospital. The fusion of local government and medical voluntarism, evident in some places in interwar Britain, was not forthcoming in Northern Ireland. In essence, the development of the Grosvenor Road medical site consolidated medical voluntarism as the major power broker in Northern Irish medicine while ensuring that other sectors, primarily the poor law and Catholic provision, remained of secondary importance.

Medical voluntarism, county infirmaries and continued independence

Outside Belfast, the picture of medical voluntarism was complex. The potential for bringing together local government and medical voluntarism was most evident in county infirmaries. Northern Ireland's seven county infirmaries (each of Northern Ireland's six counties had a county infirmary besides County Down, which had two infirmaries – one in Newry and another in Downpatrick) were semi-voluntary institutions. County councils, as already highlighted, played an important role in their financing and management. Both the city corporation and county council supported Londonderry City and County Infirmary. County infirmaries were unique to Ireland – both north and south – and no similar semi-voluntary/local authority system existed in Britain. County infirmaries were separate from poor law medicine and considered more advanced and prestigious than workhouse infirmaries. However, their pre-eminent position in provincial Ulster hospital medicine was challenged by the modernisation of workhouses into district hospitals (see Chapter 1). Threatened by these fully equipped hospitals, county infirmaries sought to re-emphasise their leading position and dissociation from the former workhouses. Competition and institutional jealousies prevailed between the sectors.

Relations between county infirmaries and district hospitals were strained in many places, undermining the potential for a more joined-up system. For example, in 1929, the Armagh County Infirmary sought funding from the county council to develop the hospital, which was opposed by many boards of guardians due to the increased burden on the county rates.[91] The county council favoured the development of the infirmary, highlighting that the hospital was staffed by the county surgeon, who had to be a fellow of the Royal College of Surgeons, in contrast to district hospitals in which no such qualifications were necessary. The Armagh County Council insisted that county infirmaries had to be the 'superior institution' in each county, and apart from district hospitals.[92] This was reflective of older perceptions of the inferiority of poor law provision. County infirmary hospitals prided themselves on providing advanced curative acute care compared to workhouse infirmaries, which traditionally catered to the long-term, chronic and pauper sick. That it was associated with medical voluntarism also gave county infirmaries a sense of superiority over district hospitals.

There was much disconnection between the management of county infirmaries and district hospitals. This was evident in towns where both institutions existed. In Lisburn, for example, the former workhouse was modernised into the Lisburn and Hillsborough District Hospital in the 1920s, independent of the Antrim County Infirmary, also located in the town. This led to much overlapping of provision. The 1927 Commission of Local Government Administration complained that the two hospitals had 'practically identical functions'. Such duplication, according to the Commission, only came about because of the operation of two different structures.[93] As set out in Chapter 1, the Commission recommended the creation of a county hospital scheme to merge the management of district hospitals, workhouse infirmaries and personal public health provision. However, this did not extend to county infirmaries, and the Commission merely recommended consultation with local authorities in the development of county hospital systems. It was slow to recommend concrete plans for a more systematic approach, fearing that an arbitrary transfer of power to local authorities would be inimical to county infirmaries' voluntary nature.[94] Officials remained reluctant to overly interfere with the voluntary sector, leaving much ambiguity over the place of county infirmaries in any joined-up organisation.

Throughout the 1930s, county infirmaries resisted any plans for the creation of a hospital structure in which their status was devalued. During the late 1920s and early 1930s, some focus on creating a health system based on counties, similar to that established in the Free State, was mooted. In 1932, representatives of county infirmaries argued that in any reformed system, their institutions should be the leading hospital in each county, with district and cottage hospitals acting in a secondary capacity. They also argued that district hospitals should not be elaborately or expensively equipped to ensure the ascendancy of county infirmaries.[95] The Ministry of Home Affairs floated a rearranged hospital scheme to create regional hospitals irrespective of county boundaries, which were increasingly seen as archaic and an inefficient means of organising hospital services.[96] This was fiercely and successfully opposed by county infirmaries which felt the measure threatened their status, arguing that infirmaries should be recognised as the leading institution in any hospital scheme.[97] By the late 1930s, no county (or regional) hospital system had emerged. While multiple factors, such as government indecision and inaction prevented any chance for real reform, opposition from county infirmaries to schemes that may have diluted their prominence was influential, indicating the strength of the sector.

Collaboration between semi-voluntary county infirmaries and local authority district hospitals, many of which were in the same town, was unattainable in the 1920s and 1930s. Institutional loyalties, notions of hospital hierarchies and perceptions of inferior provision in workhouse infirmaries permeated much thinking among advocates of county infirmaries. The medical advancement of district hospitals was met with resistance and jealousy by county infirmaries which feared their place in any reformed structures. In turn, county infirmaries in provincial Ulster maintained their independence. An inchoate voluntary health system did emerge around some hospitals on the Belfast Grosvenor Road complex. However, this was not extended to medical voluntarism in the rest of Northern Ireland, where resistance to local authority provision stymied collaboration. Instead, provincial hospitals remained largely independent of each other and other sectors, ensuring the persistence of an *ad hoc* and disjointed system.

Although voluntary hospitals sought to maintain their independence from local authority provision, their strength was evident in multiple ways. The sector demonstrated an impressive capacity to grow. As depicted in Table 3.1, the number of beds in the voluntary sector grew from 1,523 to 2,311 between 1921 and 1940. Voluntary hospitals, mostly through non-government income, successfully upgraded existing hospitals, built new institutions, advanced standards of care and embraced scientific developments. The Grosvenor Road complex was brought about by the coming together of multiple hospitals and medical education and research on one site. These successes were undoubtedly significant and point towards a sector that was often vibrant, expanding and innovative during the interwar years. This picture corrects common perceptions about the overall failure of pre-NHS healthcare in Northern Ireland.

Contribution schemes: a vehicle for working-class participation and increased democratisation?

Another positive feature of medical voluntarism was the role of the working classes in the financing and management of hospitals. While the focus on upper and middle-class-run medical institutions can distort our understanding of charitable experience and underplay the role of the working classes, much historical work on British medical voluntarism has challenged this interpretation.[98] Instead, working-class hospital contribution schemes have been identified as key to the finances of voluntary hospitals in interwar Britain, helping to stave off potential financial catastrophe during an era of spiralling costs and decreasing charitable donations.[99] Heralding a new era of mutualism, self-help and quasi-insurance, contribution schemes diluted older philanthropic terms of entitlement, which were often predicated on reciprocity and notions of the deserving and undeserving poor.[100] Membership of a scheme bestowed subscribers with entitlements to access voluntary hospitals. These schemes had the potential to replace the voluntary ethos of paternal charity and philanthropy controlled by the wealthier classes with greater democratic accountability and new avenues of user participation in hospital governance.[101] The historians Doyle and Hayes have argued that contribution schemes brought about a transfer from elite philanthropy to cross-class mutual income, which freed hospitals from their dependence on the wealthy, thus ensuring their transformation to community resources for all.[102] Yet such positive accounts have to be tempered by the lack of work on contribution schemes' social, cultural and political makeup, operation on a day-to-day level and extent of politicisation.[103] It has been contended elsewhere that the change that contribution schemes brought to voluntary hospitals was more a reformulation of the philanthropic principles underpinning medical voluntarism, in which notions of deference and social class differentiation were highly influential than a radical transformation.[104] This is the first study to consider voluntary hospital funding in Northern Ireland, the role of contribution schemes, and how these impacted the democratisation of voluntary hospitals and changing notions of entitlement to care.

In Northern Ireland, working-class activity was central to generating income in many voluntary hospitals. Long-standing sources of funding from middle- and upper-class philanthropy such as bequests, donations, gifts and yearly subscriptions provided important revenue streams for Northern Irish voluntary hospitals. For example, the Royal Victoria received £6,553 in subscriptions and £4,428 in donations and bequests in 1941 (see Table 3.3). Working-class involvement in this type of philanthropy was also evident. For example, in 1932, the Loyal Orange Lodge in the working-class and Protestant Sandy Row district of Belfast donated £500 to the Royal Victoria, for which the lodge received two life governorships in the hospital and a named bed.[105] The Orange Lodge organised the collection over two years and received support from the Women's District Lodge, indicating the prevalence of grassroots fundraising for the voluntary hospital. Working-class activity, intertwined with religious and political associational culture reflected in the Orange Order, was evident in voluntary hospital philanthropic activity.

Table 3.3 Breakdown of income of Royal Victoria Hospital, Belfast, 1900, 1926, 1936 and 1942.

Year	*General subs*	*Donations bequests*	*Dividends*	*Working people scheme*	*Hospital Saturday Collect*	*Patients contrib*	*Local/ central gov.*	*Student fees*	*Other*	*Total*
1900	1,604	4,559	1,208	2,602	535	819	0	282	110	11,499
1926	7,207	2,263	9,937	19,067	3,602	4,312	2,334	2,415	6,646	57,783
1936	6,127	3,134	9,397	30,063	5,016	3,234	2,741	2,250	4,419	66,381
1941	6,554	4,438	10,926	41,877	7,026	4,622	4,283	3,024	13,312	90,624

Source: Annual Reports of RVH.

Similar to developments in Britain, working-class contribution schemes became central to funding many voluntary hospitals, often eclipsing all other categories of income, in the interwar years. This was particularly evident in the Royal Victoria, the country's largest and most prestigious voluntary hospital, which also had the principal contribution scheme of any institution. As outlined in Table 3.3, the Royal Victoria Hospital's revenue from the working men's contribution scheme grew from a mere £2,602 in 1900 to £41,877 of the hospital's total income of £90,624 in 1941.[106] The contribution scheme became the financial linchpin of the hospital, in which reliance on this source of income outstripped the experience of many voluntary hospitals in Britain. In 1936, 45.3 per cent of the hospital's income came from the scheme, compared to the 34 per cent average of sixty-three comparative teaching voluntary hospitals in Britain.[107] Similar schemes also made up much of the income of Belfast's other voluntary hospitals. The Mater Infirmorum Hospital, for example, received almost 34 per cent of its total income in 1944 from this source.[108] By the early 1940s, Belfast's leading voluntary hospitals were reliant on working-class contribution schemes for their financial survival. This was a drastic transformation in these hospitals' funding model, moving from middle- to upper-class charity to income generated directly from the working classes.

Outside Belfast, contribution schemes varied from hospital to hospital. Schemes developed in some of the more industrialised areas. In an example of the voluntary character of county infirmaries, the County Antrim Infirmary received between £500 and £600 annually from the hospital's Working People's Committee. Most contributors came from the more industrialised areas of the county, such as Ballymena and Lisburn, indicating that contribution schemes were largely for the industrialised working classes.[109] Other hospitals had smaller schemes. For example, the Londonderry City and County Infirmary's management complained about the lack of income from workers' contributions. In 1930, it reported that the institution's financial problems would be relieved if workers' contributions were collected to the same extent as in Belfast's Royal Victoria.[110] However, by 1939, the institution received a mere tenth of its total income from this source.[111] Multiple factors undermined workers' contributions in provincial Northern Ireland. County infirmaries invariably served areas with a largely rural population.

Many were employed in agriculture, which was not conducive to the organised weekly payment into schemes associated with industrial workplaces and characteristic of urbanised areas. Also, many workers outside Belfast subscribed to the contribution schemes of the large city hospitals to the detriment of local hospitals. By 1938, 18 per cent of all the Royal Victoria's patients came from outside Belfast, many of whom were members of the hospital's contribution scheme.[112] Subscribers from up to twenty-four provincial towns from across Northern Ireland reportedly contributed to the hospital's scheme.[113] Worker contribution schemes were less significant to hospitals in provincial Northern Ireland, and the large sums generated by the working classes were mostly confined to the Belfast voluntary hospitals.

The increased importance of working-class contribution schemes to the finances of some hospitals often impacted the social relations surrounding hospitals. In many British industrial cities, social collegiality between the working and upper classes was a feature of voluntary healthcare.[114] This was also evident in Northern Ireland and, in some instances, in the elite-dominated management of voluntary hospitals. The management of the County Antrim Infirmary and the Working People's Committee reportedly enjoyed 'cordial and happy relations'.[115] The leadership of the Royal Victoria regularly congratulated the Working Men's Committee, which organised the contribution scheme, for generating large sums. This was easily politicised to emphasise the pan-class nature of Ulster unionism, evidenced during an annual meeting of the Royal Victoria in 1927, when the Northern Ireland Prime Minister and leader of unionism James Craig approbated the worker's scheme and stated:

> co-operation between rich and poor, between employer and employee was something which should be encouraged in every possible way and in every path of life. The stability of the country was very like the hospital ..., whilst the working classes and rich pull together for the one end of making that the premier hospital in the Empire if possible, in exactly the same way ... that close co-operation between the working class and employer through the country would bring Ulster to the very top pinnacle in the Empire.[116]

In this context, working-class contribution schemes provided the leaders of unionism with examples of class unity during a period of economic depression and increased social disquiet. Framing contribution schemes and medical voluntarism around social collegiality, unionism and the Empire helped to stave off political threats from organised labour and NILP, which, as highlighted in Chapter 2, were highly critical of the Ulster Unionist Party's social conservatism and inaction. Medical voluntarism allowed the Northern Irish political and social establishment to highlight the benefits of a socially hierarchical and patrician unionism.

The degree to which those involved in Northern Irish contribution schemes and wider working classes shared the unionist leadership's sentiments is less clear. Voluntary hospitals were managed by governors who were traditionally from elite social groups with the capacity to make the necessary financial contributions and the time to serve on committees.[117] However, the sheer financial importance of contribution schemes by the interwar years ensured that working-class subscribers had a greater voice in the management of voluntary hospitals. In many British hospitals, contribution schemes acted as a vehicle for working-class voluntarism and the democratisation of voluntary hospital management.[118] For example, a strong degree of worker influence was evident in the running of voluntary hospitals in numerous Yorkshire cities.[119] This resonated with mutualistic approaches to social provision through the pooling together of workers' resources, which is also evident in the co-operative, trade union and friendly societies movements.[120] Participation in the charitable activity of voluntary hospitals allowed many from the respectable working classes to enhance their social status and interact with the wealthier classes.[121] The proposition that contribution schemes brought about greater democratic involvement in the running of Northern Irish hospitals needs to be questioned.

At one level, the financial strength of contribution schemes did give worker representatives greater input and participation in hospital management. The Antrim Infirmary's Working People's Committee regularly visited the hospital to examine conditions. After multiple visits in 1930, the committee reported that they found 'everything in good order and [had] no ground whatsoever for complaint' and thanked the hospital for treating patients who worked in the local mills and factories.[122] The committee regularly communicated with the board of management and raised money through not only a contribution scheme but also sports days.[123] Reportedly, the committee's members maintained a 'lively and intelligent' interest in the hospital's management.[124] Similarly, the Mater Hospital's Working Men's Committee was an active body that met regularly and pressed employers in Belfast, highlighting businesses that failed to facilitate collections.[125] The Mater's Working Men's Committee also held three life governor positions, which ensured that they had a role in the management of the hospital.[126] In this instance, the contribution scheme allowed greater worker participation in the hierarchy of the hospital and membership among its governors. Yet the extent of patient democratisation evident in British medical voluntarism was never overly apparent, and hospitals' leadership remained primarily drawn from middle- to upper-class subscribers and governors.

The largest contribution scheme in Northern Ireland was organised by the Royal Victoria's Working Men's Committee. The scheme was as much about traditional employer patronage as it was about working-class mutualism, organisation and representation in hospital management. Unlike much mutualistic activity, membership of the scheme was less participatory, and many members had little, if any, involvement beyond paying their dues.[127] Charles Payne, a shipyard manager in Harland and Wolff shipbuilding company, described how new employees merely filled out a subscriber's slip on appointment, indicating that membership was largely functional.[128] Contribution schemes were attractive to employers for maintaining a healthy workforce and an efficient preservation of human capital.[129] The leadership of the Royal Victoria Working Men's Committee was static, with the key officeholders remaining for long periods, which was a sign of the lack of engagement by many of the subscribers.[130] The committee was less involved in working-class culture, often a characteristic of mutualistic activity, than similar schemes in English cities, where charity football matches and gala events were common.[131] The contribution scheme for the Royal Victoria was less associated with working-class activism, identity and culture, which further weakened its potential to bring greater democratic management and accountability to the hospital.

The involvement of the Working Men's Committee in the management of the Royal Victoria Hospital was not reflective of its financial importance. Voluntary hospitals were run by multiple committees, of which the board of management was the most powerful. These committees shaped the rules, oversaw finances and dictated policy. Boards of management were made up of governors – elected from subscribers – and medical staff who were ultimately responsible for the running of the hospital.[132] The Royal Victoria Hospital's thirty-five-person Board of Management had a mere two representatives from the Working Men's Committee. These included William Lavery, a shipwright by trade, who was the long-standing secretary of the Working Men's Committee.[133] His presence did stand for some form of patient and working-class representation on the board of management. Yet this participation should not be overemphasised. Working-class contributions far exceeded other financial contributions from life governors and subscribers, but the role of the Working Men's Committee in the hospital's management paled in comparison. Despite the hospital rhetoric of social collegiality and platitudes about the value of working-class contributions to the hospital, echoed by unionist leaders eager to highlight pan-class political unity, its lay management remained dominated by the middle to upper classes looking to affirm their social status. The social hierarchy of the hospital continued, ensuring the persistence of its long-standing charitable ethos. Similar power structures existed in other voluntary hospitals in which the potential for greater democratisation was never fully realised in Northern Ireland.

Entitlement to voluntary care

One facet of hospital management in which contribution schemes did bring about change in Northern Ireland was related to the terms of entitlement and access to healthcare. For much of the nineteenth and early twentieth centuries, voluntary hospitals were mostly used by the poor and working classes, who often had to receive subscribers' letters from hospitals' wealthier patrons to gain access. For example, in 1920, admission to the Belfast Incorporated Maternity Hospital was gained on application to the matron, with a letter signed by a subscriber to the hospital.[134] Reflective of paternal charity and patronage, these terms of entitlement were often imbued with middle- and upper-class notions of deservingness, neediness and poverty.[135] Such ideas were challenged by the emergence of contribution schemes, which offered working-class subscribers greater entitlement based more on the weight of their financial contributions than charity. Membership of a hospital's contribution scheme helped workers access care in voluntary hospitals free from paternalist frameworks of the deserving and non-deserving poor.

The working men's committees of voluntary hospitals also challenged admission policies on behalf of their members. For example, in 1926, the Royal Victoria's Working Men's Committee complained to the hospital's management that subscribers were struggling to access the facility. In 1930, the committee again complained that its members were kept on waiting lists for a considerable time. On this occasion, the medical staff regretted the 'unavoidable delay' and instructed the house surgeons to facilitate subscribers 'as far as possible'.[136] Membership of the contribution scheme did not lead to automatic access to care, but members could rely on the Working Men's Committee to represent their needs to the hospital's management. These schemes bestowed entitlement and rights on the working classes, which were largely non-existent previously. In this sense, contribution schemes led to a transformation in the power dynamics surrounding entitlement. Many patients were no longer passive recipients of charity but active participants whose communal contributions ensured enough financial clout to negotiate with and influence hospital management.

Contribution schemes were not without difficulties. Entitlement often differed from hospital to hospital, resulting in uneven access to voluntary healthcare across Northern Ireland. For example, in the Royal Victoria, contributors were entitled to preference for intern treatment, except in cases that were urgent or nominated by the hospital's subscribers.[137] Contrastingly, members of the Mater Infirmorum's contribution scheme were admitted free to the hospital on the 'production' of a subscriber's ticket from their employers.[138] Although the hospital maintained it had an 'ever-open door', preferential treatment was afforded to workplace subscribers and 'the holder of a subscriber's line [was] attended to first'. Like the Royal Victoria, workers in Harland and Wolff were the largest contributors to the Mater's workplace scheme. Smaller contributions came from sectors, workplaces and organisations synonymous with the Catholic population, such as the Barman's Committee, a largely Catholic occupation in Belfast and the nationalist newspaper the

Irish News.[139] The varying terms of entitlement ensured that access was uneven across institutions, and many had to subscribe to multiple hospitals. Competition also existed between individual contribution schemes. In 1939, attempts in Belfast to establish a unified city-wide contribution scheme, like those in many British cities, was opposed by the Royal Victoria Working Men's Committee because of potential threat to that hospital's income.[140] No such measure was introduced. The multitude of contribution schemes accentuated not just workers' entitlement but also the overall unity and strength of the schemes.

Voluntary hospitals were also significantly challenged by the increased demand for beds from patients beyond poor and working-class patients. By the 1930s, better-off people, attracted by voluntary hospitals' increasingly scientific progress and effective treatment, sought access to this healthcare. Such patients traditionally received medical care privately from general practitioners or private surgeries and nursing homes – these care regimes are beyond the remit of this study. Furthermore, the changing face of the workforce and increase in white collar workers, including those employed in the nascent bureaucracy of the devolved administration, increased the need for hospital care for office workers who were not usual patients of voluntary institutions.

Concerns about the greater demand for hospital services were evident in the Royal Victoria, where the management was suspicious that better-off people who were ineligible for membership sought to join the hospital's contribution scheme. The medical staff refused to allow some government employees to contribute under the scheme, such as members of the Royal Ulster Constabulary. Medical staff emphasised that they gave their services freely because the hospital was a charity, and members of the police force were not considered 'charitable patients'.[141] In 1932, the medical staff believed the treatment of 'government servants in a voluntary hospital' as a 'dangerous precedent'.[142] Cases of abuse of the scheme surfaced. In 1937, controversy arose when a woman was denied admission to the hospital as a 'subscriber' after it emerged that her husband – an official in the Department of Education – had a wage of eight hundred pounds per annum.[143] The hospital authorities believed the case was a 'flagrant violation of the scheme' although not an isolated one.[144] Contribution schemes were originally designed for the industrialised working classes. The workers' contributions never covered the full cost of their treatment, which was still considered, particularly by the medics, as a form of charity. Better-off people were not entitled to such charity, although membership of the contribution scheme helped to secure access to the hospital, leading to cases of abuse.

Many voluntary hospitals were unable to keep pace with demand from new, better-off patients. Voluntary hospitals in Northern Ireland were slow to develop private provision to meet more middle-class demand. This contrasted with south of the Irish border, where many voluntary hospitals built private wings and wards and became increasingly reliant on patient fees.[145] The Royal Victoria feared the development of a 'pay block' would threaten the institution's charitable status and the private practice of medics. It was not until 1938 that a dedicated private wing – Musgrave Nursing Home – was finally opened. Other hospitals had similar challenges. In 1938, legislation had to be passed in Stormont to allow the Royal Hospital for Sick Children to build a private wing and provide treatment to young patients from families who were not traditional recipients of medical relief.[146] Provision for paying patients in the Belfast voluntary hospitals was slow to emerge, which illustrated medical voluntarism's incapacity to meet the hospital needs and demands of much of the population.

Outside Belfast, the county infirmary and cottage hospitals were more willing to embrace payment from patients. These hospitals could not rely on well-funded contribution schemes or the large bequests and legacies that sustained the Belfast voluntary hospitals. In turn, many became increasingly reliant on patients' fees and contributions. This was evident, for example, in the Londonderry City and County Infirmary, which received a mere £196 in contribution schemes compared to £1,194 from private patients in 1929.[147] While not all county infirmaries had such an enormous gulf, they still garnered much income from paying patients. The County Antrim Infirmary received close to £700 from the hospital's contribution scheme, while £550 came from private patients. Cottage hospitals were also increasingly reliant on patients' fees. In 1931, the income for Hopefield Cottage Hospital in Portrush was £2,535, of which £2,095 came from paying patients. These fees were not always reflective of wholly private medicine and often represented a contribution by the patients towards the medical costs. However, patient payment for voluntary hospital treatment made up a far more significant proportion of the income of hospitals outside Belfast.

The contrasting terms of entitlement to medical voluntarism created much unevenness in provision across Northern Ireland. The rights of the poor, working classes, white-collar and wealthier middle-class patients varied between individual hospitals and urban and rural areas. This led to inequitable access to medical services, which undermined the effectiveness of voluntary hospitals and highlighted the sector's incapacity to provide coherent and aligned provision.

Conclusion

Medical voluntarism during the 1920s and 1930s tells us much about the interconnecting themes of this work. A key objective of this monograph is to examine the stakeholders that shaped the trajectory of health services and policy in Northern Ireland. Medical voluntarism had emerged as the most powerful force in health policy by the early 1940s. The creation of the Grosvenor Road medical complex through the coalition of three voluntary hospitals and Queen's University was an impressive example of locally driven health system-building, which mirrored developments in some interwar British cities and further afield in the United States. This early attempt at the fusion of health services was reflective of the coalescing of academic, medical and hospital forces under medical voluntarism. This was tied to the dominant unionist political establishment in Northern Ireland and drew substantial support from the aristocratic and middle-to-upper-class social elite. Medical voluntarism beyond the Grosvenor Road complex proved dynamic, and growth in hospital beds and expertise was evident across Northern Ireland. During an era when central government remained weak, medical voluntarism filled the void and led medical developments and policy innovation in Northern Ireland.

Drawing on another central theme of this work, the role of politics in healthcare, medical voluntarism was explicitly political. Most voluntary hospitals and many in the medical profession were interwoven with Ulster unionism, Protestantism and the Northern Irish establishment. Catholics and nationalists or progressive and labour-orientated health movements had marginal involvement or influence. Most pressing was the isolation of the Mater Hospital – Catholic-run and the second largest general voluntary hospital in Northern Ireland – from the evolving medical voluntary power base. Mutual distrust and suspicion stymied the potential for collaboration, ensuring that political and religious divisions undermined Northern Irish healthcare. The religious and political divides which pervaded Northern Irish society became embedded in voluntary healthcare during these years.

Medical voluntarism was not just reflective of nationalist/Catholic and unionist/Protestant divisions but also embodied the Ulster Unionist Party's attempts to offset the political challenge from rising social discontent and the Northern Ireland Labour Party. The socially hierarchical nature of medical voluntarism and its apparent pan-class support in many ways mirrored the paternalist Ulster Unionist Party and Northern Ireland government. Medical voluntarism and its ethos of independence and self-reliance sat easily with a unionist body politic that was patrician, socially conservative and favoured negligible state intervention. Medical voluntarism's building of new hospitals, growth in bed numbers and development of increasingly sophisticated provision allowed Ulster unionism to challenge criticisms of social inaction from the political left.

From a health management perspective, another key theme of this work, medical voluntarism, did help to bring about a more joined-up structure in the Belfast Grosvenor Road complex. Other healthcare providers, such as local authorities, were not involved which undermined the potential for a coordinated system. This was also evident outside Belfast where county infirmaries, threatened by the newly developed district hospitals, failed to merge services, often leading to duplication and overlapping of services in many towns. Another gap in voluntary provision was the inconsistency in entitlement to care across hospitals, leading to patchy patient coverage in which sections of the population, primarily those outside the poor and working classes, struggled to access voluntary hospitals.

Key themes from Section 1

The exploration of healthcare in the 1920s and 1930s provides many insights into the development of health policy in Northern

Ireland. Firstly, a mixed economy of healthcare was evident in Northern Ireland, which provided medical and hospital care. Made up of municipal, poor law and voluntary sectors, this mixed economy made some significant gains and progress throughout the period. Where local poor law reform was enacted, district hospitals often emerged as leading institutions that garnered much local pride and loyalty, providing for not just the poor but a broader social spectrum. Medical voluntarism was also at the forefront of achievement and progress, best demonstrated in the Grosvenor Road complex, which brought about the increased academisation of hospital medicine, two new hospitals and a nascent joined-up health system. Belfast's voluntary hospitals grew in tandem with urban health structures across the UK and further afield in what can be viewed as positive interwar healthcare developments.

The strength of stakeholders in Northern Irish healthcare is a key theme that emerges from this analysis of the interwar years. This was specifically true of medical voluntarism. In Northern Ireland, the sector was centrally tied to the ruling Ulster unionist political and social elite and leading medical professions. It was easily interwoven with a socially hierarchical and conservative Ulster unionist body politic whose interests were tied to elite medicine, academia, the middle- to upper-class management of voluntary hospitals and the social elite. In many ways, medical voluntarism was the embodiment of the Northern Irish unionist establishment, which dominated the country's political, social and economic life during this period.

How political circumstances framed policy is another theme evident in interwar Northern Irish healthcare. While the political power of the dominant Ulster Unionist Party in Northern Ireland helped to shape the strength of medical voluntarism, politics also ensured that socialist-inspired municipal healthcare was far less influential. Although the deepening economic crisis in the interwar years created social instability and led to gains for the Northern Ireland Labour Party, this did not translate to progressive and socialist local authority health services, evidenced when Belfast Corporation's vision for health centres and enhanced maternity and child welfare became unstuck. Such policies failed to succeed in a Northern Irish medical landscape dominated by the upper echelons of the medical profession, voluntary hospitals and the Ulster Unionist Party. Medical voluntarism and socialist-inspired municipal provision were two contrasting and competing visions and cultures of healthcare. In Northern Ireland, socialist-inspired healthcare could not replicate the successes in local authority healthcare in some places in Britain, illustrating how contrasting political contexts shaped health policies.

Political divisions also hampered progress in other areas of healthcare. The nationalist–unionist divide impeded health reform in numerous circumstances. As portrayed in Chapter 1, localised interwar poor law reform was often shaped by the political and religious outlook of poor law unions. The experience of revolution, subsequent nationalist disenchantment from local government and poor law administration, followed by much political bitterness, undermined reform in many areas in the early decades of Northern Ireland. In turn, a multitiered poor law emerged. Areas with majority unionist and Protestant populations, primarily in the eastern half of Northern Ireland, saw the development of new district hospitals while many places that were predominantly Catholic and nationalist remained reliant on substandard and often stigmatising workhouse infirmaries. In a similar trend, voluntary cottage hospitals existed in largely unionist areas while nationalist regions did not witness the emergence of this layer of provision. The unionist-nationalist divide negatively impacted health provision in Belfast, seen through the increased isolation of the Catholic Mater Hospital from the broader voluntary hospital model. These factors further alienated an already embittered and despondent minority, who also suffered from many other disadvantages and discrimination in the Northern Irish state.

Another central theme that emerges from this analysis of 1920s and 1930s is the lack of central government direction and involvement in healthcare. This was painfully evident when the government unwaveringly refused to increase central government funding for local authority maternity and child welfare despite the large number of infant deaths. The inability to bring about poor law reform across Northern Ireland was another significant failure and pointed towards inertia in central government policymaking. The lack of a dedicated health department further weakened the capacity of the Northern Irish government to develop health policies. The government, on an economic cliff-edge from the depression and shaped by an Ulster unionist ideological opposition to state interventionism, failed to provide the lead in developing hospital provision. The vacuum created by central government non-intervention facilitated the embedding of medical voluntarism as the most potent force in Northern Irish medicine. The lack of central government direction also led to local authorities developing healthcare independent of broader planning, which led to an embedded localism and loyalty to individual hospitals. Such authorities were also key drivers and stakeholders in hospital policies.

A combination of political divisions, weak central government action and multiple influential stakeholders ensured fragmented health structures in Northern Ireland. Although shoots of collaboration were evident in some public health fields such as venereal disease, there was minimal attempt to develop hospital services systematically. Instead, voluntary, municipal and poor law hospital services remained independent of each other. This was evident in Belfast, where the Grosvenor Road medical site was an example of coalition-building between three voluntary hospitals and Queen's Medical School. Still, it excluded the Catholic Mater Hospital, Northern Ireland's second largest general voluntary hospital, and Belfast Workhouse. Outside Belfast, county infirmaries were threatened by the emergence of district hospitals and lobbied for their pre-eminence over the former workhouses. While district hospitals undoubtedly enhanced provision for local populations, they also fostered a localism in health policy, which opposed attempts at coordination. Fragmentation, competition between sectors, duplication and overlap of services became embedded in Northern Ireland.

Other problems further weakened health services by the late 1930s. There was an apparent geographical inequality in hospital provision, and the south and west of Northern Ireland had few voluntary or district hospital beds. This aggravated political and religious tensions and created regionally imbalanced hospital structures. Other divisions also existed. The persistence of long-term and chronic patients in underfunded workhouses, while acute patients were treated in better-equipped district hospitals, created further inequalities in treatment of different types of patients. Despite successes in voluntary healthcare, access to the sector remained patchy. Greater demand for hospital services diminished the capacity to provide for growing numbers of patients from higher up the social scale who had limited or no historic access or entitlement to voluntary provision. This was particularly evident in Belfast's voluntary hospitals, which struggled to provide for greater demand from more middle-class patients. Hospitals outside Belfast were quicker to adapt to these new patients, but such provision was invariably offered at a cost. Indeed, the financial health of many provincial hospitals became increasingly reliant on fully or semi-private patients, which weakened access for non-paying patients. Access to hospital care varied not just from sector to sector but also from hospital to hospital, resulting in highly complex, varied and inequitable access and entitlement.

Notes

1 Doyle, *The Politics of Hospital Provision*, see Chapter 7.

2 D. S. Lucey and V. Crossman, 'Introduction', in Lucey and Crossman (eds), *Healthcare in Ireland and Britain*, pp. 1–28.

3 J. Wright, *The 'Natural Leaders' and Their World: Politics, Culture and Society in Belfast, c. 1801–1832* (Liverpool: Liverpool University Press, 2012), esp. Chapter 5; A. Jordan, *Who Cared? Charity in Victorian and Edwardian Belfast* (Antrim: W. G. Baird, 1993); O. Purdue, *The First Great Charity of this Town: Belfast Charitable Society and its Role in the Developing City* (Dublin: Irish Academic Press, 2022); A. Sneddon, 'State intervention and provincial health care: The county infirmary system in late eighteenth-century Ulster', *IHS* 38:149 (May 2012), 5–21.

4 G. Weisz, *Divide and Conquer: A Comparative History of Medical Specialization* (Oxford: Oxford University Press, 2006); for an example of the growth of specialist voluntary hospitals in a British city, see J. Reinarz, *Health Care in Birmingham: The Birmingham Teaching Hospitals 1779–1939* (Woodbridge: Boydell Press, 2009), esp. Chapters 2, 3, 4 and 5.

5 P. Grace, 'Patronage and health care in eighteenth-century Irish county infirmaries', *IHS*, 41:159 (May 2017), 1–21.

6 F. P. Montgomery, 'The future of the hospitals', *UMJ*, 11:2 (November 1942), 116.

7 Northern Ireland Regional Hospitals Council [hereafter NIRHC], *The Red Book: A Plan for the Hospital Services of Northern Ireland* (Belfast: The Northern Ireland Regional Hospitals Council, 1946), p. 83.

8 J. Neville, 'Cottage hospitals and their communities', in Lucey and Crossman (eds), *Healthcare in Ireland and Britain*, p. 117.

9 S. Cherry, 'Change and continuity in the cottage hospitals c. 1859–1948: The experience in East Anglia', *Medical History*, 36:2 (1992), 281.
10 D. Birrell and A. Murie, *Policy and Government in Northern Ireland* (Dublin: Gill and MacMillian, 1980), pp. 110–13.
11 A. J. Willcocks, *The Creation of the National Health Service* (London: Routledge and Kegan Paul, 1967), pp. 30–1.
12 J. F. Harbinson, *The Ulster Unionist Party, 1882–1973: Its Development and Organisation* (Belfast: Blackstaff Press, 1973), pp. 191–202.
13 *BN*, 19 March 1937.
14 Harbinson, *Ulster Unionist Party*, p. 201; 'Obituary of Prof. Johnstone', *UMJ*, 8:1 (1939), 50.
15 Harbinson, *Ulster Unionist Party*, p. 202.
16 *Ibid.*
17 R. Hawkins, 'Barbour, Sir John Milne', in *DIB*, https://www.dib.ie/biography/barbour-sir-john-milne-a0365 (accessed 20 November 2024); he sat for the Antrim (1921–29) and Antrim South (1929–51) constituencies; for his chairmanship, see *Lisburn Standard*, 18 May 1923.
18 *NW*, 18 August 1934.
19 *NDHCDI*, 20 May 1931.
20 *Portadown News*, 30 September 1933.
21 See E. P. Kaufmann, *The Orange Order: A Contemporary Northern Irish History* (Oxford: Oxford University Press, 2007), p. 15; G. Walker, *A History of the Ulster Unionist Party: Protest, Pragmatism and Pessimism* (Manchester: Manchester University Press, 2004), p. 74; O. Purdue, *The Big House in the North of Ireland: Land, Power and Social Elites* (Dublin: University College Dublin Press, 2009), pp. 211–22.
22 Finlayson, *Citizen, State, and Social Welfare in Britain*, pp. 249–50.
23 Purdue, *The Big House in the North of Ireland*, p. 187.
24 RVH, *Annual Report: 134th for the Year 1926* (Belfast: RVH, 1927) p. 15.
25 RVH, *Annual Report: 135th for the Year 1927* (Belfast: RVH, 1928).
26 *BN*, 24 May 1929. The countess was married to the Earl of Clanwilliam, an Irish peer.
27 RVH, *Annual Report: 150th for the Year 1942* (Belfast: RVH, 1943), p. 16.
28 *BN*, 16 August 1948.
29 *BN*, 3 July 1948; *BN*, 1 January 1951.

30 K. Waddington, 'Subscribing to a democracy? Management and the voluntary ideology of the London Hospitals, 1850–1900', *English Historical Review*, 118:476 (April 2003), 367.
31 Webster, *The National Health Service*, p. 5.
32 For an excellent historiographical outline see Doyle, *The Politics of Hospital Provision*, pp. 170–1.
33 Fox, *Health Policies, Health Politics.*
34 S. Sheard, 'The roots of regionalism: municipal medicine from the Local Government Board to the Dawson Report', in Lucey and Crossman (eds), *Healthcare in Ireland and Britain*, pp. 237–53.
35 For Leeds and Sheffield, see Doyle, *The Politics of Hospital Provision*; M. Gorsky, 'The Gloucestershire extension of medical services scheme: an experiment in the integration of health services in Britain before the NHS', *Medical History*, 50:4 (2006), 491–512; Gorsky, '"Threshold of a New Era"', 247–67.
36 Gorsky, 'Threshold of a New Era', 249–50.
37 Reinarz, *Health Care in Birmingham*, p. 247.
38 J. V. Pickstone, *Ways of Knowing: A New History of Science, Technology and Medicine* (Manchester: Manchester University Press, 2000), p. 163.
39 For an outline of Sir William Crawford's career, see 'Death of Sir William Crawford', *Irish Times*, 13 May 1922.
40 QUB Library, Belfast, QUB3/2/1/1/10, QUB Senate minutes, 26 November 1924.
41 QUB Library, QUB3/2/1/1/10, QUB Senate minutes, 13 May 1925.
42 QUB Library, QUB3/2/1/1/12, QUB Senate minutes, Vice Chancellor Report for 1925–6, p. 125.
43 A. Greer, 'Agriculture and rural policy since 1914', in Kennedy and Ollerenshaw (eds), *Ulster Since 1600: Politics, Economy, and Society*, p. 280; Greer, *Rural Politics in Northern Ireland: Policy Networks and Agricultural Development Since Partition* (Aldershot, 1996), p. 16; QUB Senate minutes, 26 November 1924, pp. 171–2.
44 QUB Library, QUB/3/2/1/1/12, QUB Senate minutes, 21 November 1928.
45 G. Jones, 'The Rockefeller Foundation and medical education in Ireland in the 1920s', *IHS*, 30:120 (1997), 566.
46 P. Froggatt, 'The "Connexion" between the Royal and Queen's 1849–1949: Alliance or special relationship', *UMJ*, 67:1 (1998), 117.
47 QUB Library, QUB/3/2/1/1/12, QUB Senate minutes, 23 November 1927.
48 S. Sturdy and R. Cooter, 'Science, scientific management, and the transformation of medicine in Britain, *c.* 1870–1950', *History of Science*, 36:4 (1998), 421–66; P. F. Pérez, *The Emergence of Modern*

Hospital Management in the World, 1880s–1930s (Bingley: Emerald Publishing Ltd., 2021); Pickstone, *Ways of Knowing*, p. 183.
49 Doyle, *The Politics of Hospital Provision*, p. 50.
50 Reinarz, *Health Care in Birmingham*, p. 234.
51 Sturdy and Cooter, 'Science, scientific management and the transformation of medicine', 441–3.
52 A. Flexner, *Medical Education in Europe: A Report to the Carnegie Foundation for the Advancement of Teaching* (New York: The Carnegie Foundation for the Advancement of Teaching, 1912), pp. 59–60.
53 A. Hull, 'Hector's House: Sir Hector Hetherington and the academicization of Glasgow Hospital medicine before the NHS', *Medical History*, 45:2 (2011), 211–12.
54 QUB Library, QUB/3/2/1/1/12, QUB Senate minutes, 11 July 1928.
55 *BT*, 19 November 1931.
56 PRONI, MIC514/1/1/22, RVH Board of Management Committee minute book, 16 July 1928.
57 T. W. Moody and J. C. Beckett, *Queen's Belfast, 1845–1949: Volume II* (Belfast: Faber & Faber for the Queen's University of Belfast, 1959), p. 505.
58 'Queen's University Institute of Pathology', *UMJ*, 2:3 (July 1933), 151–2.
59 *BT*, 17 January 1928; *BT*, 18 February 1931; *BT*, 21 October 1933.
60 RVH, *Annual Report: 136th for the Year 1928* (Belfast: RVH, 1930), p. 17.
61 RVH, *Annual Report: 137th for the Year 1929* (Belfast: RVH, 1931), p. 42.
62 *BT*, 24 February 1930.
63 *BT*, 15 March 1932; *BT*, 25 November 1932.
64 *BT*, 8 June 1929.
65 QUB Library, QUB3/2/1/1/13, QUB Senate minutes, 11 October 1933, p. 109.
66 NPHT, *Survey of the Hospital Services*, p. 37.
67 Gorsky, 'Gloucestershire', 494.
68 Jones, 'Rockefeller', 566, 571.
69 L. Kelly, *Irish Medical Education and Student Culture, c.1850–1950* (Liverpool: Liverpool University Press, 2017), pp. 214–16.
70 F. Prochaska, *Christianity and Social Services in Modern Britain: The Disinherited Spirit* (Oxford: Oxford University Press, 2006), p. 11.
71 B. M. Wall, *Unlikely Entrepreneurs: Catholic Sisters and the Hospital Marketplace, 1865–1925* (Columbus, OH: Ohio State University Press, 2005).

72 NPHT, *Survey of the Hospital Services*, p. 71.
73 The two that opposed the measure were Rev. J. McCaughan, president of St Malachy's College and a crown nominee, and Mr J. B. Moore, a co-opted member and former consultant at the Mater; see Froggatt, 'The "Connexion" between the Royal and Queen's 1849–1949', 119.
74 M. Elliot, *The Catholics of Ulster: A History* (London: Penguin, 2001), p. 386.
75 Martin, 'Why have a Catholic Hospital at all?', p. 103.
76 Jones, 'The Rockefeller Foundation and medical education in Ireland in the 1920s', 570.
77 Lucey, *The End of the Irish Poor Law?*, pp. 153–5.
78 P. Fernández Pérez, *The Emergence of Modern Hospital Management and Organisation in the World 1880s–1930s* (Leeds: Emerald Publishing, 2021), p. 110.
79 *Report of the Irish Public Health Council*, p. 19.
80 PRONI, CAB9/D/61/1, Cabinet Secretariat, Ministry of Education Files, Possibility of Northern Ireland receiving a grant from the Rockefeller Trust for the erection of a state laboratory, Livingstone, QUB to P. M. Craigavon, 2 December 1931; J. B. Lyons, 'Irish medicine's appeal to Rockefeller, 1920s', *Irish Journal of Medical Science*, 166:1 (1997), 54.
81 PRONI, CAB9/D/61/1, Pollock to P.M. Craigavon, 5 December 1931.
82 Gorsky, 'Threshold of a New Era', 266.
83 Gorsky, 'Gloucestershire', 493; Doyle, *The Politics of Hospital Provision*, p. 29.
84 For Manchester see J. V. Pickstone, *Medicine and Industrial Society: A History of Hospital Development in Manchester and its Regions, 1752–1946* (Manchester: Manchester University Press, 1985), p. 322.
85 NIRHC, *The Red Book*, p. 77.
86 *NW*, 10 August 1932.
87 McCormick, 'Venereal disease', p. 194.
88 For example, during 1919 over three thousand Wasserman tests and three hundred other tests were carried out in the Royal Victoria Hospital laboratory, see M. G. Nelson, 'Thomas Houston and the founding of clinical pathology at the RVH, Belfast', *UMJ*, 63:2 (October 1994), 229.
89 McCormick, *Regulating Sexuality*, p. 127.
90 PRONI, LA/7/9DA/27, Belfast County Borough Medical Officer of Health Report, 1937, p. 20.
91 *Portadown News*, 5 April 1929.
92 *Portadown News*, 16 March 1929.

93 *Departmental Commission on Local Government Administration*, pp. 101–2.
94 *Departmental Commission on Local Government Administration*, pp. 115–16.
95 *BN*, 29 February 1932.
96 *BN*, 29 December 1931.
97 *BN*, 13 February 1934.
98 Prochaska, *Christianity and Social Services in Modern Britain*, p. 21.
99 S. Cherry, 'Beyond National Insurance. The voluntary hospitals and hospital contributory schemes: a regional study', *Social History of Medicine*, v (1992), 455–82.
100 Cherry, 'Accountability, entitlement and control issues and voluntary hospital funding', 215–33.
101 G. C. Gosling, '"Open the other eye": Payment, civic duty and hospital contributory schemes in Bristol, *c.* 1927–1948', *Medical History*, 54 (2010), 475–94; M. Gorsky, and J. Mohan with T. Willis, *Mutualism and Health Care: British Hospital Contributory Schemes in the Twentieth Century* (Manchester: Manchester University Press, 2006). p. 2.
102 Hayes and Doyle, 'Eggs, rags and whist drives', 712–40.
103 Among the rare exceptions is B. M. Doyle, 'The economics, culture, and politics of hospital contributory schemes: The case of interwar Leeds', *Labour History Review*, 77:3 (2012), 292.
104 G. C. Gosling, *Payment and Philanthropy in British Health Care, 1918–49* (Manchester: Manchester University Press), pp. 8–9.
105 *NW*, 22 February 1932.
106 RVH, *Annual Report: 108th for the Year 1900* (Belfast: RVH, 1901); RVH, *Annual Report: 134th for the Year 1926*; RVH, *Annual Report: 149th for the Year 1941* (Belfast: RVH, 1942).
107 Gorsky *et al.*, 'The financial health of voluntary hospitals in interwar Britain', 549.
108 Diocese of Down and Connor Office, Belfast, Mater Infirmorum Hospital Uncatalogued Archive, *Annual Report for 1944.*
109 *Lisburn Standard*, 26 April 1935.
110 *BN*, 29 January 1930.
111 *Derry Journal*, 27 January 1939.
112 *BN*, 31 March 1938.
113 *BN*, 21 April 1933.
114 See Doyle, 'The economics, culture, and politics of hospital contributory schemes'; *ibid.*, 'Labour and hospitals in three Yorkshire towns: Middlesbrough, Leeds, Sheffield'; 'Power and accountability in the voluntary hospitals of Middlesbrough 1900–1948', in A. Borsay and

P. Shapely (eds), *Medicine, Charity and Mutual Aid: The Consumption of Health and Welfare in Britain, c.1550–1950* (Aldershot: Ashgate, 2007), pp. 207–24.

115 *Lisburn Standard*, 26 April 1935.

116 *NW*, 19 March 1927.

117 Waddington, 'Subscribing to a democracy?', 367.

118 Gorsky *et al.*, *Mutualism and Health Care*, p. 2.

119 Doyle, 'Power and accountability in the voluntary hospitals'; 'Labour and hospitals in three Yorkshire towns', 374–2.

120 Doyle, 'The economics, culture, and politics of hospital contributory schemes', pp. 302, 313.

121 Prochaska, *Christianity and Social Services in Modern Britain*, p. 22.

122 PRONI, HOS7/3/1/A/5, County Antrim Infirmary Governors, Committee of Management minutes, 21 January 1931.

123 PRONI, HOS7/3/1/A/5, County Antrim Infirmary Governors, Committee of Management minutes, 21 June 1933.

124 *BT*, 13 February 1929.

125 *BN*, 7 May 1925; *BN*, 10 November 1928.

126 Diocese of Down and Connor Office, Belfast, Mater Infirmorum Hospital Uncatalogued Archive, Mater Infirmorum Hospital Workers Maintenance Committee, *Mater Infirmorum Hospital Belfast: Workers Maintenance Committee's Report for 1942* (Printed by the Irish News [hereafter *IN*], Belfast, 1942), p. 20.

127 Gorsky *et al.*, *Mutualism and Health Care*, pp. 106–14.

128 RVH, *Annual Report: 131th for the Year 1923* (Belfast: RVH, 1924), p. 17.

129 Gorsky *et al.*, *Mutualism and Health Care*, p. 19.

130 William Carson remained chairman of the hospital's Working Men's Committee for over fifteen years until his death in 1936; Royal Victoria Hospital Working Men's Committee, *Report of the Royal Victoria Hospital Working Men's Committee, 1936* (Belfast: The Committee, 1937), p. 4.

131 Doyle, 'The economics, culture, and politics of hospital contributory schemes'; Hayes and Doyle, 'Eggs, rags and whist drives', 712–40.

132 Waddington, 'Subscribing to a democracy?', 361.

133 *BT*, 13 May 1943.

134 PRONI, HOS 2/2/9/23, copy of *Belfast Incorporated Maternity Hospital, Annual Report with Statement of Accounts and Lists of Subscribers, Year Ending 31st December 1920* (Belfast, 1921).

135 J. Reinarz, 'Investigating the "Deserving Poor": Charity and the voluntary hospitals in nineteenth-century Birmingham', in Borsay and Shapely (eds), *Medicine, Charity and Mutual Aid*, pp. 111–33.

136 PRONI, MIC514/1/2/3, RVH medical staff minute book, 31 October 1930.
137 RVH, *Annual Report…1923*, p. 12.
138 *Mater Infirmorum Hospital Belfast: Workers Maintenance Committee's Report, 1942*, p. 24.
139 *Mater Infirmorum Hospital Belfast: Workers Maintenance Committee's Report, 1942*, back page.
140 *NW*, 27 April 1939.
141 PRONI, MIC514/1/2/3, RVH medical staff minute book, 18 October 1932.
142 PRONI, MIC514/1/2/3, RVH medical staff minute book, 17 May 1932.
143 PRONI, MIC514/1/2/3, RVH medical staff minute book, 6 July 1937.
144 PRONI, MIC514/1/2/3, RVH medical staff minute book, 18 March 1938.
145 By the mid-1930s £149,283 (56.7 per cent) out of a total of £262,916 in ordinary income for voluntary hospitals came from patient fees in southern Ireland; see Irish Free State, *The Hospitals Commission First General Report* (Dublin: Stationery Office, Saorstát Éireann, 1936), p. 125.
146 The National Archives, Kew, HO 45/17681, Belfast Hospital for Sick Children (Incorporated) Act (Northern Ireland), 1938.
147 *BN*, 29 January 1930.

Section 2

4

Reform, regionalisation and the creation of the National Health Service

The 1940s were a monumental period of transformation for Northern Ireland's healthcare, culminating in the introduction of a comprehensive and universal service under the 1948 Health Services Act, which was part of the UK's National Health Service. Exploring the evolution of medical planning in 1940s Northern Ireland, the chapter argues that interest groups, mainly voluntary hospitals and consultant medical elite, were key to shaping the new service. It is shown that medical voluntarism and the power base that coalesced on the Grosvenor Road site succeeded in eking out significant concessions from the Northern Irish government. This protected the interests of medical voluntarism but weakened the role of the central state and undermined integration, which was a key motivation of the NHS.

This chapter builds on existing scholarship on the establishment of the welfare state and NHS in Northern Ireland, which has concentrated less on the role of the medical profession and more on politics and religious divides. Following the 1942 Beveridge Report and the experience of war, the socially conservative Ulster Unionist Party was forced to engage with social issues in the 1945 general election. It is viewed that the growth of non-unionist parties, mainly the Northern Ireland Labour Party, brought an unprecedented degree of political pressure for social reform upon the newly elected unionist government.[1] Much of the focus on the birth of the welfare state, including health service reform, in Northern Ireland has been on unionist unease at introducing Westminster's post-war socialist reforms, which led to faltering debates concerning Northern Ireland's constitutional status.[2] The success of William Grant,

Northern Ireland's first Minister of Health and Local Government, in overcoming opposition in Ulster unionism and bringing about a reformed, universal health system through successive legislation has been stressed. In this analysis, Grant's adroitness in dealing with the medical profession, compared to the acrimony surrounding Aneurin Bevan's negotiations with the BMA in Britain, is viewed as critical.[3] Furthermore, the crisis in Belfast's local politics surrounding the dissolution of the administrations of the Belfast Board of Guardians and Belfast Corporation's Tuberculosis Committee, following a scandal at Whiteabbey Sanatorium, metamorphosed into a broader political crisis and has been identified as an essential factor in bringing about health reform in Northern Ireland.[4] Historians have also focused on religious division, which led to the Catholic voluntary Mater Infirmorum staying outside the reformed health services. In this instance, Catholic unwillingness to engage with an extension of the welfare state combined with sectarian attitudes towards the hospital led to it remaining as one of the few voluntary general hospitals throughout the UK.[5]

This chapter challenges some of these interpretations and switches the focus to the dynamics that shaped the formulation of health policy and the creation of Northern Ireland's post-war health services. Its central argument is that Northern Ireland's post-1948 hospital service was born out of conflict between an emerging central state and medical voluntarism – the region's key interest group and stakeholder – made up of elite medicine, leading voluntary hospitals and many within Ulster unionism. This draws on historiographical debates on whether the NHS in Britain emerged out of a broad consensus in favour of reform or the outcome of conflict between progressive forces and more conservative and reactionary influences.[6] Hospital policy in Northern Ireland was shaped by medical voluntarism's attempts to safeguard its advantages in the new NHS in which voluntary hospitals would be subsumed by the state. Although the labour movement was far less influential in Northern Ireland than in Britain, the NHS in Northern Ireland was in many ways shaped by the conflict between medical voluntarism and the state. The former successfully agitated against much of the government's reform and ringfenced its pre-eminence in the new system. Medical voluntarism's power, which grew significantly in the interwar years, subverted the government's health policy and negatively impacted the post-1948 management of the health services.

Yet the role of central government, despite the strength of medical voluntarism, in health also grew exponentially, and these years transformed centralised state healthcare in Northern Ireland. It is posited that the central state's earlier abdication for responsibility of hospitals to voluntary and local government increasingly gave way to the emergence of central government as a key actor in health policy, funding and management. This transformation was brought about by a combination of wartime conditions, post-war planning for the welfare state and, ultimately, the introduction of a universal and nationalised health service, which necessitated the expansion of the Stormont government's health bureaucracy. The extent of government involvement that emerged in 1948 was unimaginable at the beginning of the decade. New management structures were developed, which significantly reorganised hospital and health services, although the overall aims of amalgamation were not fully achieved at this point.

Wartime, the Emergency Hospital Service and creeping state intervention

The 1940s brought much change to the health landscape in Northern Ireland, which attempted to transform the disaggregated mixed economy of healthcare described in the first section of this book. In a political climate traditionally dominated by the constitutional question, social issues came to the fore when Northern Ireland's wartime experience exposed the failures of the interwar policies. Across the United Kingdom, welfare reform, prompted by the Beveridge Report, had become a key policy objective. The state's obligation to provide medical attention to a civilian population suffering from exogenous threats of aerial attacks led to the inauguration of the Emergency Hospital Service (EHS) – later the Emergency Medical Service. This wartime reorganisation of health services has been viewed as vital to paving the way for the universal and free-at-the-point-of-contact NHS that came into effect in

1948 and specifically provided the regionalised model for the NHS Regional Hospital Boards in Britain.[7]

There remains, however, little examination of the scheme in the history of 1940s health reform in Northern Ireland. The EHS has been described in its 1950s official history (with a Northern Irish section), but understandings of its regional or local impact remain lacking.[8] Historiographical work has addressed the Northern Irish experience of the Second World War with much emphasis on the government's failure to prepare adequately for wartime conditions and the Blitz, as well as some work on public health measures.[9] The analysis presented here places the experience of the EHS in Northern Ireland as an essential step in the trajectory towards increased state involvement in health policy and management. The Emergency Hospital Service provided a framework to transform the localist and fragmented system of the 1920s and 1930s to a more centralist, harmonised model, which was a key objective of post-war reforms. In response to wartime conditions, the EHS partly reordered the management of Northern Ireland's health and represented the first systematic attempt at reorganisation of the multiple providers – voluntary, poor law and city/county corporations – of hospital provision. This represented a significant turning point for the role of the Stormont government, which failed to provide any real direction during the 1920s and 1930s. Overall, this book analyses the trajectory of Northern Ireland's health services from a disjointed and disaggregated structure into a more joined-up and centralised system – the EHS was a key juncture in this process.

It is also argued that the EHS brought fissures to the fore between voluntary hospitals and the state over issues relating to funding, control and power, which were an augur of future tensions around hospital reform. Although the EHS was a temporary measure, it altered the nexus between medical voluntarism, local authorities and central government during a key stage in health policy development.

The likelihood of war forced the British government to reorganise civil defence. By mid-1938, Whitehall's Ministry of Health established the EHS in England and Wales to provide a wartime hospital service. Under the scheme, all hospitals – voluntary and local authority – were organised into regions to deal with war-related sickness (initially confined to service personnel and war/air attack casualties, but it later included workers in the wartime economy).[10] The hospitals were run by existing authorities but within a regional framework, with the Ministry of Health deciding what role each should play.[11] The Ministry also upgraded facilities, paid hospitals for beds and coordinated medical staff, while consultants were paid full-time salaries and distributed among the regions.[12] The Ministry set performance standards, introduced national pay scales and provided eighty thousand new beds in Britain.[13] This represented a significant change in British hospitals and amounted to a unified national wartime health service funded and organised by central government.[14]

In Northern Ireland, the pending war was viewed as an opportunity to merge the existing complex hospital structure. In April 1939, the Northern Irish branch of the BMA believed that the war offered a 'great opportunity for comprehensive reorganisation' and 'closer co-operation' between hospitals.[15] Although any scheme which impinged on the independence of voluntary hospitals was likely to provoke opposition from medical voluntarism, the government sought to acquiesce concerns among the profession. In July 1939, the Northern Irish BMA recommended that a hospital officer should be appointed to develop a scheme acceptable to the hospital authorities, medical staff and ministry.[16] The Ministry of Home Affairs was anxious to placate the medical profession whose co-operation, as in Britain, was vital for the scheme's implementation and to overcome the central government's lack of medical expertise.[17] In turn, Dr F. M. B. Allen, a key medical leader of medical voluntarism and the medical profession, was appointed as the EHS's Hospital Officer. Allen was a paediatric consultant at the Royal Hospital for Sick Children, one of the three hospitals that made up the powerful voluntary Grosvenor Road medical site. He was also heavily involved in medical politics. He was the secretary of the Northern Irish BMA branch, which, according to government officials, gave him 'unusually wide contacts with[in] the medical profession'.[18] Allen had already lobbied the Ministry on the rate of payment for participating doctors in the scheme.[19] His appointment was viewed as important for smooth relations between the government and medical profession. In September 1939, the Minister of Home Affairs, Sir Dawson Bates, thanked the medical profession for their co-operation in the planning for the emergency services.[20]

The appointment of Allen ensured that the government's leading EHS official was representative of medical voluntarism and the medical elite.

The new service had to overcome the region's entrenched inability to create an integrated hospital structure. For the emergency plan to work, a greater organisation of hospitals was necessary to allow for patient flows between hospitals in the event of an attack. In September 1939, the EHS scheme was announced by the Ministry and included in that year's Civil Defence Act (Northern Ireland). The scheme, which was based on Allen's recommendations, divided Northern Ireland's hospitals into four groups to deal with casualties. The first group was to receive most patients and included Belfast's leading general hospitals. These were supported by eight voluntary hospitals in the Belfast region, which were to receive casualties and specialist cases. The second group included district hospitals, county infirmaries and cottage hospitals in counties Antrim and Down, a region that was also believed to be under threat. The third group was made up of all Northern Irish fever hospitals, mental hospitals and sanatoria, which were to receive ordinary medical cases from hospitals in the first and second groups. The final group of hospitals included four voluntary hospitals that were to be called upon only in exceptional circumstances.[21] Regardless of voluntary or local government management of hospitals, this allowed for the transfer and evacuation of patients from hospitals in danger zones to those in safer areas.[22] This wartime restructure of hospitals was the first attempt to organise Northern Ireland's disparate hospital services into a coherent system. While the interwar years witnessed some collaboration between hospitals, best evident on the Grosvenor Road site, health services were often disjointed. Radically, the EHS cut across municipal, poor law and voluntary authorities to align disparate administrative structures, hospital sectors and institutions.

The EHS also helped to address gaps in provision. Consultancy and specialist services were mostly confined to Belfast's voluntary hospitals. There was a significant omission in such provision in the rest of Northern Ireland, where local authority and provincial voluntary hospitals had more rudimentary expertise. Also, many of the sick had difficulty in accessing voluntary specialist care in which entitlement was predicated mainly on poverty, membership of a hospital contribution scheme or payment. The EHS addressed these deficiencies in multiple ways. To ensure access to consultant and specialist expertise, mobile teams were set up which hospitals in the EHS scheme could call on.[23] New procedures were developed under the EHS for specialist outpatient services, which allowed participating hospitals to send their patients to other hospitals for a second opinion or special investigation.[24] This organisation of services was previously lacking, while it also broadened the availability of specialist care in Northern Ireland beyond Belfast.

Another significant development was the central government's acceptance of financial responsibility for the EHS. This was a reversal of the state's long-standing policy on hospitals. During the 1920s and 1930s, voluntary hospitals received little, if any, state funding while central and local government were locked in intractable disputes over finances, which significantly inhibited development. The pending war and subsequent need to realign hospitals overcame such entrenched positions. Stormont officials could not expect or rely on local authorities to meet the cost of a service which was of national importance. Local authorities still had to pay 30 per cent of the cost, which differed from the entire compensation from the state that voluntary hospitals received.[25] Treatment of air raid casualties was paid on a capitation basis at a rate negotiated between Whitehall's Ministry of Health and the BHA.[26] Additional medical equipment such as beds, x-ray apparatus and operating theatre equipment was also subsidised by the Ministry of Home Affairs. This helped to upgrade many hospitals throughout Northern Ireland.[27] For example, the Ballymena Workhouse invested close to £12,000 in renovations under the scheme.[28] In Magherafelt, the guardians began renovating the workhouse as an emergency hospital in 1942.[29] When completed in 1944, the need for casualty beds had subsided with the decreased likelihood of air attacks, by which stage the guardians transformed the workhouse into a district hospital.[30] The EHS also added over one thousand hospital beds to the pre-war stock.[31] Central government finance was a radical change in the funding model of Northern Irish hospitals, which helped individual hospitals meet the costs of patient care and the upgrading of facilities from the state's coffers for the first time.

The EHS may have represented a transformation of the central state's role in healthcare, but it was ill-equipped to meet the threat of air attacks. It was assumed that Northern Ireland would not be a target for attacks, which led to the dilution of the scheme. Hospitals were initially ordered to restrict general admissions to urgent and acute cases, while institutions in danger areas were to discharge fit patients; this soon gave way, and hospitals were allowed to revert to a more liberal admission policy.[32] Although the newly established Ministry of Public Security took over the EHS in 1940 from Home Affairs, the scheme remained confined to a small number of armed-forces casualties and children under the evacuation schemes.[33] In general, there was a lack of preparedness on the part of the Stormont government for air attacks.

The desultory plans of the EHS came to the fore during and after the Belfast Blitz of spring 1941, in which the city suffered from four air attacks between April and May. An estimated fifty-six thousand homes were damaged, leaving one hundred thousand people temporarily and fifteen thousand permanently homeless.[34] There was also a mass evacuation from Belfast. Northern Ireland's hospitals were overwhelmed by the volume of casualties, which amounted to approximately 970 fatalities and 2,494 injured, the majority of which were in Belfast. Some attacks also occurred outside Belfast, such as in Newtownards and Bangor, where the hospitals in each town received the injured.[35] In Belfast, the Mater Hospital, Royal Victoria and City (workhouse) hospitals were the major casualty hospitals under the emergency plan. The emergency services were impeded by the destruction of the Ulster Hospital for Children and Women and the Belfast Hospital for Diseases of the Skin.[36] The medical response to the Blitz was broadly considered a failure and lacked the necessary hospital capacity, personnel, ambulance provision and first-aid parties.[37] The historian Brian Barton's account of the Blitz highlights its impact on hospitals. The Mater Hospital was so low on food that green peas were served for dinner.[38] Hospitals' morgues overflowed with corpses, many dismembered, leading to the smell of decomposing flesh and chaos among relatives and friends of the missing looking for their loved ones.[39] Alternative mortuaries had to be established, including the Corporation's public baths.[40] This was symptomatic of the overall inadequacy of the government's civilian planning for air attacks.

The EHS plan also proved ineffectual in dealing with the aftermath of the 1941 air attacks. While no further attacks would occur after May 1941, the continued threat ensured that many hospitals faced major disruption. Reserved beds for potential air raid casualties strained capacity, leading to the steep rise in waiting lists for ordinary patients, with only urgent cases admitted to hospitals.[41] After the April 1941 air attack, the Royal Victoria's medical staff called on the EHS to transfer some of the hospital's ordinary work to a hospital outside the city.[42] However, only casualties from air attacks could be treated under the emergency scheme and not hospitals' ordinary patients. This fault line in the emergency scheme was highlighted by Thomas Bailie, an independent unionist MP for North Down in the Stormont parliament, in November 1941, who sought to make emergency casualty beds outside Belfast available to relieve hospitals' waiting lists of ordinary patients. His calls were rejected by Lowry, secretary of the Ministry of Home Affairs, who believed the use of the scheme by the ordinary sick was illegal.[43] Hospitals struggled to combine their day-to-day functions with emergency provision for potential air attacks. Although the government's EHS plan was centred on the flow of patients between hospitals to ensure that it could withstand the stress of casualties from air attacks, it failed to address the implications of emergency provision on ordinary care.

The first state-run hospital – Central Emergency Hospital

Tensions simmered between the Ministry and hospitals over the EHS. Under increased pressure from hospitals, the government looked to expand the EHS by taking direct responsibility for emergency cases. As early as May 1941, a plan emerged to convert part of Belfast's municipal mental institution, Purdysburn, into a central EHS hospital run by the Ministry of Home Affairs. It was envisaged that this would relieve hospitals of some air raid casualty duties and free up beds for more emergency and ordinary patients. Divisions between hospitals and central government soon escalated over the funding of the proposed scheme. Hospitals were only willing to support the government's scheme if it fully met the cost of running the new emergency hospital.[44] The voluntary hospitals agitated for the government to pay all capital and excess expenditure in the proposed central hospital. The EHS Hospital Officer, Allen, vigorously supported the voluntary hospitals and informed government officials that an undercurrent of 'anxiety and criticism' existed in 'hospital and medical circles' towards the government.[45] Allen chastised the government's inertia and parsimony, and he complained that the administration was delayed by 'observance of peace-time regulation', which contradicted London's 'spirit' and 'attitude' and the prevailing determination to 'get the job done'.[46] Many within voluntary hospitals were suspicious of increased state encroachment on their independence. A surgeon in the Mater, Dr Kennedy, acknowledged that hospitals were under pressure but warned that the 'state was not the cure', and he feared 'where red tape would begin or end' with any state intervention.[47] Relations between central government and voluntary hospitals quickly became strained over the issues of control, funding and the demands of emergency services. The independence from government of voluntary hospitals was infringed upon by a nascent central government health bureaucracy struggling to cope with wartime conditions.

The government's position was partly determined by economic conservatism, which had shaped Northern Ireland's fiscal policy since its foundation. The Ministry of Finance's secretary, W. B. Spender, renowned for his austere interwar economic policies, informed the Prime Minister that Allen was merely a 'temporary officer' in the government's employment, who had little acquaintance with the 'principles of government administration' and regarded any Treasury supervision as 'irksome'.[48] Spender was critical of Allen's failure to provide a detailed estimation of the scheme's potential cost and advised the government:

> I feel it would be dangerous for a technical officer to receive the very wide financial powers which Dr Allen seems to visualise as being entrusted to him, and if I am correct in this view, I do not think the Ministry of Home Affairs officials would accord Dr Allen their support.[49]

Spender's imperiousness reflected the long-held economic conservatism ingrained within much of Northern Irish officialdom.

Such official attitudes were increasingly challenged in a broader political climate which looked unfavourably on the government's record of social inaction. The experience of the air raids had a profound impact on Northern Irish politics. The ineptness of the government's response exposed a range of social problems. It acted as a platform for growing discontent – within and outside unionism – with the government, particularly Prime Minister John Andrews, who was increasingly viewed as obdurately conservative and incompetent, and eventually forced to resign in 1943.[50] Dissent over wartime social and employment conditions threatened to bridge the political and religious divide, and the Unionist Party suffered some by-election losses, albeit to independent unionist candidates. Allen recognised this discontent during debates on the central EHS hospital, and he warned the government of the 'public outcry' if the treatment of casualties, care of the sick and welfare for the aged and infirm failed to meet demand.[51] The labour movement also pressurised the government, and, in late 1941, the Northern Ireland Labour Party MP, Jack Beattie, demanded that the EHS be extended to all citizens.[52] The experiences of war challenged the government's conservative health and welfare policies, and it was under political pressure to extend the EHS scheme.

The relationship between the Ministry and voluntary hospitals further deteriorated after the government proposed to take responsibility for five hundred beds in Purdysburn Hospital to house and treat 'casualties arising from hostile attacks' in late 1941.[53] Voluntary hospitals rejected this proposal because it excluded ordinary patients on their waiting lists, whose access to hospital care was delayed by the reserving of casualty beds. The management committees of the Royal Victoria and Royal Maternity informed the Ministry that they 'were very perturbed' over the scheme.[54] The medical staff of the Royal Victoria warned that the Ministry's plans would not ensure the treatment of the civilian sick and demanded that the hospitals would have no financial liability for the cost of civilian sick in the EHS hospital.[55] The Royal Victoria also informed the Ministry that the provision of five hundred beds was inadequate and sought an extra three hundred spaces – the failure to come to an agreement delayed the new hospital, which did not open until October 1942.[56] The decreased likelihood of an air attack led the Ministry to succumb to allowing ordinary patients on the waiting lists of the Royal Victoria and Mater hospitals to receive treatment in the new hospital.[57] Only patients requiring general medical and surgical treatment were admitted under this scheme. Patients who were subscribers to these hospitals' contribution schemes were not required to pay, but the hospital had to make a one-off payment of £1 10s regardless of the extent of treatment for each patient. Non-subscribing patients were means tested and had to pay according to their capacity. Despite these terms, the ability to transfer ordinary patients from these hospitals' ordinary waiting lists was a significant win for the voluntary hospitals. By 1947, 1,221 patients on the Royal Victoria's waiting list were treated under the scheme.[58] These negotiations illustrated the capacity of voluntary hospitals, especially the Royal Victoria, to eke out significant concessions from the government.

The establishment of the Central Emergency Hospital was a watershed moment for the state and Ministry of Home Affairs in the delivery of health services. Within three years, the emergency hospital was moved to a stand-alone hospital at Musgrave Park, a prominent former military hospital with seven hundred beds.[59] The government extended provision in the hospital to include Northern Ireland's first occupational health department, and tuberculosis provision to relieve local authority waiting lists.[60] The Ministry also created a centralised blood transfusion department for all of Northern Ireland.[61] The government now directly managed the delivery of some health services for the general population and not just wartime casualties.

The increased role of the state was also a transformation of the dynamics underpinning health policymaking in Northern Ireland. The first state-run hospital in Northern Ireland, the Central Emergency Hospital, cost the Ministry over £100,000 per annum by the mid-1940s.[62] This illustrated the government's transition away from deep-rooted financial parsimony, unwillingness to take responsibility for hospital services and indifference towards health reform. At one level, central government had now emerged as a key power broker in hospitals and health policymaking. Voluntary hospitals also had a victory of sorts; they now could draw on government resources to meet not just casualties relating to war but also the ordinary sick on their waiting lists. Yet this engagement with the state also represented the passing of medical voluntarism's apotheosis of power and independence. Traditionally the most influential stakeholder in Northern Irish medicine, it now had to engage, negotiate and cede power to central government in an augury of future relations in the post-war welfare state. Although in 1946 William

Grant (Minister of Health and Local Government) specified that the EHS provided the basis for further co-operation between the government and hospitals, the reality was a relationship based on conflict as much as consensus, as the powerful medical voluntarism had to adapt to the growing apparatus of central state administration.[63]

Hospital policy, regionalisation and post-war planning

Outside of the context of war, calls for health reform had been gaining momentum since the late 1930s. In 1938, Dr Leonard Kidd chastised the plethora of disparate government ministries and local authorities responsible for health and called for the establishment of a dedicated Ministry of Health.[64] The impact of the Second World War heralded a new emphasis on post-war reconstruction and created a renewed atmosphere for social reform.[65] The Stormont government's Planning Advisory Board set up specialist committees to investigate social services, including housing, transport and sewerage, among other areas.[66] Medical reform came to the fore in the UK's policy agenda with the 1942 Beveridge Report and the emergence of post-war planning. In Britain, proposals for health reform were put forward by diverse, often competing, interest groups such as voluntary hospitals, the right-of-centre advocacy group Political and Economic Planning, the BMA's Medical Planning Commission and the Labour Party-affiliated Socialist Medical Association.[67] The need for substantial reform and state involvement was accepted on the whole, although limited consensus emerged on how health services were to be organised, managed, funded and accessed.

The regionalisation of health services emerged as a key concept in health planning by the early 1940s. Predicated on the spatial organisation of medical services around centres of expertise, this blueprint cut across local government boundaries and promised an enhanced service.[68] At its optimum, regional health structures can act as an intermediate tier of organisations in which rationalisation and specialisation are realised.[69] This approach, as explained in the previous chapter, had some influence at a local level in Britain during the 1920s and 1930s but was not implemented nationally. In 1937, the BHA – a representative body of voluntary hospitals – set up the 1937 Sankey Commission which recommended the regional organisation of such hospitals across Britain, although it ignored Northern Ireland. Responses to the Second World War across the United Kingdom introduced the regional organisation of health services through the EHS, which had evaded politicians and planners for the previous two decades.[70]

The place of regionalisation of hospital services has had different interpretations in the historiography of the NHS' establishment. Much debate has prevailed on whether the UK's NHS emerged from a broad consensus in favour of reform or the outcome of conflict between progressive forces in the form of the labour movement and more conservative and reactionary influences. Regional health policies are viewed by some as the apogee of rational and technocratic health planning, promoted by an evolving consensus among government officials, think tanks, medical profession and hospitals, which ultimately led to the NHS in 1948 and its regionalised structures.[71] Multiple historians, such as Klein and Fox, have identified this consensus in 1940s British health policy. In contrast, other works have stressed the confrontation between progressivism, represented by the labour movement and SMA, and more conservative forces, which were key to bringing about the NHS. From this perspective, the conflict between the Labour government and interest groups led to concessions on such a scale that the NHS could only be imperfectly realised, which perpetuated existing inefficiencies and inequities and undermined one of the NHS's founding principles to create a consolidated system.[72]

In relation to Northern Ireland, as already highlighted in Chapter 3, a regional hierarchy of sorts had developed in Belfast during the interwar years around the Grosvenor Road medical site. A coalition of multiple leading voluntary hospitals and Queen's University's Medical School developed an interrelated model, propelled by an emerging consensus around medical voluntarism. This, however, was far from an apolitical technocratic endeavour and was the embodiment of a medical voluntarism that was Belfast-based, socially hierarchical and tied to not just an academic and medical elite but also a politically dominant Ulster unionism. This was also predicated on minimal central government encroachment on the independence of medical voluntarism; such independence had become increasingly unrealistic by the 1940s as the central state assumed greater responsibility for health, as evidenced by the experience of the EHS.

One of the biggest proponents of regional health policies in the UK was the Nuffield Provincial Hospitals Trust (hereafter Nuffield Trust). Established in 1939 as a wealthy and influential academic and medical pressure group, the Nuffield Trust was committed to the regionalisation of health services, which ultimately favoured voluntary hospitals. During the wartime planning years in Britain, the Nuffield Trust developed a close partnership with the Ministry of Health, resulting in the Hospital Surveys, popularly known as the 'Domesday Books'. These analysed the medical needs of specific regions and proposed a hierarchical organisation of services.[73] The surveys, which were published in 1945, drew attention to the unevenness and deficiencies of a system born with geographic disparities.[74] They recommended the creation of regions that transcended the boundaries of local authorities, redistribution of consultants from large cities and reorganisation of services for the chronically ill.[75] The focus on regionalisation benefited voluntary hospitals whose consultant staff dreaded the prospect of coming under local government and being reduced to the rank of public health employees.[76] It contrasted greatly with other models of healthcare promulgated by the labour movement and SMA, wherein power was to be exercised by democratically elected local authorities under the Ministry of Health.[77] The Nuffield Trust's regionalisation policy *prima facie* protected the interests of medical voluntarism and embedded voluntary hospitals' pre-eminence and independence from central and local government.

Many within Northern Irish medicine welcomed the Nuffield Trust. Queen's University's Vice-Chancellor, Lindsay Keir, was a strong advocate of the Trust. Since the 1930s, Keir was a key figure in the academic-voluntary hospital nexus which developed around the Grosvenor Road medical site in Belfast. On the recommendation of the Prime Minister, Keir was appointed as the Northern Irish representative on the Trust's Board after approaches from its chairman, William Goodenough.[78] In October 1942, Keir was appointed chairman of the Northern Ireland Regional Hospitals Council, established under the auspices of the Nuffield Trust to develop a regionalisation plan for Northern Ireland's hospitals.[79] The Council was stocked with medical representatives from the BMA and BHA

– the voluntary hospital lobby group which established a Northern Irish branch in 1942.[80] The creation of a regional council contrasted with experiences in Britain, where local authorities, fearful of regionalisation, successfully resisted such plans.[81] Local government had less influence in Northern Ireland and did not offer similar resistance. In 1942, the leading medical figure Dr Frank Montgomery – consultant radiologist in the Royal Victoria and Queen's University academic – welcomed the work of the Nuffield Trust in a presidential address of the Northern Irish branch of the BMA on the future of health services in the region.[82] The Trust's apparent alignment with the interests of medical voluntarism ensured that the body was supported by the academic-voluntary nexus, which was the primary medical interest group in Northern Ireland.

The Regional Hospitals Council appointed a three-person team to survey the province's hospitals. All the surveyors were from outside Northern Irish medicine and were firm proponents of regionalised health policies. The triumvirate included the Director General of the Army Medical Services, Lieutenant General William P. MacArthur, whose career was in Britain despite his Northern Irish family connections.[83] The other surveyors were Dr Duncan Leys, the consulting physician for the northern counties in Scotland, who participated in the Nuffield Trust's survey of Scottish hospitals, and Dr Stanley Barnes, a senior British medical academic figure and dean of the Faculty of Medicine in the University of Birmingham.[84] Stanley was key to the establishment of the Birmingham Hospitals Centre, an amalgamation of the city's voluntary hospitals in 1938 on a united hospital greenfield site next to the university, which was an exceptional case of interwar voluntary hospital collaboration.[85] The surveying team's background ensured that a regionalised health system would be put forward by the Trust.

The 1944 surveyors' report called for widespread reorganisation and reform. It advised for the establishment of a Belfast Hospitals Centre, connected to the medical school, which would provide the leading and specialist hospital services for the whole of Northern Ireland.[86] Unsurprisingly, the surveyors identified the Grosvenor Road medical site for further development as the Hospitals Centre. It called for the site's substantial development, including the building of new dental and eye, ear and throat hospitals, and the expansion of the Royal Victoria to provide new regional specialities in psychiatry, neurosurgery, metabolic disease and cancer treatment.[87] A second hospital grouping in Belfast, based at Purdysburn, was planned to give medical provision to the city, while the poor law City Hospital was to be downgraded and ultimately 'evacuated'.[88] A hierarchical structure was proposed for hospitals outside Belfast. Nine provincial 500-bed hospitals were to be established to provide comprehensive hospital services for a population catchment area of around 100,000. These hospitals were to be fully merged with the Belfast Hospital Centre, which would receive patients in need of more specialist services.[89] Polyclinics, or cottage hospitals, were to provide minor surgical facilities and convalescent care outside Belfast. The surveyors also stressed the lag in hospital services compared to Britain, and the need for a heavy capital programme and the increase in specialists and consultants.[90]

The surveyors' report was presented to the Regional Hospitals Council and formed the basis of the Council's subsequent report, known as *The Red Book*. The Council endorsed Nuffield's recommendations and contended that it provided 'the best foundation for a properly coordinated hospital service for the future'.[91] These ideas were presented through the lexicon of technocratic and scientific expertise, free from the influence of stakeholders, whether political, sectoral or local. In many ways, the proposals were the embodiment of the logical hierarchy of hospital services, which had gained a consensus among many medical planners, medics and voluntary hospitals in Britain.

Radical changes in the management of health services were also proposed. Both the surveyors and *The Red Book* adumbrated a reformed administration made up of a central hospitals body responsible for overall policy and harmonisation of ten area committees.[92] The surveyors recognised that such proposals represented a 'revolutionary' change in management which 'cut across many of the institutional and personal rivalries which have naturally developed in the past'; they, however, optimistically believed that 'men of goodwill [would] rapidly' adjust to change.[93] The Council was similarly optimistic and believed such committees would allow for the 'frankest exchange of views' but 'old ideas of boundaries, functions and tradition' would be discarded in favour of 'welding' hospitals into a single coordinated service'.[94] The proposals promised a major restructuring of Northern Ireland's hospital services. They envisaged a sea change in organisational structure, aimed at eradicating the tensions and divisions that permeated Northern Irish hospitals. They were predicated on the belief that consensus would be achieved by an emerging technocracy that would overcome the inherent fissures and interest group power that characterised Northern Irish hospital management.

The proposals' claims to be free of stakeholder bias were weak. In many ways, the report perpetuated the power of medical voluntarism in Northern Ireland, which was to be further strengthened in the reorganised health service. In contrast, the role of local and central government was marginalised. The Grosvenor Road site in Belfast was to be consolidated into the centre of Northern Irish medicine while local authority medicine in the city, notably Belfast City Hospital, was sidelined. The proposed new hospital framework proposed a radical restructuring of services outside Belfast, which dispensed with local authority boundaries. Although neither the surveyors' nor the Council's reports expressed which hospitals would be the leading institutions, the voluntary county infirmaries could be confident that their interests would be protected. Shaped by regional health policies, the proposed structures would cement the power structures which had evolved since the interwar years.

Politically, the plans resonated with the social conservatism of the Ulster unionist government. Many within Ulster unionism were distrustful and suspicious of the socialist welfare proposals that emanated from the labour movement in Britain.[95] In contrast, the Trust was a non-government, endowed and elitist body which encompassed many of the leading medical and academic figures in Britain. It sat easily with the leadership of Ulster unionism while also appealing to their British and imperial sentiment. This was evident in 1944 when William Grant, the Minister of the newly established Ministry of Health and Local Government (MHLG), stated:

> when an organisation such as the Nuffield Trust decided to interest itself in the hospital services of our country, we feel that we are sharing in the wide and deep fund of solid British experience, and we know that, yet another link is being forged in that great chain which binds us to the Empire.[96]

The Nuffield Trust's attractiveness to Ulster unionism was partly explained by its association with voluntary hospitals, which had long been affiliated with conservative pillars of local communities in Britain.[97] It was far more palatable to mainstream Ulster unionism than other pressure groups promoting medical reform, such as the SMA. It helped assuage unionist anxieties over condoning British Labour Party socialist health reform. The Trust's focus on regional policies and management structures with meagre government control was also in keeping with much unionist political opinion. The Trust's proposals gave the veneer of technocratic, apolitical and modernising scientific approaches. Still, they were in many ways reflective of existing power structures and the medical, political and social elite in Northern Ireland.

The proposals, however, were unrealistic for multiple reasons. Northern Irish healthcare prior to the 1940s was far from the technocratic force championed by the proponents of regional policies. The proposals failed to fully appreciate the entrenched localism, institutional loyalties and divisions that permeated Northern Irish healthcare. The proposal to downgrade and ultimately close Belfast City Hospital ignored that institution's medical advancement and was quietly dropped by the Regional Hospitals Council.[98] Outside Belfast, the objective of merging hospital administrations across voluntary and local government represented a major challenge. As depicted in section one of this book, the semi-voluntary county infirmaries and local authority district hospitals developed independently from each other during the interwar years, and relations were marked by sectoral rivalry and competition. The Mater Hospital was glossed over with no direction on how to accommodate its Catholic and nationalist affiliations in a proposed system in which the unionist and Protestant elite would inevitably dominate. The difficulties in surmounting the multiple interest groups inherent in Northern Irish hospitals were not recognised in the proposals, which naively predicted that these challenges would wash away in favour of technocratic solutions.

The plans envisaged limited, if any, central government involvement. While this was popular with medical voluntarism and many within Ulster unionism, it did not reflect the increasing necessity for greater state action. More significant central government funding, responsibility and direction in health policy and the management of health services were inevitable. Still, the Nuffield Trust model of regionalised health failed to emphasise the role of the state. The experience of the Emergency Hospital Service was an augury of the tensions which could envelop government and hospital relations, particularly concerning funding and hospital independence. While the regionalisation of health represented a consensus among voluntary hospitals, academic medicine and many within unionism, it failed to account for the imminent fissures that had shaped healthcare to that point.

Select Committee on Health Services and policy proposals

The proposed negligible role of government envisaged by the Nuffield proposals was attenuated by increased criticism of state inaction. In 1942, Dr William Lyle, recently elected Unionist Party MP for Queen's University, launched an attack on the record of the Minister of Home Affairs, Dawson Bates, in healthcare.[99] In January 1943, the beleaguered Northern Irish Prime Minister, John Andrews, who was soon to be replaced, established a select committee to examine the region's health services. The Select Committee focused on all areas of healthcare, including hospitals, primary care and environmental services. Within an atmosphere of reform, the findings of the Select Committee were likely to have a real impact, unlike previous inquiries such as the 1927 Local Government Administration Commission, whose recommendations were largely ignored.

The Select Committee took sixty-seven days of evidence and heard from over 140 witnesses involved in the health services. It allowed the key professional, local authority, political and central government groups a platform to air concerns, draw battle lines and agitate for any change. The ten-man Select Committee was composed of Stormont MPs primarily drawn from the Ulster Unionist Party, many of whom were also medical professionals. It was chaired by Howard Stevenson, the leading Royal Victoria surgeon and Unionist Party MP who represented the multiseat Queen's University constituency. In contrast, two other Unionist Party MPs and medics – Dr George Doughan and Dr William Lyle, who represented the Central Armagh and Queen's University constituencies, respectively – also sat on the committee. Most other committee members were Ulster Unionist Party MPs, although the NILP's Harry Midgley and John Campbell, a Nationalist MP for North Belfast, were also members.[100] The committee heard evidence from an array of medical representatives, including the BMA, BHA, Medical Practitioners' Union, Royal Victoria Hospital and Royal Maternity Hospital, among others.

The interests of medical voluntarism were widely articulated and highly influential, which was unsurprising considering its strong representation among the Select Committee and witnesses that gave evidence. Although *The Red Book* was not yet published, in 1943, the newly elected and third Prime Minister of Northern Ireland, Basil Brooke, directed the Nuffield Trust to keep the Select Committee's chairman abreast of the 'intentions and extent of the survey'.[101] Regional health policies were also evident in Lindsay Keir's evidence on orthopaedic services when he called for a central, longer-stay hospital in Belfast which would monitor and provide personnel to local clinics throughout Northern Ireland.[102] The BHA articulated the interests of voluntary hospitals at the Select Committee. Initially established in Britain in 1884, the BHA was the representative body of voluntary hospitals and emphasised the traditional virtues of voluntarism.[103] Its main priority was to avoid subservience to local authorities and improve state grants to voluntary hospitals.[104] Its secretary, R. W. Harland, pushed for state grants for nurses in voluntary hospitals at the Select Committee.[105] Similarly, Prof. Lowry of the Royal Maternity Hospital called for increased state loans for capital projects and support for poorer patients in voluntary hospitals. Lowry also promoted private practice and paying patients, which mostly benefited consultants and voluntary hospitals. Averring medical voluntarist ideals, he maintained that voluntary effort was not 'dead', pointing to the voluminous philanthropic funding generated for the Royal Maternity in the early 1930s while ignoring the sector's financial subsidence.[106] Most committee members were receptive to the interests of medical voluntarism. The independent Unionist MP Thomas Bailie believed it was not the committee's wish for the state to 'displace voluntary effort'.[107] Ulster Unionist Party MP Samuel Hall-Thompson warned that any increased government authority was the 'thin wedge' of voluntary hospitals becoming 'state-aided'.[108] The committee's interim report in July 1943 recommended that the state fund 50 per cent of nurses' salaries, which the government quickly introduced.[109] This represented a significant financial contribution by the Northern Irish government to the running of voluntary hospitals. Its final report in February 1944 proposed other measures that favoured voluntary hospitals, including state funding for teaching hospitals and protection of voluntary hospitals' benefactions.

In contrast to medical voluntarism, the influence of policies from the labour movement or local government over the committee was negligible. Local authorities feared that if their boundaries were irrelevant, as proposed under regional policies, their obsolescence in healthcare would be hastened.[110] In Britain, the SMA sought a local authority health service and opposed the pre-eminence and independence of voluntary hospitals. In Northern Ireland, the capacity for progressive local authority health policies was modest, as painfully illustrated by the failure of Belfast Corporation to develop maternity and child welfare in the early 1930s (see Chapter 2). A branch of the SMA was established in Belfast, and under the NILP, the pamphlet *Health in Belfast* was published in 1943, which heavily criticised the government's record.[111] Despite some electoral success by the NILP, the general weakness of the labour movement in Northern Ireland undermined the SMA's influence in policymaking. This was evident when the SMA's policy of establishing local authority primary care health centres – a key ideological divergence between the labour movement and the medical profession in Britain – received little attention during the proceedings.[112] The political weight of local authorities was greatly reduced after the dissolution of the Belfast Board of Guardians in 1939 and the Belfast Council's TB Committee in 1941 over corruption and maladministration controversies.[113] Instead, the case for local authority healthcare at the Select Committee fell to minor local authorities such as the Carrickfergus Urban District Council.[114]

The capacity of either the SMA or local government bodies to influence policymaking and act as a bulwark to regionalisation and deterioration of local authority power was minimal in Northern Ireland. Much of the Select Committee's proceedings and findings were shaped by the medical profession and voluntary hospitals. At the same time, the quiescence of other interest groups, including local government and the labour movement, limited their sway.

The proceedings and findings of the Select Committee portrayed the influence of medical voluntarism over hospital policymaking in Northern Ireland.

The Select Committee's headline recommendation was the establishment of a central government ministry dedicated to health services. The Northern Irish government under Basil Brooke quickly set up the MHLG in July 1944 and appointed William Grant as its maiden minister. Grant was previously the Minister for Public Security (1941–43), when he gained experience in running the Emergency Medical Service. Grant was representative of the trade unionist strand in Ulster unionism and approached reform with a genuine passion that stemmed from his working-class background.[115] Grant set about introducing significant reforms of public health and tuberculosis prior to developing legislation for the whole of the health services.[116] Tuberculosis reform led to the creation of the Northern Ireland Tuberculosis Authority. This sweeping measure established a joint authority to administer services to ensure uniformity of provision throughout the province.[117] Historians view the creation of the Ministry as a key milestone in Northern Irish health policy, brought about by a general appetite and aspiration for reform, representing the trajectory towards greater central government oversight of health, which was irresistible to even the most conservative elements of unionism.[118]

The Ministry, however, was far from a radical development. It finally brought Northern Ireland in line with Britain and the Irish Free State, where central government health departments had existed for over twenty years. Also, the Select Committee attached a major caveat that weakened the power of the Ministry in hospital policymaking – it recommended that an advisory council to the Ministry be appointed to act as the 'authority to settle hospital policy for the region'.[119] Subsequently, the Health Advisory Council was set up in late 1944, which was primarily made up of leading medical voluntary figures in Northern Ireland. Stevenson, the chair of the Select Committee and consultant surgeon, headed up the new Council. Most of the twenty-person Council were medical professionals, including BMA leaders Frank Montgomery and Ian McClure – the latter was a gynaecologist in the Royal Maternity and a future Ulster Unionist Party MP.[120] These figures were staunchly opposed to the nationalisation of health services envisaged under Westminster's 1944 White Paper, which radically proposed a universal, free-at-the-point-of-contact health service directed by the Ministry of Health and under the management of local government. In December 1944, McClure claimed that 'in Northern Ireland there was no evidence that either the people or the doctors wanted the White Paper. They did not want to lose their freedom'.[121] Much of Northern Irish health policymaking and reform was in the hands of doctors who were against the radical reforms promised by Westminster.

In contrast to the White Paper's focus on local government, the Health Advisory Council believed regionalisation was 'the best modern thought' on hospital organisation.[122] It also differed from the Westminster White Paper regarding authority and decision-making responsibilities between the government and individual hospitals. While London sought a far more significant role for central and local government, the Advisory Council wished to minimise state bureaucracy. It maintained that hospitals should be managed independently by their existing boards of management.[123] The Health Advisory Council aimed to enhance the influence of the medical profession and voluntary hospitals in shaping policy while greatly diminishing the role of the new Ministry of Health and Local Government. This was intended to give medical voluntarism much influence but lessen the power and sway of politicians and civil servants.

A consensus had emerged among key medical stakeholders and policymakers in Northern Ireland, which focused on a regionalised health service and ensured the independence of hospitals. This represented the coalition of interests of the medical elite, academic medicine and medical voluntarism, which had coalesced to emerge as Northern Ireland's most potent medical interest group. The blueprints and proposed policies developed by successive bodies, including think tanks, government inquiries and expert advisory groups, promoted a new structure that cemented this coalition's position and promulgated a small central government with little power. Many within government acquiesced to these proposals, which fitted the socially conservative, small state and non-interventionist principles that permeated much of Northern Irish officialdom.

The trajectory of health policy in the UK took a major change of direction with the 1945 landslide election of the Labour Party and the appointment of the socialist doctor and son of a Welsh coal miner, Aneurin Bevan, as Minister of Health. The coalition government's 1944 White Paper was dismissed and replaced by Bevan's proposals for a nationalised health service, leading to the March 1946 National Health Service Bill. Nationalisation involved the state taking full command of all hospitals, which took many by surprise in not just Northern Ireland but also in Britain. This drastic policy step change has been described as the most decisive action regarding hospitals ever taken in a western nation.[124] Bevan also committed to a regionalised structure, which helped to overcome hospital and elite consultant opposition and their fear of the ignominy of municipalisation.[125] He also offered consultants multiple financial incentives, famously claiming to have 'stuffed their mouths with gold'. These were attractive to hospital medical staff and senior medics who were rescued from their honorary status and offered full or part-time contracts.[126] Bevan also conceded to the continuation of pay beds and permitted teaching hospitals to keep their endowments for teaching and research purposes, which was another concession to the medical elite.[127] In a further significant concession, the prestigious voluntary teaching hospitals were allowed to preserve some of their independent administration, and each was granted its own board of governors, which directly reported to the Ministry, thereby avoiding subservience to the regional hospital boards.[128] These compromises undermined regional planning, perpetuated divisions in the health service and gave the medical elite professional advantage but helped Bevan stave off potential opposition.[129]

The nationalisation of health services, especially voluntary hospitals, in Northern Ireland, however, was far from straightforward. The historical literature on Northern Ireland has not considered how the seemingly irrevocable positions of medical voluntarism and state authority shaped the health services introduced in 1948. Historians have long noted that the election of the Labour government and its nationalisation programme was anathema to many within Ulster unionism. Debate within the Unionist Party took place on whether Northern Ireland should adopt Dominion status to avoid the socialist welfare state, which many believed was being foisted on an unsupportive and socially conservative Northern Ireland. It is broadly assumed, however, that these critical voices were faced down, and the social legislation in London was replicated in Northern Ireland.[130] William Grant, as Minister of Health and Local Government, is viewed by historians as being key to the successful introduction of the NHS in Northern Ireland.[131] He has been lauded for his political adroitness in avoiding the 'hyperbole and acrimony' in Britain between the medical profession and Bevan that dominated the introduction of the NHS.[132] Grant's favourable reputation is predicated mainly on his avoidance of the conflict regarding general practice that enveloped negotiations between Bevan and the BMA in Britain. Yet, such a positive perspective is weakened by the lack of analysis on the tensions surrounding proposals to nationalise hospitals. Conflict between Grant and voluntary hospitals threatened to derail the reforms in Northern Ireland, ultimately compelling the former to make significant concessions. These embedded many of the pre-existing inequities and inefficiencies that the reforms aimed to address.

A nationalised health service for Northern Ireland? – concessions and dilution of state influence

Hospitals were a far more challenging issue for William Grant than general practice. The prospect of nationalising hospitals under the direct authority of the Ministry greatly exceeded the role of central government envisaged in the multiple blueprints for a reformed health service in Northern Ireland. Instead of a small central government compliant to the interests of medical voluntarism, Bevan's NHS Bill placed the state at the core of the management of hospitals while eroding the independence of medical voluntarism. This threatened the consensus in much of Northern Irish healthcare that sought to protect voluntary hospitals. A further complication was that the state's takeover of voluntary hospitals was inextricably linked to the socialism of the Labour Party in Britain, which many within Ulster unionism implacably opposed.

To overcome conflict between central government and medical voluntarism, Grant devised a new central authority with responsibility for hospitals and policymaking. This body (eventually established as the Northern Ireland Hospitals Authority in 1948) had executive power and administrative responsibilities for the hospital services but was free from central government oversight. The

Minister of Health and Local Government appointed members of the Authority, but it was not an agent of the Ministry and free of ministerial supervision. Ownership of hospitals would also pass to the new body and not the Ministry. While funding the Hospitals Authority, the government would have little influence over the management, direction of policy or control over hospitals. The creation of this central authority was more in keeping with the consensus that had emerged in Northern Irish policymaking than Bevan's nationalisation plans. It was reflective of the proposals developed by the Nuffield Trust, Regional Hospitals Council, Select Committee on Health Services and Health Advisory Council, which all favoured some organisation under a single body, run not by government but existing medical power brokers and largely independent of the state and civil service. This new central authority was a major compromise to the key stakeholders in Northern Irish hospitals. The new structures proposed by Grant were far from trivial or merely the minutiae of administrative reform. They represented the state's potential abdication of power to the dominant stakeholders in Northern Irish hospitals. Remarkably, not only was the new authority loosely accountable to the government, but the government's own capacity for centralised hospital policymaking was limited.

Grant's central authority was not just a concession to medical voluntarism but also an attempt to assuage disquiet within Ulster unionism regarding the socialist tendencies of the London-orientated welfare state. Grant maintained that the scheme did not amount to the nationalisation of hospitals which many within unionism saw as socialism. He informed the cabinet that the Northern Irish Ministry would 'promote' a joined-up health service which, he claimed, differed from British legislation where Westminster's Ministry of Health would 'provide' such services.[133] Soon after the Health Services Bill's publication in 1947, he stated publicly that 'nationalisation and socialism' were not amenable to Northern Ireland. He claimed the Bill was superior to the English measure because it did not establish a state 'bureaucratic organisation'. He also claimed that he allowed the 'professions to hammer out the details' of the scheme.[134] The Northern Irish government reiterated its unionist and conservative values while promoting the legislation. The Northern Irish Prime Minister Basil Brooke distanced the measure from the 'London socialist government'. Brooke acknowledged that Stormont was subordinate to Westminster but maintained that Northern Ireland could modify legislation to make it 'more acceptable to the Ulster people'.[135] While recapitulating the terms of the Bill at a grassroots meeting of the Antrim Unionist Association, Brooke declared that he was 'not a socialist' but a unionist first, then a conservative and reasserted: 'in Ulster [they] were definitely not following the [hospital] nationalisation policy of the Labour government in Great Britain'.[136] The dilution of central government involvement in the new services was partly shaped by political pressure from within unionism. The creation of a central body, free of central state oversight, allowed the government to present the new services as different from the nationalisation evident in Britain, where regional hospital boards and teaching hospitals were directly under central government. This undoubtedly helped to make the new services more palatable to medical voluntarism and much of Ulster unionism. Still, it was also inimical to the power of central government, which, after all, was funding the services. The state now had financial responsibility for health services but curtailed power in their management or policy direction.

Grant's confidence that voluntary hospitals would welcome the Bill was misplaced. Despite his assurances that hospital management would maintain much independence from the state, the establishment of a central body with wide-ranging powers over finance, property and policy frightened many within medical voluntarism, who feared their power would be eroded. Medical voluntary criticism centred on four issues, including the power of the ministry, independence of individual hospital management, pay beds and endowments. While voluntary hospitals had long been a powerful force in Northern Irish medicine, they were further strengthened by the establishment of a regional branch of the BHA in 1942. This representative body had much experience of lobbying on behalf of voluntary hospitals in Britain, where it denounced Bevan's plans for hospital nationalisation as state confiscation.[137] At a BHA branch meeting in early October in Belfast, attended by the association's general secretary, J. P. Wetenhall, and numerous Unionist Party MPs and voluntary hospital representatives, the Bill was heavily criticised.[138] The Association later claimed the proposed legislation 'virtually [gave] the Ministry of Health dictatorial powers' over the Hospitals Authority.[139] In a submission to the government, the BHA demanded that the Hospitals Authority remain 'truly autonomous and not subject to constant direction by the Ministry', concluding with a passionate plea for the continuation of voluntarism:

> voluntary effort has still a large contribution to make in the hospitals of the future. Every effort should be made to encourage and foster that public spirit and disinterested lay and medical service which has so long maintained the notable and outstanding achievements of the voluntary hospitals.[140]

Medical and lay opposition was also widespread. In a private letter to Grant in late October, Allen (a leading medical figure, formerly the EHS Officer) was scathing about the proposed legislation. He complained that the more he 'look[ed] at it [Health Services Bill] the more convinced ... [he was] that the medical profession should never have been involved in any way in its construction'.[141] He heavily criticised the infringement of the proposed Hospitals Authority over individual institutions' autonomy and threats to their endowments. Another vocal supporter of medical voluntarism was Herbert Quin, chairman of the Royal Victoria Hospital, and Ulster Unionist Party MP for Queen's University. A barrister, Quin was representative of the lay, non-clinical leadership of medical voluntarism that was politically unionist and drawn from the professional and business classes. He informed a meeting to protest Grant's Bill that they 'did not want state control or direction in running the [Royal Victoria] hospital'.[142] He subsequently complained in Stormont that 'ministerial control ... [was] too dominating'.[143] Evidently, many were not convinced of Grant's claims that the new central authority was the panacea to state control and nationalisation. Conflict and tensions between Grant and medical voluntarism dominated the introduction of the health services.

Another source of tension was the introduction of a lower management tier, which threatened the independence of individual hospital administrations. As in Britain, hospital management committees were to be established with the responsibility of managing groups of hospitals in a defined geographical area to allow for greater harmonisation, avoidance of duplication and enhanced efficiency.[144] Sitting under the central authority, hospital management committees were key to the hierarchical model promoted by hospital planners, in which individual hospital authorities would come together, breaking down long-held institutional loyalties and fiefdoms. This highly idealised vision of inter-hospital harmony, unsurprisingly, proved unrealistic, and any hint of infringement on local power faced opposition. A. F. Wilson, an Ulster Unionist Party MP for the Belfast Windsor constituency in the Stormont parliament, feared that integration would lead to the exodus of those involved in existing hospital administrations.[145] The BHA also pressed the government on the matter. It approved 'in principle' the regionalisation originally proposed in *The Red Book* but sought to preserve each hospital's character, retain the local management of hospitals and guarantee that management committees would be composed of existing hospital authorities. It also wanted assurances that individual hospitals would have 'complete professional freedom … [and] be empowered to appoint and employ their own lay and nursing staffs'.[146] This foregrounded the tensions at the heart of medical reform. Any attempt to bring about a more planned, balanced and efficient system inevitably impinged on the independence of individual hospitals and their management. Such encroachment was invariably met with opposition from many hospitals.

Resistance to increased state involvement was based on multiple factors. Firstly, criticism was reflective of the interests of the management, both clinical and lay, of individual voluntary hospitals, which had come to form the bedrock of medical voluntary administration. Drawn from the unionist middle and upper classes, participation in voluntary hospitals was central to this group's civic and political role in society, conferring prestige, patronage and power locally and nationally. A more organised, centrally administered health service was a clear threat to these philanthropic and voluntary spheres. Secondly, opposition to the amalgamation of hospital management also represented a local and institutional loyalty which shaped popular attitudes to Northern Irish hospitals, fostered by the *ad hoc* and disaggregated development of healthcare since the nineteenth century. As outlined in earlier chapters, this localism became embedded in the interwar decades. The creation of an increasingly centralised and technocratic state posed a threat to these philanthropic, local and institutional interests.

Grant was forced to make further concessions and assurances about the diminished role of the state and institutional and local independence. He reiterated in Stormont that the Ministry would 'have nothing to do with the control of hospitals'.[147] He rejected claims that the new service was a state monolith and insisted: 'we are not seeking to provide for a soulless uniformity and rigid adherence to set rules in every matter'.[148] During the first Stormont debate on the Bill, Grant further committed to a continuation of existing management and maintained that hospitals would be administered 'very largely [by] the people who are running them now. I do not want to make a violent break with tradition'.[149] Grant regularly claimed that the pre-NHS voluntary ethos would be perpetuated in the new service. Praising the voluntary hospitals, he outlined that it was the government's 'sincere hope that the voluntary spirit and interest will be maintained and strengthened to make the new scheme the success we all desire'.[150] Further amendments were added to the legislation, including requiring appointments to the central authority and hospital management committees to be made only after consultation with representatives of voluntary hospitals.[151]

The creation of a central body independent of ministerial stewardship was a significant concession to medical voluntarism that was not afforded voluntary hospitals in Britain. The undermining of the central government's role ensured that the power of existing medical stakeholders was assimilated into the new structure. This diminished the government's capacity to influence and manage the health services, which were, paradoxically, to be publicly funded. Commitments to maintaining existing local and institutional hospital management weakened the new system's ability to align or tackle inefficiencies, which was a key driver of reform. This illustrated the strength of medical voluntarism and the limitations of central government in the health policymaking process in Northern Ireland.

The power of interest groups further eroded other aspects of the proposed health legislation. The government also ceded to the issue of paying beds on account of pressure from the medical profession and some within Ulster unionism. The consultant elite sought the continuation of private and pay beds in hospitals. Grant feared that coterminous private and public beds attenuated the universalism at the core of the new services and informed the cabinet that they undermined 'the principle of free treatment for all'. He worried that private patients would get preferential access to state-funded hospitals while public patients would be placed on waiting lists.[152] Grant conceded to allow private beds but sought restrictions that included fixing fees at a ceiling, ensuring the availability of pay beds tied to public waiting lists, and limiting the practice to existing hospitals and not permitting it in any new facilities.[153] Medical opposition emerged to Grant's proposed restrictions. The medical leader, Allen, chastised the threat to pay hospital beds as 'class legislation of the worst type'.[154] Political opposition was also evident. At a cabinet meeting, two government ministers, Samuel Hall-Thompson and Roland Nugent, sought the continuation of hospitals' private wings, such as Royal Victoria's Musgrave Nursing Home.[155] Backbench unionist MPs aired stringent criticism. Hugh Minford, the Ulster Unionist Party MP for Antrim, attacked the 'socialist tendencies' of the proposals, arguing that any restriction on pay beds would undermine entry to the profession.[156] In the face of such condemnation the proposed regulations were removed, and pay beds were permitted in existing and new hospitals.[157] Grant reserved much 'personal misgivings' about this concession.[158] This highlighted the weakness of central government in the design of the health services. The influence of the medical profession, aligned with strands of Ulster unionism, was key to shaping health policy in this instance.

Another major strength of voluntary hospitals threatened by the encroachment of the state was the use of endowments. Endowments were a lucrative source of voluntary hospital finance that local authority hospitals did not enjoy. They allowed voluntary hospitals much financial independence and capacity to invest in capital projects, new specialisms and research. They were also reflective of the socially hierarchical and paternal ethos of medical voluntarism. Significant restrictions existed on hospital use of endowments under the NHS in England and Wales, which in many cases were pooled or reallocated to support broader objectives; only teaching hospitals could keep their endowments and for teaching and research purposes only.[159] Grant, wary of voluntary hospital backlash, committed to not directly impacting hospital endowments but believed that it was 'obviously improper' for hospitals with such funds to get the same amount of state funding as other hospitals without endowments. The proposed legislation had a 'special arrangement' for adjusting the state grant in accordance with income from endowments, which a purposely established Hospital Endowments Commission would arbitrate.[160] This proposal promised to address financial inequities between voluntary and local authority hospitals and within more rural and peripheral regions in Northern Ireland, where medical voluntarism was weak.

The threat of reduced public funding for voluntary hospitals prompted a fierce backlash from the representatives of medical voluntarism and many within unionism. The *Belfast News-Letter* newspaper editorialised that this essentially amounted to government 'confiscation' of endowments.[161] The Unionist Party MP for the East Down constituency, Colonel Gordon, took 'extreme exception' to the encroachment on endowments.[162] Quin complained that hospital endowments were to be offset against the cost of funding hospitals at a meeting of the Royal Victoria's Ex-Patients Guild. He espoused the voluntary hospital ethos of independence and individualism by declaring: 'nothing was going to stand in the way of making the Royal Victoria the number one hospital in the United Kingdom'.[163] Similar to the government's forfeit on pay beds, it also conceded on endowments despite Grant's objections.[164] Although a significant difference from the NHS in Britain, endowments were effectively allowed to remain with hospitals free of any restrictions or impact on state funding (as outlined in Chapter 5, endowments were to be passed to hospital management committees which oversaw groups of institutions, but they could only be used for the benefit of hospitals for which they were originally intended).[165] This concession further strengthened the place of these hospitals, which could now enjoy the full benefits of state funding along with income from endowments. Such private income also ensured these hospitals had much financial independence from the Hospitals Authority. The protection of endowments further illustrated the strength of medical voluntarism during the negotiations for the new health service and the weakness of the central government.

Conclusion

The concessions to medical voluntarism ensured that the Health Services Act was passed, which came into force on the appointed day of 5 July 1948, along with two separate NHS acts for Scotland and England and Wales. Simultaneously, a universal, free-at-the-point-of-contact service was introduced across the United

Kingdom. The new health service brought a revolution in entitlement. Universalism removed the need to pay medical fees, contribution scheme subscriptions, or prove entitlement through poverty to medical relief or deservingness for charitable care. The management and organisation of health services were also radically altered. The establishment of the Hospitals Authority in Northern Ireland, unique in a UK context, was a major transformation of hospital management. A centralised health bureaucracy was, for the first time, responsible for the organisation and policy development of hospital services in Northern Ireland. The lower tier of hospital management committees had the potential to realise more efficient organisation of hospital services at a regional and local level, removing local authority boundaries and divisions between voluntary and rate-aided hospitals. All hospital services were to be funded by the state – the London government committed to funding 80 per cent of the excess cost of health and welfare services introduced – in an unprecedented commitment by central government to developing health services.[166] Following on from the experience of the Emergency Hospital Service, a more connected and centralised health service was realised in 1948.

Yet, the introduction of the health services was greatly shaped by the power of medical voluntarism. A coalition of voluntary hospitals, elite consultants and many with Ulster unionism sought meagre state control, pre-eminence of voluntary hospitals, and institutional independence from unifying organisational structures. A consensus had emerged in Northern Irish policymaking among planners, hospitals, medics, politicians and government officials to preserve the interests of medical voluntarism through regionalisation, evidenced in the blueprints proposed by multiple bodies, including the Nuffield Trust, Health Advisory Council and the Select Committee on Health Services. While nationalisation threatened this consensus by elevating the role of the state in the management of health services, the power of medical voluntarism, which feared the socialistic tendencies of the welfare state, somewhat succeeded in protecting the sector's interests. The creation of the Hospitals Authority, free of ministerial supervision, government commitments to the maintenance of individual hospital independence, voluntary hospitals' access to endowments and preservation of pay beds were all significant concessions that went further than what Bevan offered hospitals and medics in Britain. These concessions embedded many of the existing inequities, inefficiencies and power structures into the new system. Central government was left in the paradoxical position of having financial responsibility for healthcare services but no real power over policy, management or direction of services.

These findings contribute to the historiography of the introduction of the NHS in Northern Ireland. Most accounts have praised the role of William Grant in successfully introducing the welfare state in line with the rest of the United Kingdom. Still, this chapter's analysis indicates the importance of medical voluntarism in shaping the services. Similarly, the assumption that unionist opposition to nationalisation and welfare policies was largely ineffectual is also challenged.[167] Instead, middle- to upper-class unionists, long proponents of medical voluntarism, successfully protected key aspects of the sector's power in the new service while simultaneously attenuating the role of the state and central government. A combination of political and medical pressure diluted many of the founding principles of the NHS in Northern Ireland. This allowed unionist politicians to, somewhat justifiably, claim that the nationalisation of hospitals did not occur in Northern Ireland. In this sense, Northern Ireland's adoption of health services differed from Britain's, something which has not been appreciated by historians of Northern Ireland or the NHS overall. Finally, these findings also depict that the hospital services in Northern Ireland were based on conflict and tensions between central government and medical voluntarism. These findings challenge wider historiographical arguments that the NHS emerged out of a consensus between stakeholders and government based on logical, scientific-based organisation of health services. Instead, medical voluntarism forced significant concessions from Grant and the Northern Irish government, which in many ways subverted the new service.

Notes

1 P. Ollerenshaw, *Northern Ireland in the Second World War: Politics, Economic Mobilisation and Society, 1939–45* (Manchester: Manchester University Press, 2013), p. 215.

2 S. Wichert, *Northern Ireland since 1945* (Essex: Longman, 1991), p. 43.

3 Martin, 'Social policy and social change since 1914', p. 315; Privilege, 'The Northern Ireland government and the welfare state', 459.

4 Privilege and Jones, 'Crisis and scandal', 51; Jones, *Captain of All These Men of Death*, p. 192.

5 The failure to integrate the Mater into Northern Ireland's health services is comprehensively covered in the historiography, see Privilege, 'The Northern Ireland government and the welfare state', 453–7; Martin, 'Why have a Catholic Hospital at all?', pp. 101–15.

6 Key works in this historiography include Webster, 'Conflict and consensus'; Klein, *The New Politics of the NHS*; for a brief outline of this historiographical debate, see Gorsky, 'The British National Health Service 1948–2008', pp. 441–3.

7 C. Webster, *The Health Services Since the War. Vol. 1: Problems of Health Care: The NHS before 1957* (London: HMSO, 1988); *ibid.*, *National Health Service: A Political History*, pp. 6–7; R. M. Titmuss, *History of the Second World War: Problems of Social Policy* (London: HMSO, 1951), pp. 487–501; Stewart, 'Health care systems in Britain and Ireland', pp. 76–7.

8 C. L. Dunn (ed.), *The Emergency Medical Services, Volume 2: Scotland, Northern Ireland and Principal Air Raids on Industrial Centres in Great Britain* (London: HMSO, 1953); the EHS has been outlined for some localities, see Pickstone, *Medicine and Industrial Society*, pp. 296–9.

9 Ollerenshaw, *Northern Ireland in the Second World War*, pp. 29–30; for public health, see L. McCormick, 'Venereal diseases in Northern Ireland during the Second World War', in M. H. Preston and M. Ó hÓgartaigh (eds), *Gender, Medicine and the State in Ireland, 1700–1950* (New York: Syracuse University Press, 2012), pp. 221–35.

10 B. Harris, *The Origins of the British Welfare State: State and Social Welfare in England and Wales, 1800–1945* (Basingstoke: Palgrave Macmillan, 2004), p. 287.

11 V. Berridge, *Health and Society in Britain since 1939* (Cambridge: Cambridge University Press, 1999), p. 13.

12 Fox, 'The National Health Service and the Second World War', p. 42.

13 N. Hayes, 'Do we really want a National Health Service? Hospitals, patients and public opinions before 1948', *English Historical Review*, 127:526 (2012), 638.

14 Titmuss, *Problems of Social Policy*, p. 62.

15 *NIHoCD*, 22, 18 April 1939, p. 955.

16 PRONI, BG/23/P/3, Magherafelt Board of Guardians, Ministry of Home Affairs Memorandum on Emergency Hospital Service, 15 November 1939.

17 Titmuss, *Problems of Social Policy*, p. 76.
18 PRONI, CAB/9/CD/37/1/P/46–7, Cabinet Secretariat, Civil Defence, Hospital accommodation in event of wartime emergency, Cabinet Memorandum on Dr Allen, 13 June 1941.
19 PRONI, CAB/9/CD/37/1/P/90, Irwin to Holmes, Cabinet Secretary, 10 July 1939.
20 *NIHoCD*, 22, 4 September 1939, p. 1900.
21 'Emergency Hospital Service for Northern Ireland', *BMJ*, 2:4170 (23 September 1939), 189.
22 Titmuss, *Problems of Social Policy*, p. 75.
23 PRONI, BG/23/P/4, Magherafelt Board of Guardians, EHS Circular, 26 November 1940.
24 PRONI, BG/23/P/2, Magherafelt Board of Guardians, EHS Circular, 30 April 1941.
25 'Emergency Hospital Service for Northern Ireland', 190.
26 *Ibid.*
27 A. S. MacNalty (ed.), *The Civilian Health and Medical Services: Vol. II* (London: HMSO, 1955), pp. 371–2.
28 *BO*, 15 May 1942.
29 *Mid-Ulster Mail*, 31 January 1942.
30 *Mid-Ulster Mail*, 15 January 1944.
31 Ministry of Health and Local Government [hereafter MHLG], *Report on Health and Local Government Administration in Northern Ireland during the Period 1 April 1938 to 31 December 1946* (Belfast: HMSO, 1948), p. 25.
32 PRONI, BG/23/1, Magherafelt Board of Guardians, EHS Circular, 4 September 1939.
33 Dunn, *The Emergency Medical Services*, p. 136.
34 For the Blitz see S. Douds, *The Belfast Blitz: The People's Story* (Belfast: Blackstaff Press, 2011); B. Barton, *The Blitz: Belfast in the War Years* (Belfast: Blackstaff, 1989).
35 B. Barton, *The Belfast Blitz: The City in the War Years* (Belfast: The Ulster Historical Foundation), pp. 326–7.
36 Dunn, *The Emergency Medical Services*, p. 136.
37 Ollerenshaw, *Northern Ireland*, p. 160; Barton, *The Belfast Blitz*, p. 33.
38 Barton, *The Belfast Blitz*, p. 258.
39 *Ibid.*, p. 271.
40 *Ibid.*, p. 273.
41 RVH, *Annual Report: 149th for the Year 1942* (Belfast: RVH, 1943), p. 282.

42 PRONI, MIC514/1/1/24, RVH Management Committee minutes, 23 April 1941.
43 *BN*, 13 November 1941.
44 PRONI, MIC514/1/1/24, RVH Management Committee minutes, 3 September 1941.
45 PRONI, CAB/9/CD/37/1, Cabinet Secretariat, Civil Defence, Hospital accommodation in event of wartime emergency, Purdysburn Reserve Hospital, 25 July 1941.
46 *Ibid.*
47 *Irish Weekly and Ulster Examiner*, 7 June 1941.
48 For an outline of Spender's career see P. Maume, 'Spender, Sir Wilfrid Bliss', in *DIB*, www.dib.ie/biography/spender-sir-wilfrid-bliss-a8206 (accessed 24 November 2024).
49 PRONI, CAB/9/CD/37/1, Purdysburn Reserve Hospital, W. B. Spender to Prime Minister.
50 Edwards, *History of the Northern Ireland Labour Party*, pp. 22–4.
51 PRONI, CAB/9/CD/37/1, Purdysburn Reserve Hospital, 25 July 1941.
52 *NIHoCD*, 24, 12 November 1941, pp. 2233–4.
53 PRONI, MIC514/1/1/24, RVH Management Committee minutes, 17 December 1941.
54 PRONI, MIC514/1/1/24, RVH Management Committee minutes, 7 January 1942
55 PRONI, MIC514/1/1/24, RVH Management Committee minutes, 15 April 1942.
56 PRONI, MIC514/1/1/24, RVH Management Committee minutes, 7 October 1942.
57 *BN*, 14 June 1943.
58 PRONI, FIN/18/26, Hospitals: Musgrave Park, MHLG to MoF, 19 June 1947.
59 *NW*, 9 March 1945.
60 *NW*, 27 October 1944.
61 *BN*, 15 June 1943.
62 *BN*, 6 March 1946
63 *BN*, 5 March 1946
64 Kidd, 'A Ministry of Health for Northern Ireland', 229–40.
65 Ollerenshaw, *Northern Ireland in the Second World War*, pp. 202–5; Martin, 'Social policy and social change', p. 315.
66 J. Ditch, *Social Policy in Northern Ireland between 1939–50* (Aldershot: Avebury, 1988), p. 72.
67 Harris, *The Origins of the British Welfare State*, p. 295.

68 For an outline of the development of pre-1940s regional policies, see Mohan, *Planning*, pp. 45–55; Fox, *Health Policies, Health Politics*.
69 M. Lambert, 'A history of the intermediate tier in the English NHS: Centre, region, periphery', *Social Policy and Administration*, Early View (2024), 14.
70 Webster, *The National Health Service*, p. 6.
71 Gorsky, 'The British NHS', 441–3.
72 Webster, 'Conflict and consensus', 115–51.
73 G. McLachlan, *A History of the NPHT 1940–1990* (London: NPHT, 1992); Mohan, *Planning*, p. 78; Fox, *Health Policies, Health Politics*, p. 99.
74 M. Powell, 'Hospital provision before the NHS: A geographical study of the 1945 Hospital Survey', *Social History of Medicine*, 5:3 (1992), 412.
75 Hayes, 'Do we really want a National Health Service?', 628.
76 Powell, 'Hospital provision', 491; Webster, *The National Health Service*, p. 10.
77 J. Stewart, '"For a Healthy London" the Socialist Medical Association and the London County Council in the 1930s', *Medical History*, 41:4 (1997), 431.
78 PRONI, CAB/9/B/253, Cabinet Secretariat, Nuffield Provincial Hospitals Trust, 29 April 1940.
79 NIRHC, *The Red Book*; Lawrence, 'The health services', 299.
80 NIRHC, *The Red Book*, foreword.
81 Fox, *Health Policies, Health Politics*, p. 97; McLachlan, *A History of the NPHT*, p. 35.
82 F. P. Montgomery, '"The Future of the Hospitals": Presidential address delivered before the Northern Ireland Branch of the BMA', *UMJ*, 11:2 (1942), 123.
83 MacArthur was originally from County Down, educated at Queen's University, Belfast, and was an Irish language speaker, see 'Lieut.-General William P. MacArthur: Obituary', *BMJ*, 2:5405 (8 August 1964), 389.
84 'Regionalisation of Scottish Hospitals', *BMJ*, 2:4166 (9 November 1940), 653; 'Surveys of Hospital Services', *BMJ*, 2:4310 (14 August 1943), 209.
85 'Stanley Barnes: Obituary', *BMJ* 2:4938 (17 August 1955), 567; Reinarz, *Health Care in Birmingham*, p. 184; S. Barnes, *The Birmingham Hospitals Centre* (Birmingham: Stanford & Mann, 1952).
86 NPHT, *Survey of Hospital Services*, p. 5.
87 NPHT, *Survey of Hospital Services*, pp. 35–6.

88 NPHT, *Survey of Hospital Services*, pp. 45–6.
89 NPHT, *Survey of Hospital Services*, pp. 27–32.
90 A. T. Elder, 'The Health Services of Northern Ireland', *British Journal of Preventive and Social Medicine*, 7 (1953), 106.
91 NIRHC, *The Red Book*, foreword.
92 NPHT, *Survey of Hospital Services*, pp. 40–1.
93 NPHT, *Survey of Hospital Services*, p. 30.
94 NIRHC, *The Red Book*, p. 21.
95 Privilege, 'The Northern Ireland government and the welfare state', 440.
96 *BN*, 16 November 1944.
97 M. Rintala, *Creating the NHS: Aneurin Bevan and the Medical Lords* (London: Routledge, 2003), p. 7.
98 NIRHC, *The Red Book*, p. 13,
99 Ollerenshaw, *Northern Ireland in the Second World War*, p. 172.
100 Privilege, 'The Northern Ireland government and the welfare state', 443.
101 PRONI, CAB/9/B/253, Cabinet Secretariat, Nuffield Provincial Hospitals Trust, Note 8 June 1943.
102 Northern Ireland House of Commons Select Committee on Health Services, *Special Interim and Final Reports of the Select Committee on Health Services in Northern Ireland together with Proceedings of the Committee and Minutes of Evidence and Appendix* (Belfast: HMSO, 1944), p. 477.
103 Mohan, *Planning*, p. 84.
104 Gorsky *et al.*, *Mutualism and Health Care*, p. 157.
105 *Select Committee on Health Services*, pp. 552–6.
106 *Select Committee on Health Services*, pp. 497–9.
107 *Select Committee on Health Services*, p. 501
108 *Select Committee on Health Services*, p. 499.
109 *Select Committee on Health Services*; *NIHoCD*, 26, 20 July 1943, p. 1395.
110 Webster, 'Conflict and consensus', 133.
111 Privilege, 'The Northern Ireland government and the welfare state', 441.
112 Webster, 'Conflict and consensus', 117.
113 Privilege and Jones, 'Crisis and scandal', 51.
114 *Select Committee on Health Services*, pp. 181, 185.
115 Martin, 'Social policy and social change', p. 315; Grant was formerly chairman of the Belfast District Shipwrights' Association and a founding member of the Ulster Unionist Labour Association, see D. Ferriter, 'Grant, William', in *DIB*, www.dib.ie/biography/grant-william-a3575 (accessed 20 November 2024).

116 This included the 1946 Public Health and Local Government (Administrative Provisions) Act and Public Health (TB) Act (Northern Ireland) which established the Northern Ireland Tuberculosis Authority to provide tuberculosis provision.
117 Jones, *Captain of All These Men of Death*, pp. 217–18.
118 Privilege and Jones, 'Crisis and scandal', 50–1.
119 *Select Committee on Health Services*, p. 80.
120 Health Advisory Council, *First Annual Report of the Health Advisory Council* (Belfast: HMSO, 1946).
121 'BMA Annual Representative', *BMJ*, 2:S147 (16 December 1944), 149.
122 Health Advisory Council, *Health Advisory Council*, p. 11.
123 *Report on Health and Local Government Administration in Northern Ireland during the period 1 Apr 1938 to 31 Dec 1946* (Belfast: HMSO, 1948), pp. 36–7.
124 Rintala, *Creating the NHS*, p. 49.
125 Webster, *The National Health Service*, pp. 17–18.
126 Webster, *The National Health Service*, p. 26.
127 Mohan, *Planning*, p. 84.
128 Webster, *The National Health Service*, p. 36.
129 K. Waddington, *Medical Education at St. Bartholomew's Hospital, 1123–1995* (Woodbridge: Boydell & Brewer, 2003), p. 291.
130 Walker, *A History of The Ulster Unionist Party*, pp. 104–5.
131 Ferriter, 'Grant, William'.
132 Privilege, 'The Northern Ireland government and the welfare state', 459.
133 PRONI, CAB/4/723/5, Cabinet Secretariat, Cabinet Conclusions: Health Services Bill, Notes by the MHLG drawing attention to some points of importance or of difficulty, 10 July 1947.
134 *BN*, 4 September 1947.
135 *BN*, 21 October 1947.
136 *BN*, 14 November 1947.
137 Finlayson, *Citizen, State, and Social Welfare*, p. 270.
138 *BN*, 3 October 1947.
139 *BN*, 8 October 1947.
140 PRONI, CAB/9/C/65/1, Cabinet Secretariat, Ministry of Labour/Health and Social Services C Files, Health Services for Northern Ireland: recommendations of the BHA NI Branch, October 1947.
141 PRONI, CAB/9/C/65/1, Cabinet Secretariat, Ministry of Labour/Health and Social Services C Files, Health service in Northern Ireland: proposals, Dr F. M. B. Allen to Sir Robert Grandsen, Stormont Castle, 20 October 1947.

142 *BN*, 3 October 1947.
143 *BT*, 9 October 1947.
144 Mohan, *Planning*, p. 229.
145 *BT*, 9 October 1947.
146 PRONI, CAB/9/C/65/1, Cabinet Secretariat, Ministry of Labour/Health and Social Services C Files, Health Services for Northern Ireland: recommendations of the BHA NI Branch, October 1947.
147 *NIHoCD*, Health Services Bill, 31, 9 October 1947, p. 1765.
148 *BN*, 25 November 1947.
149 *NIHoCD*, Health Services Bill, 31, 24 September 1947, p. 1460.
150 *NIHoCD*, Health Services Bill, 31, 24 September 1947, p. 1464.
151 *BN*, 30 October 1947.
152 PRONI, CAB/4/720, Cabinet Secretariat, Conclusion Files, Memo to the Cabinet Submitted by the Minister of Health and Local Government, 10 June 1947.
153 *Ibid.*
154 PRONI, CAB/9/C/65/1, Health service in Northern Ireland: proposals, Dr F.M.B. Allen to Sir Robert Grandsen, Stormont Castle, 16 October 1947.
155 PRONI, CAB/4/723, Cabinet Secretariat/Cabinet Conclusions, Health Services Bill, 10 July 1947.
156 *BT*, 19 November 1947.
157 PRONI, CAB/9/C/65/1, Cabinet Secretariat/Cabinet Conclusions, Health Services Bill, Health Services Bill, L. G. P. Freer, MHLG to Sir Robert Gransden, Stormont Castle, 12 November 1947.
158 *BN*, 20 November 1947.
159 Rintala, *Creating the NHS*, p. 102.
160 PRONI, CAB/4/723/5, Cabinet Secretariat/Cabinet Conclusions, Health Services Bill, Notes by the Minister of Health and Local Government drawing attention to some points of importance or of difficulty, 10 July 1947.
161 *BN*, 8 October 1947.
162 *BT*, 9 October 1947.
163 *BN*, 13 October 1947.
164 PRONI, CAB/4/733, Cabinet Secretariat/Cabinet Conclusions, Health Services Bill, 30 October 1947.
165 PRONI, CAB/9/C/65/1, Cabinet Secretariat, Ministry of Labour/Health and Social Services C Files, Health Services Bill, L. G. P. Freer, MHLG to Sir Robert Gransden, Stormont Castle, 12 November 1947.
166 Ditch, *Social Policy in Northern Ireland between 1939–50*, p. 106.
167 Walker, *A History of The Ulster Unionist Party*, p. 107.

Section 3

5

Limitations of reform: division, fragmentation and resistance

Introduction

Northern Ireland enjoyed multiple benefits from the 1948 Health Services Act. A universal, free-at-the-point-of-contact health service was established that provided for the entire population, regardless of political, religious or social background. As will be explored later in this book, Northern Ireland's health services were marked by a substantial growth in doctors, primarily consultants and specialists, and an expansive hospital building programme. Modernisation was at the core of the Hospitals Authority's aspirations. It sought to provide a planned and integrated service based on scientific knowledge and planning during an era of organisational and managerial revolution, when governments increasingly believed progressive social reform would be achieved through the adoption and application of expertise. This new technocracy aspired to value-free decision-making and depoliticised public administration.[1] Yet the new structures were also marked by much continuity from the pre-1948 era in Northern Ireland. The lexicon of modernity belied the persistence of the power of traditional power brokers, including unionist, medical and local stakeholders and weakness of central government. Furthermore, religious and political divisions, which pervaded Northern Irish society, led to much acrimony and recalcitrance to processes of modernisation. The strength of these forces hamstrung the capacity of the central government or the Hospitals Authority to address the system's idiosyncrasies and inefficiencies inherited from the pre-1948 era. For much of the post-war period, hospital policy was shaped by conflict and tensions between a modernising centre and stakeholders looking to protect their position.

The creation of the NHS in 1948 failed to bring about a genuinely streamlined service anywhere in the UK. Fragmentation was baked in at the outset, which was evident in the siloing of primary and secondary care in the tripartite system of hospitals, general health services and local authority provision. A similar structure was introduced in Northern Ireland. The Northern Ireland General Health Services administered primary care including general practice, dentistry and pharmacies; the Hospitals Authority was responsible for hospital and specialist services; local authorities inherited environmental and public health from the pre-1948 framework – the Northern Ireland Tuberculosis Authority, in operation between 1944 and 1959 when the Hospitals Authority subsumed it, was another layer to the health services.

As outlined in the previous chapter, the Hospitals Authority was established as a statutory board, and it was not an agent of the Ministry of Health and Local Government. The high level of autonomy enjoyed by the Hospitals Authority contrasted with the NHS's regional hospital boards in Britain, which were under the control of central government. In England and Wales, teaching hospitals completely avoided the regional tier of organisation and were under the direct authority of the Ministry of Health. In Northern Ireland, the Ministry's role was restricted to appointing the members to the Hospitals Authority. It had minimal, if any, role in policy development or the delivery of services, which were the responsibility of the Hospitals Authority. Ownership of hospitals lay with the Hospitals Authority, while in England, the Ministry of Health held possession. The Hospitals Authority was also charged with medical and dental research, which in England was in the hands of the Ministry of Health.[2] In Britain, the relationship between the Minister of Health and the RHBs was often tense. The centre attempted to enforce stricter regulations, chiefly financial ones, on the periphery, while the latter frequently complained of too much bureaucratic oversight by the former.[3] In the Scottish NHS, regional hospital boards were subject to even greater central government power than in England and Wales.[4] In Northern Ireland, the Stormont parliament did have ultimate power by approving the Hospitals Authority's annual budget while also ensuring that there was no excessive or extravagant spending of public money, although central government was mostly kept at arm's length. In 1953, the Deputy Chief Medical

Officer of Northern Ireland, A.T. Elder, described how the overriding power of the Ministry of Health and Local Government was rarely used.[5] The newly established Ministry's lessened function in health was evident in the reduction of senior medical staff from seven in 1947 to three in 1949.[6] The Ministry also divested the only central state-run hospital, Musgrave Park, which had acted as the EHS Hospital described in the previous chapter, to the Hospitals Authority. In essence, the Hospitals Authority took full responsibility for hospital services while the role of central government in policy and management became even more diminished.

The Hospitals Authority membership and continuation of traditional elites

The traditional power brokers in Northern Ireland hospitals, including representatives from the medical profession, the former voluntary hospitals and Ulster unionism dominated the composition of the Hospitals Authority. In turn, nationalist and working-class interests were by and large sidelined. Membership of the Hospitals Authority carried much influence, as evidenced by the body's annual budget, which grew to twenty-seven million pounds by 1965, when it also employed a staff of eighteen thousand.[7] While the Minister appointed members independently, the 1948 Health Services Act protected the place of medical and hospital representatives. No less than one-third of members had to be medics, while at least three had to have experience in mental hospitals. At least a quarter of members had to be appointed after consultation with representatives of former voluntary and rate-aided hospitals. These were concessions granted during the negotiation of the Health Services Act and ensured that medical interest groups had a greater voice than on the RHBs in Britain.

Inevitably, the composition of the Hospitals Authority was populated by the interest groups that dominated pre-1948 health services. Ostensibly, Grant was sensitive about the perceived biases of the Authority's members. He stressed that their appointments were based on individuals' 'knowledge, ability and experience, who were to serve the people of Northern Ireland and not merely represent a section of the people'.[8] The medical stakeholders, however, were evident in the Ministry's nomination and selection of the Authority's membership. Medical interests were well represented on the thirty-two-person Authority. Two BHA nominees, Dr F. P. Montgomery and William McKinney, were appointed as chairman and vice-chairman, respectively. Montgomery was a consultant radiologist in the Royal Victoria since 1940 and was appointed to Queen's Medical School in 1938. He had a record in health reform and sat on the Health Advisory Council, chairing its hospitals committee.[9] Of the remaining thirty, seventeen were proposed by either the BHA or BMA. The BHA nominated leading medical and hospital representatives such as Dr W. B. Allen, Herbert Quin and the body's secretary, M. P. Sinclair.[10] These were key proponents of the medical profession and voluntary hospitals who agitated, often in a bellicose manner, for concessions from the government during the 1940s health debates and reforms. Allen and Ian McClure, another prominent BMA member, were selected, although some of the more combative nominees, such as Quin or Sinclair, were not appointed. Many of the key individuals who lobbied the government for their sectional interests during the negotiations surrounding the Health Services Bill now sat on the new Authority.

Socially and politically, the Hospitals Authority membership was made up of the middle and upper classes who have long been identified as the prime groupings in the leadership of Ulster unionism and the Northern Irish establishment.[11] As outlined in Chapter 3, this group was representative of the socially hierarchical, paternalist elite, which had dominated the leadership of medical voluntarism prior to 1948. For example, the Authority's vice-chairman, McKinney, was a Belfast businessman whose background was rooted in industry, medical voluntarism and civic activity. A director of his Dunmurry-based family business, Lilliput Laundry and Dye Works, McKinney was appointed in 1931 to the Royal Victoria's Board of Management, subsequently becoming the hospital's honorary secretary. His voluntary work was not confined to hospital administration; he also sat on the board of Belfast Saving's Society.[12] Other members had similar backgrounds. Marcia Mackie – one of six women appointed to the Authority, who would later become its chairman – was from one of the major industrialist families in Northern Ireland. An American, she married the chairman of James Mackie & Sons, the largest textile engineering company in Northern Ireland. Prior to joining the Hospitals Authority, she was the president of the Ladies Guild of the Royal Maternity.[13] She also had a unionist background and was once the president of the Greenisland branch of the Carrickfergus Unionist Association.[14] Julia Boyd, another upper-class female member of the Hospitals Authority, also had a background in unionist politics and public life. She was president of the Women's Unionist Council in Derry/Londonderry and sat on the executive committee of the Ulster Unionist Party while also running a textile manufacturing firm.[15] This social and political elite, which permeated the leadership of voluntary hospitals prior to 1948, persisted in the management of the NHS in Northern Ireland. The Hospitals Authority may have represented a new organisational structure but was, in many ways, a continuation of the power of stakeholders that dominated Northern Irish hospitals prior to 1948.

The Hospitals Authority adopted the rhetoric of modernisation, but it often embodied the ethos and spirit of medical voluntarism, if not the organisation or financing. In a continuation of traditions of voluntary administration, membership of the Authority was honorary. This was evident when Allen wrote to Grant to accept the invitation to sit on the body. He was concerned that the work would be 'onerous', above all considering his 'good many commitments', but he accepted on account of it being 'well worth doing'.[16] In Britain, the once proud tradition of voluntarism was viewed as increasingly amateurish in the post-war years and anathema to new modes of hospital management in the NHS.[17] However, traditions of voluntarism continued in Northern Ireland, mainly facilitated by nominated, non-elected boards and honorary bodies such as the Authority. Strands of voluntarism remained key to the administration of the new health services in a continuation of older trends.

In contrast to the strength of the interests of the former medical voluntary sector, working-class and labour interests were not facilitated. During the Northern Irish cabinet's consideration of the 1948 Health Services Bill, government ministers debated whether to remunerate members of the bodies and committees that would manage the new service. Brian Maginess, the Minister of Labour and National Insurance, insisted there was a 'public interest' in the involvement of workers' representatives in health management and that 'no obstacles' should be placed in the way of their participation. The cabinet, however, decided against paying committee members which inevitably undermined the capacity of many workers to devote their time to participate in the running of the new service.[18] Similarly, officials in the Ministry had little regard for working-class representatives and warned Grant that workers' contribution schemes would be 'importunate' in seeking appointments to the Authority.[19] Although these schemes played a key role in the funding of voluntary hospitals, as outlined in Chapter 3, Grant did not seek nominations from such bodies.

Similarly, trade unions were poorly represented on the Authority. The Irish Trade Union Congress wrote to the Ministry complaining of the lack of workers' representatives on the Authority, highlighting the role contribution schemes played prior to 1948, stating that 'the subscriptions from workers ... in the past have [been] of inestimable value to the hospitals in Northern Ireland'. It also maintained that the majority of patients treated in hospitals were wage earners and should be represented on the Authority.[20] The Northern Irish government did not recognise the Dublin-based Irish Trade Unions Congress until 1964, but other unions were also not represented.[21] The National Union of General and Municipal Workers complained to the Ministry about its lack of representation, despite the fact that the union supported the 'large majority of employees in hospitals engaged in general and domestic work'.[22] The lack of elected and local authority representatives further diminished the potential of working-class involvement or greater democratic influence. Only four members were nominated by the Rate Aided Hospitals Association. At the same time, a mere three Stormont MPs and two county councillors were selected, indicating the lack of elected voices on the Authority.[23] On the whole, the Authority was socially conservative and hierarchical, drawn predominantly from leading medical professionals and the paternalistic social elite of the former voluntary hospital administrations and unionist establishment.

There was also a lack of nationalists and Catholics appointed to the Hospitals Authority. Cahir Healy, MP for Stormont's Fermanagh South constituency, was one of the few nationalists and Catholics appointed. In 1955, Healy complained that only four of the thirty-two-person Authority were Catholics.[24] Many geographical areas with large nationalist populations were also underrepresented. The

Newry Chamber of Commerce complained to Grant that the town had no representative, although, it argued, there were many from the area with the necessary experience and skills.[25] Located close to the border with the south, Newry was a predominantly politically nationalist and Catholic town and often excluded from the wider public life of Northern Ireland. The lack of Catholic representation on the Authority continued throughout the 1950s and 1960s. Like most Northern Irish government bodies, nationalists were largely underrepresented. The management of the health services, especially the Authority, remained in the hands of the political, social and medical elite with little input or involvement from much of Northern Irish society such as representatives of the working classes or the nationalist and Catholic population.

Hospital Management Committees – unionist power and nationalist isolation

The Hospitals Authority was the upper tier of hospital management and was appointed by the Minister, making political appointments partly unsurprising. The lower tier of administration – hospital management committees – were charged with amalgamating the management of multiple hospitals to bring about greater coordination and efficiency, a key objective of the new service. The Authority appointed hospital management committees after consultation with various stakeholders in a process in which former voluntary hospital representatives had significant influence. As the lower tier of hospital management, HMCs were powerful bodies with responsibility for many workers, both lay and clinical, and substantial budgets and expenditure. Such resources brought much local power and patronage to those in control.

Inevitably, hospital management committees were drawn from the same narrow social and political background as the Hospitals Authority, mainly a unionist and Protestant middle to upper class. At a conference on Northern Ireland's health services in 1957, the director of the Nuffield Foundation, Farren-Brown, believed that hospital management committee members were drawn from 'business or the professions', and there was a lack of working-class representation to articulate the 'interests, needs and wishes' of patients from that social background.[26] In some areas of Northern Ireland, hospital management committees were vestiges of the old patrician ruling class, such as the Tyrone and Fermanagh HMC, which the Duchess of Abercorn chaired.[27] In 1953, the Omagh Rural Council complained that management committees were populated by 'people from the "Big Houses" ... who were never heard of before outside their own estates'.[28] Similar to the Hospitals Authority, lay membership of HMCs was drawn mainly from the socially conservative, middle- to upper-class unionist polity that was previously the enduring backbone of medical voluntarism.

The membership of hospital management committees often intersected with unionist politics and Protestant organisations such as the Orange Order. For much of the first half of the twentieth century, the Order's leadership was disproportionately drawn from the elite middle and upper classes of Ulster-Protestant society. However, much of its rank-and-file membership came from the rural and urban working classes.[29] The nexus between elite unionism, Protestantism and hospital management was widely evident. For example, Thomas Bailie a one-time independent unionist MP who became an Ulster Unionist Party MP for North Down, was chairman of the North Down Hospital Management Committee, member of the Orange Order and prominent businessman in Bangor, County Down.[30] Similarly, the North-West Hospital Management Committee was chaired by J. H. Welch; he was also a prominent local unionist and business owner, acting as treasurer of the Londonderry and Foyle Unionist Association while also one of the owners of the Welch, Margetson & Co shirt manufacturers.[31] The chairman of the Mid-Ulster Hospital Management Committee, S. G. Davison, was another example of the overlap between Protestantism, unionist politics and hospital management. A lifelong unionist, he also sat on the executive committee of the South Derry Unionist Association and was a member of the Orange Order.[32] Hospital management committees were an important source of local power and influence for the unionist local elite and an extension of their control over public administration.

Conversely, hospital management committees, like the Hospitals Authority, had few Catholic members. An analysis of 478 members of HMCs in 1960 undertaken by the Catholic chaplain of Queen's University, Fr Michael Kelly, revealed that only 58, or 12 per cent, were Catholics. However, almost 35 per cent of Northern Ireland's population were that religion.[33] As late as 1972, only 72 out of 436 members of HMCs were Catholic.[34] Kelly rejected the often-aired government's defence that appointments were based on merit alone, which inferred that there were not enough suitably qualified Catholics, and wrote:

> let no one tell me that it is impossible to get Catholics to serve on management committees and do good work ... Having been in intimate contact with twenty years of Catholic graduates from Queen's University I can assure those responsible that, in any area, and from the ranks of those graduates alone I could fill their committees ... this present position, I suggest, is simply a boycott of Catholics ... [and] extends across all Northern Ireland and every hospital type.[35]

Nationalists were particularly aggrieved at their lack of representation on hospital management committees in areas with majority Catholic populations, including counties Fermanagh and Tyrone, and the region of south Down. In the Northern Ireland Senate, a nationalist named P. J. O'Hare complained that only four of the eighteen members of the Fermanagh HMC were nationalists. However, the county had thirty-two thousand Catholics compared to twenty-four thousand Protestants. He contended that the members were appointed purely on political grounds, demanding that nationalists in Fermanagh be shown 'justice and fair play' in relation to hospital management.[36]

Nationalists easily politicised the lack of Catholic representation. Constitutional nationalist politics in Northern Ireland during this era is largely viewed as having failed to move beyond constitutional grievances and being marked by disorganisation, division and periods of abstentionism from the Westminster and Stormont parliaments, often to the detriment of their political movement.[37] Despite this, nationalists and Catholics in some regions were better organised and challenged unionism, often impacting hospital management. This was evident in the southern part of County Down where nationalists controlled local government, including the Newry Board of Guardians, which prior to its dissolution in 1948 managed the former workhouse, Daisy Hill Hospital. Nationalists also governed multiple other local authority bodies in the region including the urban and rural district councils in Newry and Kilkeel. Nationalist-run local authorities, like their unionist counterparts, often distributed local authority housing and employment on a political and sectarian basis, although on a whole the weight of discrimination fell far more on Catholics than Protestants throughout Northern Ireland.[38] The region was also the focus of much nationalist political organisation and opposition to the Northern Irish state, views which found expression in the Newry-based newspaper, the *Frontier Sentinel*. This newspaper was part of a syndicated network of Catholic-nationalist newspapers in south and west Ulster, which also included the *Fermanagh Herald* and Omagh-based *Ulster Herald*.[39] The Anti-Partition League, a relatively ephemeral rank-and-file northern nationalist organisation, held 'monster meetings' in Newry during the late 1940s to protest partition. After the League's dissolution in the 1950s, another nationalist body, the Irish Citizen Association, was active in the region, led by the Nationalist MP for the Stormont South Down constituency, Joseph Connellan.[40] He was a long-standing politician who strongly advocated nationalist participation on public boards and worked hard in Stormont to ensure his constituency received its fair share of public expenditure.[41] The nationalist body politic in the south Down area was well organised with a strong local leadership which sought to challenge unionist power. Inevitably, hospital politics became engulfed in nationalist–unionist and sectarian tensions.

Local nationalists challenged the unionist-managed South Down Hospital Management Committee, which was responsible for the Daisy Hill, Newry General and Mourne District hospitals. Although the area had a large majority Catholic population, only five of the fifteen members of the South Down Hospital Management Committee were of that religion. Some prominent local nationalist figures, including Charles Magee, the former chairman of the Newry Board of Guardians and a leading member of the management of the Daisy Hill Hospital, were appointed to the South Down HMC. However, the committee was stacked with many unionists, such as S. M. Baird, a Newry estate agent who was also a prominent member of the South Down Unionist Association and Orange Order.[42] Tensions emerged over the religious composition of the committee. The *Frontier Sentinel* claimed that the Hospitals Authority intentionally sought to 'flout the religious convictions' of the majority of the area's population and intensify 'religious bitterness'.[43] During a 1955 Stormont debate, the Nationalist MP Cahir Healy complained about the lack of Catholics on the committee and questioned: 'did the Minister really desire the co-operation of Roman Catholic people in th[is] area?'[44] Similarly, Joseph Connellan, during a meeting of the Irish Citizen Association in Newry in 1956, hit out at 'handpicked' management committees.[45] The lack of Catholic representation on the South Down HMC became highly politicised and used by nationalists as a focal point for concerns about the sectarian and discriminatory nature of the Northern Irish state. Hospital politics became part of the wider nationalist campaign to discredit the unionist government and seek the end of Irish partition.

Political and sectarian conflict marked much hospital management in south Down as unionists wrested command over hospital administration from nationalists. The creation of the South Down Hospital Management Committee in 1948 by the Hospitals Authority represented the weakening of nationalist power in hospital management in the region. Individual hospital management committees were established initially, which ensured the continued power of Catholics in some hospitals such as Daisy Hill. However, these were abolished in 1957, meaning that the unionist-managed South Down HMC had even more authority over individual hospitals.[46] Employment practices became highly contested on the hospital management committee and nationalist and Catholic representatives claimed that politics and sectarianism dominated its hiring practices. Joseph Annett, a nationalist representative from the Mourne District Hospital, resigned from the South Down HMC in protest over alleged sectarian discrimination against Catholics in the hospital's hiring and appointment practices.[47] Nationalist frustration about their lack of influence over decision-making came to a head on the South Down HMC in 1954 when the nationalist members resigned *en masse* from the body. Charles Magee complained that all matters of 'hospital efficiency' and appointments were decided on a 'purely party vote'. Allegations of sectarianism were met with counter-accusations from unionists. Baird blatantly defended politically and sectarian motivated appointments on the basis that unionists only replicated what 'nationalists did when they had the majority'.[48] Nationalist criticism of the committee's employment practices persisted. In 1958, Connellan chastised the appointment of a Protestant pharmacist from Derry/Londonderry to the Daisy Hill Hospital over a suitably qualified Catholic candidate as an 'exhibition of bigotry'.[49] Hospital management became embroiled in tensions between nationalist and unionist members over the making of appointments.

Political and religious divisions discredited the management of hospital services in the south Down area. Unionists utilised the new management structures to bring about their greater power over hospitals and the patronage which this brought. Motivated by a combination of a loss of their power and patronage, genuine fears over the discriminatory nature of the Northern Irish state and political objectives to weaken Irish partition, nationalists boycotted and heavily criticised the management of hospital services.

Allegations of discrimination against Catholics in the hospital services persisted throughout the 1960s and 1970s and came to the fore during the Civil Rights movement and Troubles. The Hospitals Authority and government defended employment practices in the hospital services on the grounds that appointments were based on merit and not religious adherence. Such defences were far from compelling. During the early years of the Civil Rights campaign for greater equality for Catholics in Northern Ireland, the nationalist leader Eddie McAteer criticised the lack of employment of Catholics in Altnagelvin Hospital in Derry/Londonderry, where he claimed only seven out of eighty-seven non-medical staff in the hospital were Catholic.[50] The Minister of Health and Social Services, William Morgan, did undertake a confidential internal review which substantiated McAteer's claims – Catholics were only employed in lower grades such as general porters and ambulance drivers, and in those categories they were greatly outnumbered by Protestants (twenty-two of twenty-seven general porters were Protestant and twenty-one of twenty-three employees in the ambulance department were Protestant).[51] Despite the lack of Catholics employed in the hospital in a city with a majority Catholic population, Morgan fell back on the official line that appointments were made on merit alone.[52] The denial of religious bias in hiring in the face of such stark statistics lacked credibility in the minds of nationalists, Catholics and the era's Civil Rights activists. A 1988 report by the Fair Employment Agency into the religious composition of those employed by the then Western Health and Social

Area Board – an area that consisted of places with a large Catholic population including Derry/Londonderry, Strabane and Enniskillen – showed that out of 771 non-medical staff hired between 1940 and 1970, 54.3 per cent were Protestant and 39 per cent were Catholic. However, the former accounted for 58 per cent of the population.[53] This cohort did not include medics, whose better education and higher social class status ensured many doctors were Protestants. Still, it was made up of all administrative, clerical and other employees, indicating that fewer Catholics than Protestants were hired in lower grades. Catholics suffered regardless of whether positions were clinical, professional, skilled or unskilled. This discrimination mirrored similar practices of Unionist-controlled local government bodies, which used their power to make appointments in a way which benefited Protestants.[54]

The sense that the state hospital service was largely unionist and Protestant-controlled was even more pronounced in the upper echelons of hospital medicine and the medical profession. Catholics had long grievances with representation and employment in hospitals in Northern Ireland. In 1941, one writer to the Dominion Office in Whitehall complained that while 'our Catholic people always have excelled in the medical profession', they were underrepresented in the health services, including Belfast City Hospital where, it was claimed, there was not a single Catholic permanent member of staff.[55] The introduction of the Hospitals Authority did little to alleviate the lack of Catholics in senior medical posts despite the significant growth in personnel in the service and frequent nationalist criticisms. In 1960, Fr. Kelly of Queen's complained that out of seventy matrons employed by the Authority, only six were Catholic, while only a mere thirty-five out of 573 consultants were that religion.[56] The management of Northern Ireland's leading hospital, Royal Victoria, especially stood out for the lack of Catholics.[57] Fr Kelly highlighted that only four of its 135 consultants were Catholics, while its management committee was completely free of Catholics in 1960.[58] Although the educational gap between Catholics and Protestants can partly explain the preponderance of the latter in senior medical posts, the overall impression of a Protestant-managed hospital system is hard to avoid. The growth of the welfare state, generally, and post-war hospital services, particularly, brought not just benefits through greater entitlements but also growth in employment. Yet, these employment opportunities primarily benefited Protestants, ensuring that the health service exacerbated religious and political inequality in Northern Ireland.

Religious tensions at times came to the fore in the running of hospitals, particularly at a local level. The formal opening of Altnagelvin Hospital, for example, in Derry/Londonderry was boycotted by Catholics after the North-Western Hospital Management Committee insisted a Protestant prayer mark the event. The Catholic Bishop of Derry, Dr Neil Farren, who also sat on the HMC, criticised the committee for reversing a prior decision not to have any prayers that were 'against Catholic conscience'.[59] In turn, Bishop Farren informed the committee that no Catholic, besides doctors and nurses whose duties necessitated their attendance, was 'free in conscience to attend' the hospital's official opening; importantly, no longer-term boycott was extended to working or receiving care in the hospital. The opening was very much reflective of the 'Big House' unionist and Protestant nature of the Northern Ireland establishment. It was presided over by the Governor of Northern Ireland, Lord Wakehurst, and prayers were said by a Church of Ireland clergyman.[60] The controversy, however, was looked upon unfavourably by the Hospitals Authority, which had instructed the chairman of the HMC to have 'discussions locally in the hope [of] avoiding difficulties' in the lead-up to the opening.[61] The Authority often attempted to avoid religious controversies, but tensions spilled over locally. Similar tensions between Catholic religious practices and hospital management came to the fore in the region of south County Down after the Protestant-controlled hospital management committee, much to the ire of local Catholics, prohibited any religious services on the wards of hospitals, after a Catholic priest gave communion to long-stay patients in the Daisy Hill Hospital in Newry.[62] The largely Protestant management, at times, aggravated Catholic religious practices, which led to further tensions and a general sense among the nationalist and Catholic population that their beliefs were not fairly considered.

The intractability of religious divisions in Northern Irish hospital services was most controversially demonstrated in the status of the Mater Infirmorum Hospital. The hospital bitterly remained outside the health services and continued as a voluntary institution, financially reliant on a combination of patient fees, philanthropic fundraising and lotteries through pools. The Mater refused to come under the Health Services Act due to a commitment to Catholic social teaching, which opposed socialistic healthcare, along with a mistrust of the largely Protestant Northern Irish state. In contrast to Britain, where disclaimed hospitals could receive capitation payment from the NHS, Northern Irish hospitals that remained outside the Hospitals Authority could not receive any funding. As the Mater struggled financially to keep up to date with increasingly costly medical advances, the stalemate became more embittered and the focus of religious and political tensions throughout the 1950s and 1960s, which historians have widely described.[63] The result was the further fragmentation of Northern Ireland's hospital services. In 1948, the Mater was important not just to the delivery of hospital services but was also one of only two general voluntary hospitals that acted as a teaching hospital for the medical school. The Hospitals Authority was weaker without the Mater, and its isolation further hindered the divided hospital service.

In post-war Britain, there was a growing political consensus around the benefits and fundamental ethos of the welfare state and the NHS.[64] In Northern Ireland, however, the new service further embedded religious and political divisions. The continued dominance of a middle-to-upper-unionist ruling class in hospital management isolated many within Northern Irish society from participating in the running of the hospital services. Although universalism and the rapid expansion of services after 1948 brought many benefits to all of the population, the management and employment in hospitals mostly favoured unionists and Protestants and excluded many nationalists, Catholics and the labour movement. The social bonds fostered by the welfare state and the NHS in post-war Britain, where many felt a special connection with the NHS, were only partly realised in Northern Ireland.[65] Instead, the political and sectarian fissures of unionism and nationalism pervaded, ensuring a more politically divided system than in Britain. Hospital management copper-fastened unionist authority over public services, resources and employment, which furthered resentment among many nationalists and Catholics to the Northern Irish state. In these circumstances, it was unlikely that the health services could foster the social collegiality and political consensus that coalesced around the NHS in post-war Britain. These political and religious tensions also damaged the Hospitals Authority's aspirations to develop a technocratic administration based on apolitical decision-making and scientific management.

Hospital management committees and the lack of integration

Other problems came to the fore, which impaired the founding principle of the NHS to create an integrated, coordinated and planned health service. HMCs were to administratively group individual hospitals in a defined geographical area to provide structured management and day-to-day running of hospital services. Agents of the Hospitals Authority, HMCs were key to the achievement of efficiencies and lowering costs.[66] It was hoped that old demarcations between voluntary and local authority institutions, whose traditions and management differed greatly, would dissolve and the *ad hoc* disparate pre-1948 local hospital services would become integrated. Such aspirations needed the dismantling of powerful forces – primarily medical voluntarism, institutional loyalty and localism – which fuelled the disaggregated hospital system of the interwar years. Yet these influences proved difficult to overcome, and hospital fragmentation persisted after 1948.

Grouping hospitals under a single management committee was a significant challenge. Medical planners in the 1940s, as outlined in the previous chapter, had much faith in the capacity of local hospitals to come together for the greater good. The reality, however, involved defenestrating long-standing boards of governors and creating hospital groupings which cut across former boundaries, both voluntary and local government, and merging the management of hospitals whose relations were traditionally marked by rivalry rather than co-operation. The Hospitals Authority's efforts were made more difficult by the 1948 Health Services Act, which provided individual institutions with much independence. Unsurprisingly, the Authority's attempts to group hospitals led to much opposition. In September 1948, the BHA's chairman, Scott, complained to the Authority that the proposed scheme was 'not just' and went a 'long way to alienate the goodwill of the voluntary hospitals'. The BHA was concerned that individual hospital endowments would be transferred to HMCs, criticised the Authority's lack of consultation, and proposed an alternative scheme, which effectively maintained the status quo with each existing hospital committee becoming a stand-alone hospital management committee. The Authority's chair, Montgomery, attempted to assuage the BHA's concerns, insisting that endowments given to any hospital could only be used by that hospital. He was adamant, however, that the BHA's alternative scheme was 'impossible' to implement.[67] Some members of the Authority were equally as incredulous at the groupings, such as John Wilfred Haughton, member of the BHA, who criticised the process as failing to adequately consult former voluntary hospitals. He complained to the Ministry of Finance that the Authority's actions were 'dictatorial' and failed to adopt a 'democratic' approach such as allowing former voluntary hospitals to decide on groupings and appoint members to HMCs.[68] While these protests failed, they illustrated that representatives of the former voluntary hospitals opposed change from the very beginning of the new service.

Resistance from individual hospitals was also apparent. The merging of hospital administrations from Bangor and Ards under the North Down Hospital Management Committee provoked a resentful response from Bangor District Hospital. Montgomery attempted to allay the hospital's concerns, writing that individual hospitals could preserve their 'character' while acknowledging that the hospital services were developed by the 'energetic and disinterested efforts of public-spirited people', such as those involved in the Bangor Hospital.[69] Montgomery's assurances fell on deaf ears, and the hospital's former chairman, Scott, brought a legal injunction to prevent the merger. During the subsequent legal proceedings, a medic, Dr John Blakeley, complained that the Bangor and Ards hospitals 'were poles apart', emphasising social differences and maintaining that the former was a cottage hospital with a predominantly paying patient cohort. At the same time, the latter was a district hospital, largely for the working classes.[70] The Authority's plan was ultimately upheld, but the case revealed local medical recalcitrance, often based on social biases, to the consolidation of individual hospital administrations.[71]

The lobbying by hospitals and pressure groups created a far more divided system than that envisaged by the planners of the 1940s. The Hospitals Authority established thirty committees to administer a mere sixty-seven hospitals. This far exceeded the single Belfast and nine provincial authorities initially recommended by the Nuffield surveyors. The large number of HMCs undermined the principles of harmonisation, which were central tenets of health reform. Under Bevan's scheme, each 'natural hospital district' was defined as an area that would support a general hospital or combined group of hospitals, employ a comprehensive specialist staff and contain up to one thousand beds. Much fragmentation, however, persisted locally in England and Wales, and many HMCs did not reach this bed threshold, while teaching hospitals, directly under the Ministry, were outside of the regional administrative unit.[72] In Northern Ireland, even greater fissures in local hospital management were evident. The Hospitals Authority's thirty hospital management committees significantly exceeded those in similarly populated regional hospital boards in England and Scotland (see Table 5.1). A mere eleven HMCs grouped three or more hospitals; nine had only two hospitals, and eleven were single hospital entities (these were primarily mental hospitals which had their own separate HMC).

The inability of the Hospitals Authority to bring about a joined-up approach was evident across Northern Ireland. Hospital groupings in Belfast were often reflective of pre-NHS organisational structures and bore little relation to geographical considerations.[73] The

Table 5.1 Comparison of HMCs in Northern Ireland with one Scottish and two English Regional Hospital Board regions, 31 December 1953.

	Northern Ireland	*South-East Scotland*	*East Anglia*	*Oxford*
Population	1,370,932	1,136,000	1,463,000	1,458,000
Hospitals	67(a)	85	108(b)	105(b)
Beds	14,307(a)	12,677	14,584(b)	14,120
HMCs	30	16	14	16

Source: D. G. Neill, 'Some problems of integration in the hospital service of Northern Ireland (Read before the Society in Belfast on 20 April 1956)', *Journal of the Statistical and Social Inquiry Society of Ireland*, 19 (1955/56), 172.

(a) Excluding eight Tuberculosis Hospitals, which had a combined 1,000 beds, and three special care institutions with a combined 302 beds.

(b) Excluding teaching hospitals.

Belfast Hospital Management Committee (BHMC) had a combined 1,149 beds and was primarily made up of the Royal Victoria, Royal Maternity Hospital and Royal Belfast Hospital for Sick Children, centred around the Grosvenor Road site. Since the 1930s, similar traditions have marked these hospitals, which included overlapping management structures and deep links with academic medicine, as outlined in Chapter 3. No former local authority hospital was added to this group in 1948, despite Belfast City Hospital's proximity to Grosvenor Road. Belfast City Hospital was grouped with Musgrave Park Hospital and Malone Place, a small former voluntary hospital, in the South Belfast Hospital Management Committee. The failure to merge the management of the Grosvenor Road hospitals and Belfast City Hospital undermined the city's health services for much of the twentieth century. Outside Belfast, the proliferation of hospital management committees was even more prominent. Twenty-three hospital management committees existed across provincial Northern Ireland. Four committees existed in County Antrim alone, while multiple provincial committees had a single hospital, including Tyrone and Fermanagh, Mid-Ulster and South Tyrone.[74] The high number of hospital management committees illustrated the difficulties in overcoming institutional and local loyalties which shaped hospital politics and management in Northern Ireland.

In a further blow to integration, institutions were permitted to maintain individual hospital committees responsible for their day-to-day activity, including the power to appoint staff, prepare estimates and incur costs. In a joined-up service, many of these activities would have been carried out by collaborative management, which, it was believed, would create efficiencies and savings. By 1954, twenty-four individual committees in eight HMCs existed, which further diluted the coordination of hospitals.[75] Individual committees embedded institutional power and were a bulwark to the harmonisation of services. Belfast's leading former voluntary hospitals, including the Royal Victoria, Royal Maternity and Royal Hospital for Sick Children, all maintained individual committees, indicating their power and commitment to traditions of independence reminiscent of their voluntary past. Outside Belfast, most hospitals with individual management committees were former voluntary cottage hospitals and local authority district hospitals, predominantly located in counties Antrim, Armagh and Down.

As set out in the first section of this book, during the interwar years these predominantly unionist local authorities and voluntary hospitals, often motivated by localism, institutional pride and traditions of independence, developed increasingly modernised and popular hospitals but lacked organisation between areas and sectors. The continuation of these hospitals' management structures allowed them much power and independence.[76] No individual hospital management committee persisted in counties Tyrone, Derry/Londonderry or Fermanagh, where earlier hospital reform was limited. Unlike in eastern areas, where the district hospital movement predominated, localism and institutional loyalty were less evident, and the loss of individual hospital independence after 1948 proved less intractable. In this sense, many of the interwar patterns of hospital development became ingrained in the new system. The ideal of creating an aligned administration was only partially achieved, and fragmentation persisted, albeit to a lesser extent than prior to 1948.

Former voluntary hospital disenchantment, local opposition and increased politicisation of hospital policies

The new structures may have been shaped by concessions from government to assuage the fears of hospitals of increased centralisation, but many institutions, such as the Royal Victoria, splenetically resented the groupings. Despite the major concessions ceded in the 1948 Health Services Act by the government, the former voluntary hospitals remained highly critical. They viewed the Hospitals Authority and hospital management committees as curtailing their independence and agility while also undermining the 'spirit' of voluntarism. This was evident in 1950 when the Hospitals Authority sought the views of hospital management committees to gauge the success of the new scheme.[77] In reply, the Royal Victoria disabused the framework, believing that hospital management committees were overly cumbersome, delayed decision-making and 'killed' individual hospitals' sense of responsibility. The hospital decried the new structures for 'impair[ing]' medical voluntarism, claiming that it was increasingly challenging to replace many who had served the hospital voluntarily. Unrealistically, the hospital proposed to resile the new model and grant individual hospitals greater independence.[78]

Disaffection continued when membership of hospital management committees came up for reappointment in 1951. The chairman of the Belfast HMC, Herbert Quin, also chair of the Royal Victoria and a unionist politician, who at this stage was a senator in the Northern Ireland upper house, stepped down in protest along with other leading members including R. Byers and F. Bell (treasurers of the Royal Maternity and Royal Victoria, respectively). Quin complained that hospital management committees were 'not the proper set up'.[79] Attempts to create a more unified hospital organisation were central to the dissatisfaction of former voluntary hospitals. This was alluded to when the 1955 Tanner Committee, reviewing Northern Ireland's health services, commented that prior to 1948, these hospitals were accustomed to making their own decisions and found their 'present subordination in a general system irksome'.[80] The former voluntary hospitals remained the most prestigious and powerful medical institutions in Northern Ireland; however, their position, independence and traditions were threatened by the creation of new management structures in the form of the hospital management committees and the Hospitals Authority. This key stakeholder in Northern Irish hospitals increasingly objected to the Authority's centralising and reforming agenda. Although these protestations were partly motivated by these hospitals' narrow self-interests, they also resonated with wider concerns that the increasing technocracy of the NHS diluted local initiative.

Another major complaint of former voluntary hospitals was the lack of funding from the Hospitals Authority, which further threatened their prominence in Northern Irish medicine. As highlighted in Chapter 4, the 1940s medical planners envisaged that the Grosvenor Road site – developed during the 1930s through the coalition of numerous voluntary hospitals, academic medicine and Ulster unionist political support – would be further upgraded as Belfast's and Northern Ireland's leading medical facility. In the years after 1948, these aspirations were not shared by the Authority, which was unwilling to commit substantial funding for the expansion of these hospitals. While the Authority did introduce an ambitious capital expenditure programme, as described in Chapter 6, this largely sought to address regional disparities in provision outside Belfast. Worryingly for Belfast's former voluntary hospitals, the Authority's efforts in Belfast focused on developing other hospitals. Its early major investment was in the new Ulster Hospital in Dundonald, which addressed the long-identified gap in provision in the east of the city. More inimical to the prominence of former voluntary hospitals in Belfast was the commitment to develop Belfast City Hospital. When the Health Services Act was introduced in 1948, this former poor law hospital lagged behind the more prestigious voluntary hospitals and, at one stage, was even earmarked for closure by the Nuffield surveyors. The Authority, however, was committed to its development and by 1963 pledged almost £1,400,000 to the hospital.[81] The lack of Authority investment in former voluntary hospitals drew much criticism. In 1963, Albert Grant, the chairman of the Royal Victoria Hospital and Belfast Hospital Management Committee, complained about the lack of funding and publicly stated:

> Unless the Hospitals Authority is prepared to give us more money both for revenue and capital purposes, there is no doubt that the present high standard of service being offered to the public by this group will have to deteriorate.[82]

In 1963, the *Belfast Telegraph* warned against funding 'new hospitals and departments', which led to 'undue economies in the old'.[83] The level of funding sought was not, however, forthcoming. There was a sense that the Hospitals Authority was overly focused on building new hospitals, fostering nascent specialities and building up services outside Belfast to the detriment of older, former voluntary institutions.

Regardless of the underfunding from the Hospitals Authority, these former voluntary hospitals did witness some expansion during this period. Medical education grew. The introduction of joint appointments, in which Queen's University and the Authority shared the cost of medical faculty, facilitated the growth of the medical school and the teaching hospitals.[84] Departments of Physical Education and Physiotherapy and Child Health were established in the Royal Victoria and Royal Belfast Hospital for Sick Children, respectively.[85] By the early 1960s, a new dental school and microbiology building had also been constructed at Grosvenor Road.[86]

These former voluntary hospitals often relied on their funds for redevelopment. Access to endowments or 'free funds,' a major concession won during negotiations in the 1940s, facilitated the expansion of these hospitals. By the mid-1950s, the Royal Victoria and Royal Belfast Hospital for Sick Children expended £137,000 and £113,500 on building projects. These were fully financed by philanthropic funding.[87] Evoking the philanthropy of earlier medical voluntarism, two new operating theatres in the Royal Victoria were funded by the ex-patients' guild.[88] While these projects provided some upgrades to the hospitals, they were piecemeal efforts, leaving the main buildings of the Royal Victoria Hospital and the Royal Maternity Hospital in need of significant modernisation. The 1950s may have witnessed a boom in hospital building in Northern Ireland, but the Hospitals Authority's focus was on other hospitals; in turn, the major redevelopment of the Grosvenor Road medical complex envisaged by the medical planners of the 1940s was not forthcoming.

The former voluntary hospitals won major concessions during the negotiations surrounding the 1948 Health Services Act, which were designed to maintain their power, influence and pre-eminence. However, as the Hospitals Authority and hospital management committees became more embedded, the former voluntary hospitals increasingly challenged and criticised the new organisational structures. Anxiety among this key stakeholder was based on their perceived loss of independence and power in a system which sought coordination across hospitals; their fears were exacerbated as substantial funding went to other hospitals and areas as the Authority sought to develop a more comprehensive service across Northern Ireland. This represented a shift in the equilibrium of hospital medical power and influence in Northern Ireland, where the former voluntary hospitals' position as the traditional powerhouse in Northern Irish healthcare was eclipsed by the Authority. It also illustrated that the Authority commitment to develop services in underserved areas overrode loyalty to individual institutions or the former voluntary hospitals, despite that many of its members were drawn from that sector.

Localism was a significant force in Northern Irish hospital organisation. This was evident in the 1920s and 1930s, when individual local authorities, spurred on by local civic pride, rivalry with neighbouring regions and institutional loyalty, among other factors, substantially invested ratepayers' money in local hospital services. These hospitals had little concern for wider regional planning of services. Theoretically, the Hospitals Authority and hospital management committees were to act as an antidote to the fragmentation of services. Yet, greater organisation invariably meant some form of rationalisation, including the downgrading or closing of local services and hospitals, which inevitably provoked opposition. Local political passions were often stirred up by the threat of hospital closures or changes to functions in Northern Ireland; such protests were also a common feature of NHS politics in later decades throughout Britain.[89]

These tensions surfaced in the late 1950s, when the Hospitals Authority proposed the reorganisation of consultant and specialist services provided by the Mid-Antrim Hospital Management Committee. A 1957 review of consultancy services based on clinical evidence recommended the downgrading of the Massereene Hospital to a geriatric unit in Antrim town and the centralisation of surgical and gynaecological services in the nearby Waveney Hospital in Ballymena. The report was undertaken by an advisory committee composed of leading British medical experts and planners, including Sir Ernest Rock Carling and Sir Harold Boldero; both were senior medical figures who were heavily involved in the creation and implementation of the British National Health Service.[90] Other members included Mr Rodgers and Mr McAfee, two professors of surgery from Belfast.[91] Influenced by an increasingly technocratic approach to medical planning and organisation of hospital services, the Authority initially favoured the plan.[92]

The proposed changes to the Massereene Hospital, however, led to much local protest. From its modest poor law origins, Massereene had developed into a popular district hospital since the interwar years and endeared much local loyalty. Such sentiments were articulated by the *Ballymena Weekly Telegraph* when it reported: 'the people of Antrim have pride in their hospital and feel that the staff take individual and personal interest which is absent in a larger hospital'.[93] An editorial in the *Belfast News-Letter* echoed such sentiments when it demanded that the medical planners, regardless if the proposal led to greater 'hospital efficiency', to take into account the 'pride of the people in an institution that they maintained for many years before the creation of the Hospitals Authority'.[94] Multiple local bodies, including the Antrim Rural District Council and local Church of Ireland and Presbyterian congregations, called for a reversal of the plan.[95] Opposition to the plans emerged across the political and religious divide. Catholic and Protestant clergy addressed a protest meeting, where a Catholic parish priest named Rev. V. Davey stressed that the locality was 'united in any good cause and never more so than on the present occasion'.[96] Cross-religious support portrayed the depth of loyalty to the hospital in the local community, which surpassed both the technocratic logic and rationalisation tendencies of the Authority.

This local discontent also transformed into unionist political opposition at a grassroots and parliamentary level. The Muckamore branch of the Antrim Unionist Association criticised the plans.[97] The Unionist Party MP for Antrim Nathaniel Owens Minford was even more bellicose and, at a protest meeting, called for the abolition of the Hospitals Authority so that hospital policy would come directly under central government.[98] Minford tabled a motion in Stormont to this effect, which other unionist backbenchers, including Dr Robert Nixon, a Unionist Party MP for North Down, and Professor Frederick Lloyd-Dodd, a Unionist Party MP for Queen's, supported. While these unionist backbenchers acted as a vehicle for local discontent over government health policy, strong support for the Authority's status quo was also evident. Dinah McNabb, a Unionist Party MP for North Down, echoed earlier unionist disquiet over the introduction of the NHS and feared increased state interference in hospitals in which 'civil servants would think more of costs and unit charges' than patient care. The Minister of Health and Local Government, Andrews, reminded the Stormont parliament that opposition to complete state control led to the establishment of independent statutory bodies such as the Hospitals Authority in the first instance. Similar observations were made at cabinet, where the Prime Minister, Brooke, noted the reversal of the strong desire to constrain central government's role, which shaped the creation of the health services.[99] The Authority's independence from the Ministry – heralded in 1948 as a socially conservative and Ulster unionist-inspired bulwark to the perceived statism of London's socialistic welfare state – came into sharp focus when elected unionist politicians had no direct power over the proposed rationalisation of services in their constituencies.

The protests over the mid-Antrim plans were effective. The Hospitals Authority adopted a more emollient approach and backtracked. The Authority's secretary, E. H. Jones, believed that there were many advantages to centralising services but despondingly conceded that the depth of local opposition led to the shelving of the plans.[100] The force of the political backlash ensured that neither the Authority nor the Ministry had any appetite to return to the policy.[101] The Authority's capitulation was a reminder of the continued strength of localism in health policy. The creation of the Authority promised a restructuring of hospital management while addressing the duplication, inefficiencies and overlapping of services inherited from the former era of desultory local government and voluntary provision. Instead, many of the Authority's plans for greater organisation succumbed to community protest, which galvanised around traditions of localism and institutional loyalty that easily translated into wider political pressure. Many involved in the hospital services, including medics and officials in the Ministry of Health and Local Government, believed that the Authority was reluctant to implement unpopular decisions.[102] It also illustrated the shortcomings of reforms promoted by medical planners and technocrats, which were often discredited by the lack of democratic input. Failure to proactively initiate dialogue and engage with the 'public' over management proposals for radical changes has long been a feature of the NHS.[103] The mid-Antrim plans may have been based on leading expert medical opinion. Still, they did not consider the wishes of the local population and ultimately came unstuck in the face of protest.

The Massereene example also revealed growing local and popular discontent with the health services' new management structures. Criticism focused on the lack of local influence on appointments to the Hospitals Authority and hospital management committees. For example, as early as 1950, the Dalriada Hospital, formerly under the Ballycastle Board of Guardians, believed that local authorities and 'local people who ha[d] given years of service' should influence who sat on the hospital management committees. Similarly, the North Antrim Hospital Management Committee, evoking more democratic governance, sought the election of members to erode the 'present feeling of frustration'.[104] In contrast to former voluntary hospitals, local authorities had little or no influence over appointments to the bodies, leading to the alienation of many who were previously involved in hospital administration through local government. The lack of involvement of elected politicians in the management structures further fuelled local and political discontent, which criticised the technocratic, non-representative nature of decision-making in health policy.

These frustrations were articulated predominantly within the unionist community and areas, whereas nationalists, as already described in this chapter, had a different set of grievances relating to representation and discrimination. Ulster unionism was often an uneasy coalition of multiple interest groups, social classes, different Protestant denominations, and a broad political spectrum from liberalism to extreme loyalism.[105] Although the Ulster Unionist Party dominated the government between 1921 and 1972, policies were the focus of much criticism from not just independent unionism but also many within the party. Vocal backbench Ulster Unionist Party MPs often chastised government policy in a political party in which structure and discipline were loose and ambiguous.[106] Throughout the 1950s, numerous backbenchers heavily criticised the Hospitals Authority. Brian Faulkner, at the initial stages of a parliamentary career, which would lead him to become the Stormont parliament's last Prime Minister in 1971, heavily rebuked the Authority's lack of parliamentary accountability.[107] During a 1951 parliamentary debate, Faulkner attacked the 'powers we have handed over to non-elected statutory authorities' and argued that the Authority's members should be elected.[108] Similarly, in 1954, Professor Lloyd-Dodd lambasted the Authority's 'policy of centralisation' for amounting to an 'autocracy'.[109] On another occasion, Lloyd-Dodd echoed long-held unionist fears and criticised the rising costs of the welfare state, which he believed 'the UK and Northern Ireland will eventually be unable to bear'.[110] While the government easily batted off nationalist concerns about their lack of representation in the management of the health services, criticism from within the Unionist Party was more difficult to ignore. In Britain, much has been written about the post-war political consensus surrounding the NHS, where the two dominant political parties agreed about its underlying philosophy and basic structure.[111] In Northern Ireland, however, political conflict within the governing Ulster Unionist Party over hospital services shaped debate and policy.

Calls for reform

Discontentment and political pressure led to a mixed government response. In 1950, William Grant died and was replaced by Dehra Parker as the Minister of Health and Local Government; she was the sole female cabinet minister in the Northern Ireland parliament (1921–72). A staunch unionist and loyal to the party, Parker had a reputation as a capable minister.[112] She withstood early criticisms, but the setting up of the Guillebaud Committee in 1953 in Britain to examine the cost of the NHS led to calls for a similar inquiry in Northern Ireland. In early 1954, two Ulster Unionist Party backbenchers in Stormont – Lloyd-Dodd and Dr S. Rodgers (Pottinger constituency) – tabled a private member's motion that called for an inquiry into the Hospitals Authority. Parker initially rejected these calls, outlining that she would prefer to assess how the findings of the forthcoming Guillebaud Report impacted Northern Ireland.[113] Parker's 'wait and see' approach led to further backlash, and more Unionist Party MPs joined the criticism of the Hospitals Authority, with many backbenchers threatening a divisive parliamentary vote on the matter.[114]

Under significant political pressure, Parker announced the establishment of an inquiry in May 1954 into the workings of health services. Sceptical of the need for such an inquiry, she stipulated that it would be 'informal' and held in private.[115] Unlike the Guillebaud Report, the Tanner Committee did not focus on finance but concentrated on the workings and management of the health services.[116] Dr H. G. Tanner was appointed as chairman of the inquiry; an experienced medical administrator and planner, he was the former chairman of the English South-Western Regional Hospital Board (1947–53) and a central figure in the pre-NHS United Bristol Hospitals.[117] The other members of the committee included Sir George Henderson, the former Permanent Secretary (1943–53) of the Department of Health for Scotland and J. V. S. Mills, a Belfast Resident Magistrate who was formerly Northern

Ireland's Chief Crown Solicitor.[118] The appointment of Tanner and Henderson ensured the region's health services were subjected to external scrutiny by experienced British medical policymakers and planners, who were instrumental to the introduction and running of the NHS in south-west England and Scotland, respectively.

The Tanner Report was published in 1955. While it praised the expansion of services under the Hospitals Authority and rejected any charge that it was 'irresponsible or extravagant', multiple reforms to bring Northern Ireland more in line with Britain's NHS were recommended.[119] Its key finding was that the Authority and General Health Services Board should become agents of the Ministry, although calls to disband the former and place the running of the health services fully under government command were rejected.[120] Attention was drawn to how appointed boards could not be called to parliamentary or ministerial account, which contrasted with regional hospital boards in Britain.[121] Such a reform promised to provide direct parliamentary oversight of health services and greater capacity for many of the vocal Unionist Party MPs, spurred on by frustrations of interest groups such as advocates of local services and former voluntary hospitals, to shape healthcare policy.

The Tanner Report also recommended other substantial reforms to rationalise administration, which inevitably challenged the interest groups and stakeholders whose influence permeated the hospital services. It sought to reduce the high number of hospital management committees through amalgamations, believing that fewer groupings would reduce costs and enhance consolidation. The findings criticised the hospital service's administrative fragmentation by stating: '[it] seems at present to be conceived … [as] separate local units rather than as a service for the province as a whole'.[122] The disbandment of individual hospital committees, which persisted in many hospitals, was also proposed. The members were 'strongly opposed' to this layer of administration, which gave individual hospitals many management responsibilities, including the power to make appointments and budgetary authority, but diluted the power of the overall groupings of hospitals in HMCs.[123] The report considered these individual committees as 'superfluous' which bred prevarication and impeded timely decision-making, with matters being sent 'up and down the ladder and [stuck] in various stages of development, stagnation or decay'.[124]

The large number of HMCs and persistence of individual committees for some hospitals were all concessions ceded to local interest groups and individual hospitals, especially former voluntary hospitals, during negotiations to establish the health services. These helped to protect such interest groups to the detriment of a genuinely collaborative model. Conversely, attempts by the Hospitals Authority to challenge the status quo provoked interest groups, leading to political backlash that, paradoxically, resulted in the Tanner inquiry in the first instance.

The Tanner Report was even more critical of the significant privileges that the former voluntary hospitals retained relating to endowments. Although the 1948 Health Services Act said that endowments should be transferred to hospital management committees, such funds were often belatedly transferred. Even when funding was transferred to the HMC, it could only be used by the hospital for which it was originally intended.[125] The inquiry believed that endowments gave hospitals many advantages, including the capacity to undertake capital development faster and 'to more lavish standards' than non-endowed hospitals, which often had to wait longer, even when their need for redevelopment was equal if not more urgent.[126] The Tanner Report outlined that

> this system produced marked inequalities ... they mitigate against the creation of properly integrated service, specifically by enabling these hospitals with liberal private funds to maintain a much higher standard of amenity than others can achieve ... and generally by perpetuating distinctions which may have been appropriate in their day but are no longer desirable.[127]

It proposed that endowments should be used to ensure that all hospital management committees had a reasonable fund at its disposal and that transferred endowments be used to create a research trust, drawing on the practices introduced in Scotland, which helped address imbalances. Endowments undoubtedly baked older institutional inequalities into the hospital organisation, which flew in the face of the NHS's attempts to create socialised healthcare with equal access and treatment irrespective of whether one sought care in a former voluntary hospital or not. The Tanner Report identified several other systemic biases driven by interest groups that required reform. These included the overrepresentation of the medical profession within management structures, the influence of former medical voluntarism on appointments to hospital management committees, the need for a stronger voice for local authorities and the unique disadvantages faced by the Mater Hospital.[128]

Parker was willing to implement some of the proposals and quickly developed legislation which reduced the number of medics on the Hospitals Authority. This reform also stipulated that the Authority had to consult elected local authorities and not just former voluntary authorities in appointing hospital management committee members.[129] She conceded that there was a greater 'feeling' for a closer connection between elected bodies and the hospital service.[130] These measures, however, were restricted, and there was less of an appetite or capacity in government to address the major issues highlighted by the Report. Echoing medical voluntarism's politicking surrounding the 1948 legislation, the Belfast Hospital Management Committee – the grouping of the main teaching and former voluntary hospitals – vehemently protested the proposed reforms. It declared that any infringement on endowments would be a reversal of the government's 1948 'pledge'. The hospital grouping also defended the principles of medical voluntarism in a rebuke to the Tanner Report's criticisms of the advantages former voluntary hospitals enjoyed in the new service. It stated:

> hospitals have been founded and have grown and developed as individual entities with a definite corporate personality which engenders a very real devotion and loyalty on those who work therein. We cannot foresee a Ministry or a unified state service engendering any similar feelings of devotion and loyalty.[131]

Although the health services were established seven years previously, there remained much opposition to the encroachment of a centralised state service on individual hospitals, which still clung to traditions of medical voluntarism and institutional loyalty.

There was little political support for the redistribution of endowments despite the unequal advantages they bestowed on some hospitals and the fact that Northern Ireland was out of step with other parts of the UK on the matter. By October 1955, Parker apprised

Stormont of her opposition to the redistribution of charitable bequests.[132] In 1957, Herbert Quin successfully introduced legislation that allowed HMCs greater flexibility in the use of endowments. Quin claimed the legislation ensured that the government would not interfere with the voluntary funds of hospitals. The then Minister for Health and Local Government, Jack Andrews, did not oppose the legislation, insisting that it allowed endowments to be spent on services which the exchequer could not provide (the 1948 Act precluded charitable funds from relieving any health services that were to be provided by the exchequer). The passing of the legislation ended any hope for the greater distribution of endowments envisaged by the Tanner Report. Although these hospitals had given up their voluntary status, they maintained a degree of financial independence throughout the post-war period, along with a continued ability to shape hospital policy.

Neither substantial reform of the Hospitals Authority nor hospital management committees was forthcoming. The government avoided the recommendation to make the Authority an agent of the Ministry. Parker stated that while she saw merits in greater government involvement, she was 'acutely aware of the danger of travelling too far along the road of control'.[133] The issue was allowed to slide by Parker until she stood down as minister due to ill health in 1957. That year, two ministers, Daniel Dixon and Terence O'Neill (Ministers for Commerce and Finance, respectively), informed cabinet that they favoured greater parliamentary oversight of the Hospitals Authority and other statutory bodies. While the leadership of unionism was willing to consider greater government involvement, no reform was forthcoming at this stage. Jack Andrews held the well-established unionist stance when he informed cabinet that 'local administration and control were not for his Ministry'.[134] The government remained intransigent about the Tanner Report's recommendations and was marked by a diffidence in challenging local interests or the power of former voluntary hospitals.

Conclusion

The concordant behind the creation of the health services in Northern Ireland led to significant concessions to power brokers in Northern Irish hospital management. In turn, the new management structures, in many ways, reflected the pre-1948 patterns of hospital management. Membership of the Hospitals Authority and the lower administrative tier of hospital management committees was dominated by a lay middle- to upper-class and medical profession, closely tied to the governing Ulster Unionist Party, which backboned medical voluntarism prior to the introduction of the health services. Other measures, including the Authority's independence from parliament, large number of HMCs and persistence of endowments and individual hospital committees, bestowed many advantages upon former voluntary hospitals in the new service. Local and institutional loyalties also continued after 1948. In turn, fragmentation, stakeholder resistance to planning and centralisation, and continuance of the inequities and inefficiencies inherited from the interwar years marked the early decades of the NHS in Northern Ireland.

Bias against Catholics and nationalists, a feature of unionist rule in Northern Ireland, was evident in the management of hospital services. Catholics and nationalists were largely frozen out of the system's management at all levels, and discriminatory hiring practices were also evident. Further political opposition was provoked from within unionism when the Hospitals Authority pursued greater technocratic governance over healthcare management. Recalcitrant former voluntary hospitals and local influences fiercely opposed efforts at rationalisation and centralisation. In the Authority's quest for greater central planning, criticisms focused on the encroachment of the independence of hospitals, stifling of individual hospital innovation, perceived indifference to local interests and a democratic deficit in the Authority's management structures. The lack of parliamentary oversight over the Authority became heavily politicised as unionist backbenchers struggled to influence healthcare decisions which impacted their constituencies. Although consensus prevailed in Britain over the NHS, significant political discontent over health services emerged in Northern Ireland between unionism and nationalism and within unionism.

Notes

1 A. Esmark, 'Maybe it is time to rediscover technocracy? An old framework for a new analysis of administrative reforms in the governance

era', *Journal of Public Administration Research and Theory*, 27:3 (2017), 501–16.

2 Lawrence, *The Government of Northern Ireland*, p. 141; L. G. P. Freer, 'Recent tendencies in Northern Ireland administration', in F. H. Newark (ed.), *Devolution of Government: The Experiment in Northern Ireland* (London: Institute of Public Administration, 1953), p. 66.

3 Klein, *The New Politics of the NHS*, pp. 35–6.

4 Stewart, 'The National Health Service in Scotland', 40.

5 Elder, 'The Health Services of Northern Ireland', 105.

6 MHLG, *Report on Health and Local Government Administration in Northern Ireland during the Period 1947 to 1949* (Belfast: HMSO, 1950), p. 1.

7 MHSS and NIHA, *Administrative Structure of Hospital Management Committees and Hospital Committees: Report by a Joint Working Party Appointed by the Minister of Health and Social Services and the Chairman of the NIHA* (Belfast: HMSO, 1966), p. 5 [hereafter the Hawnt Report].

8 PRONI, HLG/1/5/1, MHLG, Health Services Act (Northern Ireland) 1948: NIHA Constitution, 12. January 1948.

9 *BT*, 12 August 1972; R. M. Leman, 'Fifty years – a radiographic retrospect', *UMJ*, 35:1 (1966), 1–11.

10 PRONI, HLG/1/5/1, MHLG, Health Services Act (Northern Ireland) 1948: NIHA constitution, M. P. Sinclair, Sec. of BHA to L. G. P. Freer, MHLG, 18 February 1948.

11 Birrell and Murie, *Policy and Government in Northern Ireland*, p. 188; J. E. Sayers, 'The political parties and the social background', in T. Wilson (ed.), *Ulster Under Home Rule* (Oxford: Oxford University Press, 1955), p. 69.

12 At his death in 1979 McKinney was director of his family business, the Lilliput Laundry and Dye Works in Dunmurry. See *BT*, 7 July 1966; *BT*, 21 November 1979.

13 *BT*, 12 January 1940.

14 *BT*, 10 June 1967.

15 *BT*, 18 March 1960.

16 PRONI, HLG/1/5/1, MHLG, Health Services Act (Northern Ireland) 1948: NIHA Constitution, Allen to Grant, 16 March 1948.

17 Prochaska, *Christianity and Social Service in Modern Britain*, pp. 152–3.

18 PRONI, CAB/4/920, Cabinet Secretariat/Cabinet Conclusions, Health Services Bill, 26 June 1947.

19 PRONI, HLG/1/5/1, MHLG, Health Services Act (Northern Ireland) 1948: NIHA Constitution, 12 January 1948.

20 PRONI, HLG/1/5/1, MHLG, Health Services Act (Northern Ireland) 1948: NIHA Constitution, J. McAteer, sec. of Irish Trade Union Congress to Grant, 3 May 1948.
21 B. O'Leary, *A Treatise on Northern Ireland: Volume 2: Control* (Oxford: Oxford University Press, 2019), p. 164.
22 PRONI, HLG/1/5/1, MHLG, Health Services Act (Northern Ireland) 1948: NIHA Constitution, A. G. Mengies, District Official, Belfast, National Union of General and Municipal Workers to Grant, 24 June 1948.
23 These included T. Bailie a Stormont MP, John Wilfred Haughton who was also nominated by the BHA and mental health authorities, Alexander McKay Calder, a surgeon also nominated by the BMA and John Hopkins, a councillor also nominated by the Northern Ireland Tuberculosis Authority.
24 *NW*, 1 June 1955.
25 PRONI, HLG/1/5/1, MHLG, Health Services Act (Northern Ireland) 1948: NIHA Constitution, J. C. Campbell, Sec. of Newry Chamber of Commerce to Grant, 22 June 1949.
26 *NW*, 13 September 1957.
27 For example, see *UH*, 28 September 1963.
28 PRONI, HOS1/1/185, NIHA Records, Appointment of HMCs, newspaper clipping of *IN*, 7 September 1953.
29 Kaufmann, *The Orange Order*, pp. 1, 4.
30 *BN*, 23 November 1957.
31 *BN*, 10 April 1953.
32 *BN*, 3 June 1958.
33 M. P. Kelly, *The Northern Ireland Hospitals Authority and Catholics* (Belfast: P. Quinn & Co Ltd, 1961), pp. 3–4.
34 R. M. Fields, *Society under Siege: A Psychology of Northern Ireland* (Philadelphia, PA: Temple University Press, 1977), p. 216.
35 Kelly, *The Northern Ireland Hospitals Authority and Catholics*, pp. 3–4.
36 *Irish Weekly and Ulster Examiner*, 13 January 1951.
37 For an analysis of nationalism in Northern Ireland, see C. Norton, *The Politics of Constitutional Nationalism in Northern Ireland, 1932–70: Between Grievance and Reconciliation* (Manchester: Manchester University Press, 2014), esp. Chapters 5 and 6.
38 J. Whyte, 'How much discrimination was there under the unionist regime, 1921–68?', in T. Gallagher and J. O'Connell (eds), *Contemporary Irish Studies* (Manchester: Manchester University Press, 1983), pp. 1–35.

39 J. Quinn and P. Maume, 'Introduction', in *ibid.* (eds), *Ulster Political Lives* (Dublin: Royal Irish Academy, 2009), p. 11.
40 *Frontier Sentinel* [hereafter *FS*], 26 December 1953.
41 J. Rouse, 'Connellan, Joseph', *DIB*, www.dib.ie/biography/connellan-joseph-a1945 (accessed 20 November 2024).
42 *FS*, 16 January 1954.
43 *FS*, 29 January 1949.
44 *NW*, 1 June 1955.
45 PRONI, HOS1/1/185, NIHA Records, Appointment of HMCs, newspaper clipping of *IN*, 3 September 1956.
46 *FS*, 12 January 1957.
47 *Irish Weekly and Ulster Examiner*, 22 November 1952.
48 *BN*, 7 September 1954.
49 *FS*, 22 February 1958.
50 *BT*, 4 April 1968.
51 PRONI, HOS/1/1/688, Altnagelvin Hospital – Establishment, Altnagelvin Hospital Staff, 2 April 1968.
52 PRONI, HOS/1/1/688, Altnagelvin Hospital – Establishment, W. J. Morgan, Minister of HSS to E. McAteer, MP for Foyle, 29 May 1968.
53 Fair Employment Agency for Northern Ireland, *Report of an Investigation into the Western Health and Social Services Board under Section 12 of the Fair Employment (Northern Ireland) Act 1976* (Belfast: Fair Employment Agency, 1988), p. 28.
54 Government of Northern Ireland, *Disturbances in Northern Ireland: Report of the Commission appointed by the Governor of Northern Ireland* (Belfast: HMSO, 1969), see Chapter 10.
55 The National Archives, Kew, DO 130/24, Grievances of Catholics in Northern Ireland, 3 November 1941.
56 Kelly, *Hospitals Authority and Catholics*, pp. 8–9, 12.
57 J. McKenna, F. Manzoor and G. Jones, *Candles in the Dark: Medical Ethical Issues in Northern Ireland During the Troubles* (London: The Nuffield Trust, 2009), p. 43.
58 Kelly, *Hospitals Authority and Catholics*, pp. 8–9, 12.
59 *BT*, 1 July 1959.
60 *BT*, 4 July 1960.
61 PRONI, HOS1/1/270, NIHA Records, Discussions between NIHA and Ministry of Ministry: north-west opening ceremony, 23 November 1959.
62 *FS*, 20 October 1956.
63 Martin, 'Why have a Catholic Hospital at all?'.
64 R. M. Page, *Revisiting the Welfare State* (Maidenhead: Open University Press, 2007), esp. Chapter 3.

65 J. Crane, 'Loving' the National Health Service: Social surveys and activist feelings', in J. Crane and J. Hand, *Posters, Protests, and Prescriptions: Cultural Histories of the National Health Service in Britain* (Manchester: Manchester University Press, 2015), p. 93.
66 Committee on the Health Services in Northern Ireland, *Report of the Committee on the Health Services in Northern Ireland* (Belfast: HMSO, 1955), p. 36 [hereafter Tanner Report].
67 PRONI, HOS/1/1/2, NIHA Records, Appointment of HMCs, Memorandum of meeting between NIHA and BHA, 30 September 1948.
68 PRONI, FIN/18/25/149, Health Services Bill (Northern Ireland), 1946, J.W. Haughton to MoF, 21 January 1949.
69 PRONI, HOS/1/1/2, NIHA Records, Appointment of HMCs, F. R. Montgomery to McMillian, Secretary of Bangor Hospital, 4 August 1948.
70 *BT*, 9 November 1949.
71 *BT*, 21 December 1949.
72 Webster, *The National Health Service*, p. 19.
73 D. G. Neill, 'Some problems of integration in the hospital service of Northern Ireland', *Journal of the Statistical and Social Inquiry Society of Ireland*, 19 (1955/56), 169–83.
74 Neill, 'Some problems of integration in the hospital service of Northern Ireland', 174–5.
75 Tanner Report, p. 37.
76 Tanner Report, p. 82.
77 PRONI, HOS/1/1/184, NIHA Records, Appointment of HMCs, HMC Circular, 20 March 1950.
78 PRONI, HOS1/1/184, NIHA Records, Appointment of HMCs, Summary of replies to circular.
79 *BT*, 5 January 1951.
80 Tanner Report, p. 40.
81 NIHA, *The Development of Hospital and Specialist Services/A Memorandum Prepared by The Authority, June 1961 and Revised in November 1963* (Belfast: HMSO, 1964). p. 181.
82 *BT*, 6 September 1963.
83 *BT*, 6 September 1963.
84 NIHA, *The Development of Hospital and Specialist Services*, p. 12.
85 NIHA, *NIHA Annual Report for the Year Ending 1955* (Belfast: NIHA, 1956), p. 92.
86 W. H. T. Shepherd, 'Hospital relationships', *UMJ*, 36:1 (1967), 14.
87 NIHA, *NIHA Annual Report for the Year Ending 1960* (Belfast: NIHA, 1961), p. 23.

88 *NIHA Annual Report for 1955*, pp. 28–9.
89 E. Stewart, K. Dodworth and A. Ercia, 'The everyday work of hospital campaigns: Public knowledge and activism in the UK's National Health Services', in Crane and Hand, *Posters, Protests, and Prescriptions: Cultural Histories of the National Health Service in Britain*, p. 103.
90 For a brief outline of Boldero, see 'Sir Harold Esmond Arnison Boldero', in Inspiring Physicians, Royal College of Physicians Museum https://history.rcplondon.ac.uk/inspiring-physicians/sir-harold-esmond-arnison-boldero (accessed 15 July 2024); for Carling, see Sir Ernest Rock Carling, in Parr's Lives of the Fellows Royal College of Surgeons of England Search Results for Carling, Sir Ernest Rock (rcseng.ac.uk) (accessed 15 July 2024).
91 Gray, Government and the administration of hospital services in Northern Ireland, 282.
92 *BN*, 7 November 1957.
93 *BWT*, 21 November 1957.
94 *BN*, 14 December 1957.
95 *BWT*, 21 November 1957; *BO*, 22 November 1957.
96 *LT*, 5 December 1957.
97 *BN*, 14 November 1957.
98 *LT*, 5 December 1957.
99 PRONI, CAB/4/1054, Cabinet Secretariat/Cabinet Discussion, Notice of motion – status of Hospitals Authority, 12 December 1957.
100 *BN*, 10 January 1958.
101 PRONI, HOS/1/1/270, NIHA Records, Discussions between NIHA and MHLG, Report of the Advisory Committee on Hospital Services in the Mid-Antrim Area, 29 July 1958.
102 Gray, 'Government and the administration of hospital services in Northern Ireland', 285.
103 E. Stewart, 'A sociology of public responses to hospital change and closure', *Sociology of Health & Illness*, 41:7 (April 2019), 1251–69.
104 PRONI, HOS1/1/184, NIHA Records, Appointment of HMCs, Summary of replies to circular.
105 For fissures in the unionism see P. Buckland, 'The unity of Ulster unionism, 1886–1939', *History*, 60:199 (1975), 211–23; Reid, 'Protestant challenges to the "Protestant State"'.
106 G. Walker, 'The Ulster Unionist Party and the Bannside By-Election 1970', *Irish Political Studies*, 19:1 (2004), 61.
107 For an outline of Faulkner's career see M. Mulholland, 'Faulkner, (Arthur) Brian Deane', in *DIB*, www.dib.ie/biography/faulkner-arthur-brian-deane-a3021 (accessed 20 November 2024).

108 *NIHoCD*, 35, 30 May 1951, p. 1377.
109 *BT*, 22 February 1954.
110 *BT*, 22 February 1954.
111 Klein, *The New Politics of the NHS*, p. 46.
112 B. Hourican, 'Parker, Dame Dehra', in *DIB*, www.dib.ie/biography/parker-dame-dehra-a7189 (accessed 20 November 2024).
113 *BT*, 24 February 1954.
114 PRONI, CAB4/933/3, Cabinet Secretariat/Cabinet Conclusions, Working of Health Services Act – Prof Lloyd-Dodd's motion, 15 March 1954.
115 *BN* 20 May 1954.
116 Tanner Report, p. 5.
117 Lawrence, *The Government of Northern Ireland*, p. 144.
118 Tanner Report, p. 2.
119 Tanner Report, p. 28.
120 Tanner Report, pp. 27–9.
121 'Health services in Northern Ireland', *BMJ*, 1:4924 (21 May 1955), 1266.
122 Tanner Report, p. 36.
123 Tanner Report, p. 38.
124 Tanner Report, p. 38.
125 B. Harris and R. Cresswell, 'The legacy of voluntarism: Charitable funding in the early NHS, *The Economic History Review*, 77:2 (May 2024), 568.
126 Tanner Report, p. 40.
127 Tanner Report, p. 36; PRONI, Cabinet Secretariat, Cabinet Conclusion, CAB/4/971/5, Memorandum to the Cabinet submitted by the Minster for HLG Tanner Committee on the Health Services, 3 May 1955.
128 Lawrence, *The Government of Northern Ireland*, p. 145; Martin, 'Why have a Catholic Hospital at all?', p. 100.
129 PRONI, CAB/4/973/6, Cabinet Secretariat/Cabinet Conclusions, Health Services (Administrative Amendments) Bill (Northern Ireland), 17 May 1955.
130 PRONI, CAB/4/971/5, Cabinet Secretariat/Cabinet Conclusions, Memorandum to the Cabinet submitted by the Ministry of HLG Tanner Committee on the Health Services, 3 May 1955.
131 *BT*, 30 June 1955.
132 *BT*, 26 October 1955.
133 *BT*, 26 October 1955.
134 PRONI, CAB/4/1054, Cabinet Secretariat/Cabinet Conclusions, Notice of motion – status of the Hospitals Authority, 12 December 1957.

6

The quest for modernity: centralisation, managerialism and reorganisation

Hospital policy in Northern Ireland underwent significant change in the late 1960s and early 1970s. The eruption of the Troubles in this time led to unprecedented upheaval, civil unrest and communal and political violence, which engulfed Northern Irish society and politics for decades to come. These years also witnessed major change in the management and structure of the health services in Northern Ireland, which went from being the most disaggregated and localised, marked by weak central government, to the most coordinated, integrated and centrally run of the UK's country-specific variations of the NHS. The 1972 Health and Personal Social Services (Northern Ireland) Order introduced a merged social and medical service under direct central government jurisdiction and led to the dissolution of the Northern Ireland Hospitals Authority in 1973. This far exceeded the NHS reorganisations in Britain in 1973, which focused solely on consolidating the tripartite division of health services and did not include personal social services.

This chapter argues that multiple factors brought about these reforms and shifts in power in Northern Irish hospital policy. As set forth in the previous chapters, political and religious bias, medical and hospital stakeholder power and localism diluted and fragmented the hospital services. The creation of the Hospitals Authority in 1948, however, was a significant new organisational structure that had the potential to embed the technocratic governance of health that many post-war planners sought. Some of the Hospitals Authority's early flagship projects, such as the building of Altnagelvin Hospital, were framed within concepts of modernisation and planning. The emergence of Terence O'Neill as Prime

Minister in 1963 ushered in a reforming and modernising agenda that challenged the power and influence of the traditional stakeholders in hospitals. As it discarded traditional unionist hospital policy, central government and its civil service – influenced by an emphasis on efficiency, rationality and an emerging business-orientated managerialism – increasingly asserted its role in hospital services. While such an increased technocracy helped to shift the balance of power in Northern Irish hospital policy, other factors, including the emergence of new medical specialities, such as gerontology, and the influence of social medicine also altered the dynamics of healthcare. Yet, for much of the period, the O'Neill government proved too weak to bring about substantial reforms, often succumbing to sectional interests. It was not until the exceptional circumstances of the Troubles that full reform and unification were brought about, illustrating that the crisis of the early 1970s enabled policymakers to implement long-sought changes in the management of Northern Ireland's healthcare.

Post-war growth in services

The cost of health services became a key policy concern in 1950s Britain. Earlier assumptions that the cost of healthcare would decrease as the health of the general improved with greater access to services proved wildly off the mark. Instead, the reverse occurred, and greater financial demands led to the 1951 introduction of prescription charges throughout the UK, including Northern Ireland.[1] In response to these concerns, the Enquiry into the Cost of the NHS was established in 1953 in Britain. The committee's published findings, known popularly as the 'Guillebaud Report', were heavily influenced by the health economists Richard Titmuss and Brian Abel-Smith and concluded that there was no evidence of extravagance or inefficiency in the NHS.[2] Yet, within an atmosphere of concern about the rising cost of healthcare, the 1950s in Britain witnessed scant expansion in new hospitals, and the common criticism was that doctors had to practise twentieth-century medicine in nineteenth-century hospitals.[3] There were some positive developments such as the greater regional spread of GPs and consultants and enhanced merging of hospital services. Still, the first full decade of the NHS in Britain was characterised more by consolidation rather than expansion.[4]

Northern Ireland had a different experience from Great Britain and was marked by a greater expansion of hospital services in these years. The multiple 1940s health service surveys showed that Northern Ireland's healthcare lagged behind Great Britain, and the need for an extensive capital building programme was widely recognised.[5] In 1938, London accepted the parity principle that Northern Ireland should be entitled to enjoy the same social standards and services as Britain. However, it was not until 1944 that the British Treasury agreed to financially make up the deficit in services.[6] The 1949 Social Services Agreement ensured that Westminster would fund up to 80 per cent of the excess expenditure on a range of services, including health.[7] The commitment of the UK government to ameliorate social services in Northern Ireland to wider British standards was a major boon for the Hospitals Authority. While British hospital authorities operated against the backdrop of a curb on government expenditure, the Authority was given access to substantial funds to develop Northern Ireland's hospital services to gain parity across the UK in health provision.

Any measure of medical activity in this era illustrates the rapid expansion in hospital services. Medical staffing of hospitals witnessed an exponential rise, as demonstrated in Table 6.1. The growth of consultant staff outside Belfast, where most specialist care lay, greatly enhanced the expertise in provincial hospitals. This was evident in 1949 when a consultant physician, surgeon and anaesthetist were appointed to the Coleraine and Portrush HMC, providing many patients with local consultations who would have previously received specialist treatment in Belfast hospitals. The HMC addressed subsequent bed shortages through the repurposing of a local facility into a specialist care unit, an early example of the local success that amalgamation could bring.[8] Other medical staff also grew, including junior hospital doctors, hospital registrars, dental staff and nurses. Further indicators of hospital activity witnessed similar trajectories. This is illustrated in Table 6.2 which outlines significant growth in medical services between 1949/50 and 1972. Bed numbers, admissions to hospitals and out-patients all witnessed an inexorable rise. Similar increases were evident in

Table 6.1 Medical personnel in Northern Ireland between 1948 and 1971.

	1948	*1951*	*1956*	*1961*	*1966*	*1971*
Consultants and specialists	140	203	278	338	385	447
Other medical and dental staff	342	506	649	514	698	877
Nursing staff	3,700	4,420	5,500	6,817	9,895	11,174
Total	7,400	9,150	11,224	15,224	19,940	22,528

Source: NIHA *Annual Reports*.

Table 6.2 Medical services provided by NIHA in 1949–50 and 1972.

	1949–50	*1972*
Beds and patients		
Hospital beds	13,645	18,147
Admissions to hospitals	103,520	226,284
New out-patients	289,253	529,136
Out-patient attendances	742,563	1,467,745
Procedures and tests		
Operations	83,916	180,771
Laboratory tests	313,407	2,443,094
X-rays	159,605	1,284,044
Physiotherapy	301,708	964,853
Ambulance service		
Ambulances	82	169
Ambulance mileage	1,114,614	5,616,442
Patients carried	128,000	525,206

Source: NIHA, *NIHA Annual Report for for the Year Ending 1972* (Belfast: NIHA, 1973), p. 26.

the numbers of operations, laboratory testing and x-rays while the ambulance service also experienced steep growth.

The Hospitals Authority's most expensive and ambitious endeavour was its hospital building programme. At the Authority's inception, it was estimated that twelve million pounds in capital expenditure was needed to address deficiencies and meet wider UK standards.[9] This proved to be a conservative estimate, and between 1948 and 1960, the Authority's capital expenditure amounted to close to eighteen million pounds. As evidenced in Figure 6.1, the rate of expenditure was proportionally far greater than in Britain. This funding allowed for a cornucopia of ambitious new schemes, including new hospitals in Derry/Londonderry and Dundonald on the outskirts of Belfast and the redevelopment of the Mid-Ulster Hospital in Magherafelt. In 1955, the Tanner Report noted that 'nothing approaching this scale of expansion and improvement [had] yet been possible in any hospital region in Great Britain'.[10]

This unprecedented investment in hospital services positively impacted the health of Northern Ireland's people. Its population had access to more medical expertise, increasingly sophisticated medical techniques and enhanced diagnostics. The death rates for Northern

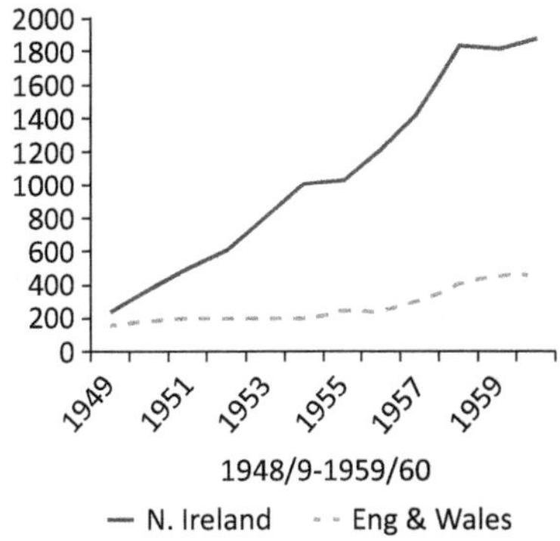

Figure 6.1 Capital expenditure on hospitals in Northern Ireland and England and Wales per 1,000 of population between 1949 and 1960

Table 6.3 Death rates per 1,000 population in Northern Ireland, England and Wales, Scotland and Irish Free State/Ireland, 1922–71.

	NI	*England & Wales*	*Scotland*	*IFS/Ireland*
1926	15.0	11.6	13.1	14.1
1937	15.1	12.4	13.9	15.3
1941*	15.2	13.5	14.7	14.6
1951	12.8	12.5	12.9	14.3
1961	11.3	12.0	12.3	12.3
1971	10.6	11.6	11.8	10.6

Source: P. Martin, 'Social policy and social change since 1914', in L. Kennedy and P. Ollerenshaw, *Ulster Since 1600: Politics, Economy, and Society* (Oxford: Oxford University Press, 2012), p. 312.
*Civilian deaths

Ireland reduced almost spectacularly, going from the highest in any country in Britain and the island of Ireland in 1926 to the lowest in 1971, as outlined in Table 6.3. Environmental, social and medical factors invariably shape population health, but the growth in healthcare undoubtedly positively impacted mortality rates.

Northern Ireland as a site of experimentation and modernity: Altnagelvin Hospital and Nuffield Experimental Unit

As explained in earlier chapters, prior to 1948, there was little, if any, central approach to planning, policy and management in healthcare. In contrast, the Hospitals Authority was a centralised body responsible for Northern Ireland's hospital services; by 1955, its annual budget of circa eight million pounds made it one of the most powerful arms of public administration in Northern Ireland.[11] The Authority became increasingly professional and drew on developing understandings of hospital administration and a commitment to planning and decision-making informed by technocratic expertise. By 1954, its headquarters had a staff of 148, which included accounts, legal and engineering teams. Along with the core staff, the Authority was run by committees responsible for developing and directing policy, the hospital building programme and making senior medical appointments while also overseeing, managing and auditing hospital management committees.[12] Reflective of the changing management of health, these structures allowed for the adoption of new techniques that espoused nascent ideas relating to modernisation, planning and efficiency. These ideas pervaded much thinking across the UK's welfare state in which planning developed in parallel with modernism in the belief that the application of knowledge through scientific methods would be a catalyst for social change.[13] This new administration was a significant step on the road to greater centralisation and the technocratic management envisaged by the architects of the NHS.

The Hospitals Authority's ambitious building programme was couched in this new commitment to scientific management, based on knowledge and expertise, and free of politics and interest group influence. This was evident in the building of the Altnagelvin Hospital in Derry/Londonderry, the Authority's flagship project. The building plans for Altnagelvin were architecturally modernistic. Unlike traditional hospital designs based on the Nightingale pavilion-style and lower-lying hospital, the new Derry/Londonderry hospital was planned as a multistorey building and tower block. Multistorey hospitals were representative of the most modern type of hospital building, advocated in the post-war world by architects, medical planners and think tanks such as the Nuffield Trust. Vertical planning was viewed as being a more economical structural design, with most wards identical in plan and stacked on top of each other, in which a central lift meant medical staff and patients had less distance to travel. They were also in keeping with progressive patient care and increased concerns about the psychological impact of surroundings on patients.[14] These hospitals provided beneficial environmental surroundings, where greater daylight and unobstructed views created a 'pleasanter atmosphere' and promoted 'cleanliness' and good ventilation, leading to a positive 'bactericidal effect'.[15] Multistorey hospitals were central to medical and social changes in patient care and reflective of the most up-to-date hospital design thinking internationally.

The commissioning of the London-based firm YRM to design the hospital was also significant.[16] This was a break from Ulster architectural tradition, in which large commissions often went to local firms that adhered to formal classicised architectural traditions, such as the local powerhouse Young & McKenzie.[17] F. R. S. Yorke, Eugene Rosenberg and Cyril Mardall established the eponymously named YRM in 1944 in London, which emerged as a key architectural firm in the nascent welfare state. YRM was the embodiment of modernism, which was predicated on the new consensus on planning in post-war Britain.[18] Modernist architecture and planning developed in common with the technocratic belief that the world could be made better by the application of knowledge through scientific principles and methods.[19] The commissioning of YRM to design Altnagelvin was a statement by the Hospitals Authority of its faith in technocratic and modernist approaches.

The multistorey hospital enjoyed special prestige in contemporary architecture and provided medical planners, designers and architects with the opportunity of endowing hospitals with a symbolic architectural modernity – like post-war Britain, the NHS hospital was to be modern, meritocratic, mechanised and efficient.[20] Altnagelvin offered the Hospitals Authority a degree of high cultural status and a place at the forefront of Britain's new architectural modernism. The newly built hospital allowed the Authority to express its new-found status. In 1956, Dr Cecil Kidd, medical adviser to the Authority and soon to be appointed Deputy Chief Medical Officer in the Ministry of Health and Local Government, claimed that Altnagelvin was a 'complete hospital' and its opening in 1960 would be 'an event of international importance in the hospital world'.[21]

The role of modernist architecture in the Hospitals Authority's hospital building programme was also reflective of the increased emphasis on medical planning, which was informed by research into hospital design and construction. In Britain, the lack of

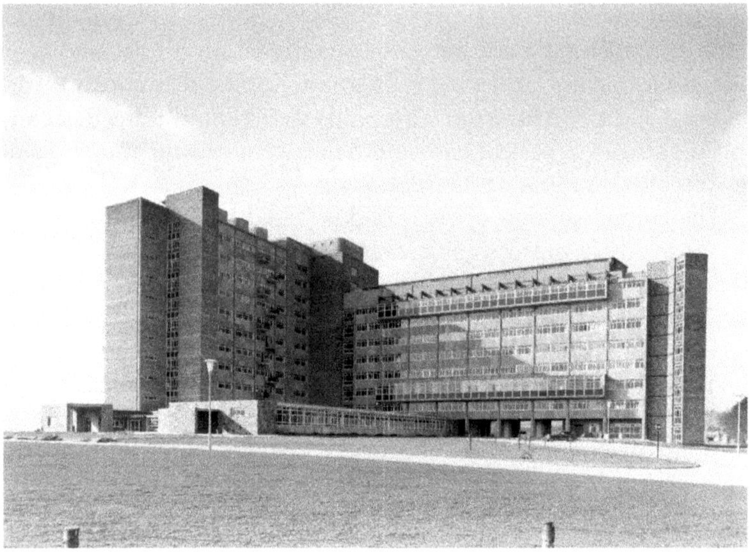

Figure 6.2 Altnagelvin Hospital, main building, Derry/Londonderry, 1960. *Source:* Photograph by Sam Lambert (London: Royal Institute of British Architects, BM/HOSP/4/A) [reproduced with permission].

hospital buildings in the 1950s meant that the Ministry of Health gave limited direction to hospital design. In turn, the Authority looked towards the Nuffield Trust in developing its hospital building programme. After the establishment of the NHS, Nuffield fundamentally reconsidered its mission, becoming an independent body dedicated to enquiry and research in all aspects of health services. Drawing on the nascent field of operations research, the Trust focused on creating efficiencies in clinical techniques and facilities, including the reorganisation of wards, clinics and practices to maximise resources.[22] The Trust undertook the 1955 study on nursing in hospitals, which applied time and motion techniques, demonstrating that much of nurses' time was inefficiently spent on administration and navigating poorly laid-out hospitals.[23] In 1949, the Trust established a collaborative research project with the University of Bristol to undertake a study into hospital design.[24] The research was interdisciplinary, headed up by architect Richard Llewelyn-Davies, and was conducted with a team that included an accountant, historian, nurse, medical doctor and statistician.[25] Llewelyn-Davies was

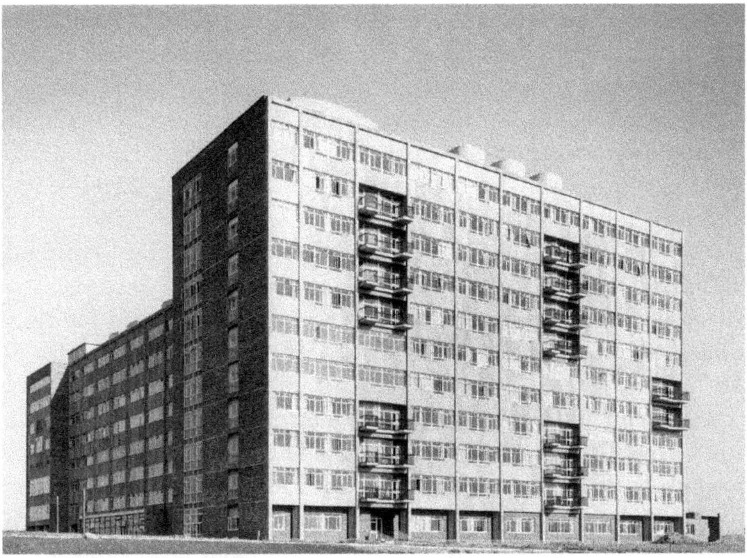

Figure 6.3 Altnagelvin Hospital, Derry/Londonderry, 1960. *Source:* Photograph by Sam Lambert (London: Royal Institute of British Architects, BM/HOSP/4/D) [reproduced with permission]

also concerned with examining the phenomenology and 'physical environment' of hospital life and how sound, colour, lighting, heating and ventilation could impact patients' treatment and therapy.[26] The study also provided a detailed examination of ward activities through visits to hospitals, observation of activities and workflow analysis.[27] The subsequent *Studies in the Functions and Design of Hospitals* became a standard reference for hospital design globally for decades.

Such new modes of management were attractive to the Hospitals Authority, which was eager to present itself as a modern and technocratic organisation. The fledgling Hospitals Authority regularly collaborated with the Nuffield Trust, eager for its hospital building programme to be shaped by the latter's experimental work on hospitals.[28] Kidd emphasised that the Authority had fully embraced the new approaches proposed by Nuffield, including the design and building of hospitals by multidisciplinary teams.[29] Echoing Llewelyn-Davies' research, Kidd highlighted the environmental benefits of sunlight, ventilation and scenic views, averring the vertical tower design as the ideal type of hospital. He maintained that the 'new approach and experiment in materials and design' had to be 'seized by all concerned in the creation of hospital buildings'.[30] Altnagelvin's multistorey and vertical tower was the embodiment of the new, modernist approaches to hospital architectural design promulgated by the Nuffield Trust and adopted by the Hospitals Authority.

Nuffield's most extensive collaboration with the Hospitals Authority related to the Nuffield Experimental Ward Unit at Musgrave Park Hospital in Belfast – the unit, or Nuffield House as it became commonly known, was part of the wider 700-bed hospital. In 1950, the Authority agreed to build at its own expense an experimental unit designed by the Llewelyn-Davies-led investigation team on the functions and designs of hospitals.[31] Experimental hospital units – another unit was established in Larkfield Hospital in Greenock, Scotland – were the third and final stage of Llewelyn-Davies' project and allowed for the testing and demonstrating of the research's earlier stages. The experimental surgical unit was opened in 1957 at a cost of £150,000. It included eighty surgical beds, two operating theatres, x-ray facilities and a central sterile supply department (CSSD) serving the entire hospital.[32] The CSSD was the first in any civilian hospital in the UK. Musgrave's Nuffield House was the basis of further research, including a 1960 *British Medical Journal* article that espoused the financial, working and medical advantages of CSSDs in hospitals.[33] Senior staff of leading British hospitals, such as London's Guy's, St Thomas's and St Bartholomew's, inspected the unit and were reportedly so 'impressed with the nursing techniques and hospital routines' that they asked to have ward sisters seconded to it.[34]

Northern Ireland was propelled to the forefront of post-war innovation in hospitals. The Nuffield Trust's research on hospital design and function influenced the subsequent period of capital development in Britain, ushered in with Enoch Powell's 1962 Hospital Plan.[35] Altnagelvin was the UK's first purpose-built post-war general hospital, and its L-shaped tower design was modified by YRM when they adopted the 'matchbox on a muffin' design for their next hospital, Hull Royal Infirmary, which became the design norm under Britain's hospital capital programme in the 1960s.[36] Northern Ireland's early hospital building programme offered British-based hospital planners, designers and architects the opportunity to experiment, test and develop ideas and approaches that would be implemented later across 1960s Britain. Northern Ireland's place at the forefront of hospital planning was not lost on the Authority, whose officials confidently and eagerly presented their activities at national and international conferences, often on invitation, such as at the International Hospital Congress.[37] Northern Ireland's newfound prominence contrasted with pre-1948 diffidence when the region's underdeveloped health services garnered little wider attention.

Modernisation emerged as a key factor in shaping health policy and management of health in Northern Ireland. Both Altnagelvin and Musgrave represented ideals of modernity, meritocracy and efficiency, which were at the helm of post-war medical planners' thinking. These increasingly technocratic approaches represented the emergence of new forms of governance and administration in healthcare in Northern Ireland. The Hospitals Authority's adoption and application of the latest expertise in relation to the design and managing of hospitals illustrated its wish to break from the older, fragmented health management, which was dominated by stakeholder influence, unionist–nationalist political divisions and the cloud of sectarianism.

Limits to modernity

The Hospitals Authority had emerged as a major new power, ostensibly based on technocratic expertise, in Northern Irish healthcare. Yet the modernising focus of the Authority was weakened by traditional stakeholders and power brokers in hospital services. As the previous chapter explained, this was evident in the unsuccessful attempts by the Authority to rationalise services, tackle the inherent inequalities that hospital endowments perpetuated or bring about real integration through reform and amalgamation of hospital management committees. Planning and modernity may have been the apotheosis of hospital management and encompassed the Authority's flagship projects of Altnagelvin and Nuffield House. Still, deep-rooted power structures and dynamics continued to shape hospital policy.

Despite the Hospitals Authority's rhetoric of modernisation relating to its hospital building programme, it often succumbed to local and individual hospital demands for capital expenditure. It failed to implement a more coherent, planned approach. The 1940s plans for a regionalised framework with the Grosvenor Road medical site in Belfast as the centre, connected to nine provincial hospitals, each with comprehensive general and specialist services, as outlined in Chapter 4, were not realised. Instead, during the early years of the Authority, funding was spread 'as widely as possible over ... many individual schemes'.[38] The Authority defended this approach on the grounds that hospitals throughout Northern Ireland needed updating. It acknowledged that proposals to develop provincial, regionally focused hospitals were 'sound in principle ... [but] difficult to progress' and would take years to come about. [39] By the early 1960s, the Authority investment in hospitals had perpetuated a localism that attenuated plans for a regionalised and hierarchical model.

Such an *ad hoc* approach was evident in the Hospitals Authority's new building programme published in 1961, revised in 1963, which outlined planned projects up to March 1972. This committed to develop as many hospitals as possible and unveiled an ambitious programme of 550 projects at a cost of fifty-two million pounds.[40] Although the programme was couched in rhetoric of planning and modernisation, the large number of projects made rationalisation unlikely. The objective of establishing large provincial hospitals was undermined by the volume of approved projects that developed many smaller hospitals. For example, Ballymena was identified as one of the locations for a large provincial hospital which would serve the mid-Antrim area. Surrounding hospitals, however, also received pledges for funding, such as Massereene, which had close to half a million pounds earmarked for development.[41] Plans for Massereene's rationalisation, quelled in the 1950s, were long forgotten in the building programme of the early 1960s. In general, the Authority's programme failed to rationalise services, including the downgrading of existing hospitals, necessary to create larger comprehensive provincial hospitals envisaged by the medical planners of the 1940s and, instead, focused on upgrading many smaller hospitals.

In Belfast, the Royal Victoria and Belfast City hospitals were earmarked for redevelopment, including a £2.8 million rebuilding of the former.[42] The Royal Victoria's redevelopment was widely supported. The *Belfast Telegraph* believed it would create 'one of the biggest hospital complexes in the UK, providing almost every conceivable kind of hospital care'.[43] Yet, there was no attempt to tackle the lack of co-operation between the two Belfast hospitals, a longstanding factor in the fragmentation of the city's hospital services.

O'Neillism and modernisation

The appointment of Terence O'Neill as Prime Minister ushered in a new phase in Northern Ireland politics. O'Neill held liberal views and famously sought to normalise relations with the Irish Republic and address some of the disadvantages suffered by the nationalist and Catholic minority in Northern Ireland. O'Neill's reformist government also embraced a rhetoric and practice of planning and modernisation, believing that economic and social progress would dissolve fissures in Northern Ireland's divided society and redress communal strife and inequality.[44] Historians have viewed O'Neill's commitment to modernisation as an attempt to present unionism as progressive to offset political pressure from the NILP, win back support of the professional classes and secure finance from Whitehall for costly modernist plans beyond the resources of the local economy.[45] During O'Neill's tenure, Stormont was able to adopt ambitious plans, sought by the 1964 Wilson Report, including the building of a new city, a new university, sixty-five thousand new homes and four new motorways, along with the introduction of an economic plan.[46] This amounted to a national planning strategy, which included a vast development programme as Northern Ireland fully embraced the post-war welfare-state modernism.[47] It also represented an unprecedented level of central government interventionism and planning in Northern Ireland. O'Neill's approach contrasted greatly with that of his predecessor, Brooke, who believed planning was a 'socialist menace'.[48]

O'Neill's government quickly turned to reforming the hospital services. The issue of the independence of the Hospitals Authority came to the fore again. Ian McClure, MP for Queen's University, leading gynaecologist and medical scion of the former voluntary hospitals, stoked controversy over the lack of funding for the Royal Maternity Hospital. During a Stormont debate in October 1964, McClure sensationally called the hospital an 'obstetric slum', claiming it suffered from overcrowding – which resulted in cancelled operations – and poor infection control. These conditions, he controversially and caustically claimed, were caused by a lack of funding from the Authority and Ministry.[49] A subsequent official inquiry denigrated McClure's comments as 'irresponsible and incorrect' but did concede that the hospital's labour wards were 'outdated' and 'overcrowded' while some nurses had 'deplorable' accommodation.[50] Unionist backbenchers in Stormont, long aggrieved at their lack of influence over the Authority (described in Chapter 5), sensed an opportunity and tabled a motion that the body was in 'neglect of the duty laid on it by parliament' and had to come under the direct control of government.[51] Prior to a parliamentary meeting of the Ulster Unionist Party, the cabinet agreed to make the Authority an agent of the Ministry. The Prime Minister, O'Neill, was in little doubt of the backbenchers' motivations, believing that they 'were only interested in the status of the Hospitals Authority and were using the Royal Maternity incident as an occasion on which to raise the question'.[52] Legislation was introduced with the 1967 Health Services Amendment Act which created a framework for joint decision making between the Authority and Ministry, with final responsibility for policy and finance resting with the latter.[53]

The Hospitals Authority's status as a statutory body, free from central government influence, was an anomaly, rooted in Ulster unionist suspicion of state action and the negotiations surrounding the creation of the NHS. While Brooke's government resisted calls for its reform, O'Neill believed Northern Ireland should fall into line with what 'had been accepted in Great Britain by both major parties' and the Authority come fully under the Ministry.[54] Norman Dugdale, a leading civil servant in the Ministry who went on to have a distinguished career, acknowledged the 'political pressure' from dissident unionist backbenchers but maintained that the 'Minister [William Craig], for quite different reasons, was largely in sympathy' with the reform.[55] This was hinted at by the *Belfast Telegraph,* which commented that the measure would not 'produce the detailed oversight of individual hospitals which some MPs may have in mind'.[56] Under the cloak of backbench unionist pressure for greater parliamentary oversight of hospitals, the government, motivated by a modernising agenda, made the Authority an agent of the Ministry; this was a major *volte-face* from well-established unionist health policy, which was antithetical to central government governance of the health services. As a result, the Stormont administration had a newfound power and responsibility over healthcare and was propelled to the fore of hospital planning and policymaking.

Regardless of unionist backbench ambitions for greater influence over hospital policy, the reform of the Hospitals Authority was in line with the O'Neill premiership's promise to bring economic and social modernisation, including a centralised and rationalised public administration, to Northern Ireland.[57] This period represented the highpoint of a new administrative rationalism, which believed that organisational change could improve government policies and, in the case of health services, bring about greater organisation and efficiencies.[58] This was evident in Northern Ireland, where ministries were reorganised in 1964. The Ministry of Health and Local Government was abolished, and the health services came under the newly established Ministry of Health and Social Services. William Craig, who at this stage of his career had a reputation as a modernising MP, was appointed as its first minister.[59] O'Neill's enthusiasm for reform was matched by a cohort of civil servants who saw much opportunity to enhance public administration through the modernisation and planning agenda while shaking off the traditional conservativism that dominated much of Northern Irish government.[60] The rhetoric of modernisation also lent the government credibility, even as it faced growing criticism for its lack of transparency and the discrimination suffered by the Catholic and nationalist minority. After assuming direct command of the Authority, O'Neill's government now had the opportunity to shape the hospital services along the principles of modernisation and rationalisation purported by its ministers and civil servants.

Northern Ireland's Hospital Plan, 1966

O'Neill's reform plans were influenced by wider UK developments in which planning surged in popularity in the 1960s. The availability of new social and economic information combined with nascent statistical, accounting and management techniques, and technological advances brought about greater confidence in the potential for state intervention to bring about modernisation.[61] The 1960s were marked by the state's attempts at long-term planning, which promised theoretical change and organisational reform that would make state spending more rational, orderly and efficient.[62] The introduction of the 1962 Hospital Plan by Enoch Powell (Minister of Health, 1961–3) represented an ambitious project of hospital expansion in England and Wales. The Plan, and its parallel in Scotland, were the first major capital programmes under the NHS to upgrade the obsolescent hospital stock in Britain.[63] This was combined with a promise that new hospitals would lead to productive efficiencies and the avoidance of uneconomic practices, leading to an overall restraint in expenditure.[64]

In an early example of the shortcomings of the supposed scientific techniques underpinning the high altar of technocratic planning, the building projects under the Hospital Plan were hopelessly underbudgeted. Estimates for new hospitals tended to understate the need for services and associated costs, which were exacerbated by problems with construction brought about by a simultaneous increase in the building of new homes, schools and universities. As early as 1964, it was apparent that the Hospital Plan in Britain would be hugely more expensive than first envisaged, and costings for many projects were 'soon consigned to the realms of fantasy'.[65] The Plan was vitiated by difficulties in making long-term projections such as forecasting bed needs for regions against unpredictable population growth, further complicated by the building of new towns.[66] Predicated on early 1960s planning, technology and architecture, the first new hospitals were inevitably outmoded by their opening in the mid-1970s.

In Northern Ireland, O'Neill's reforming central government became increasingly concerned that the Hospitals Authority was outdated, amateurish and not in keeping with modernisation. Much of the Authority's leadership dated from the pre-NHS voluntary era. In 1965, Marcela Mackie replaced William McKinney, becoming only the second chair of the Authority.[67] The appointment of a female to this prestigious position was undoubtedly significant, but Mackie's background illustrated the continued traditions of voluntarism in hospital management. This was reflected when Mackie self-deprecatingly described how she could dedicate herself to the honorary position: 'I have the time. That's my main qualification. All the other people on the Authority have their own jobs to attend to, and this is almost a full-time job'.[68] Mackie invoked an amateurism and the older medical voluntary ethos, which was not in keeping with the modernisation and rationalisation ideals that pervaded hospital management in the 1960s and the agenda of the O'Neill government.

Government concerns were evident in 1965 when the Ministry of Finance's Organisation and Methods branch undertook a review of the Hospitals Authority's administration. This gave a scathing assessment of the administration, financial management and expertise of the Authority. The Ministry highlighted numerous 'basic weaknesses' in its administrative structure, including the dearth of senior staff and insufficient coordination of its various sub-committees. It also identified the absence of a blueprint for the development of hospital services based on factors such as population and trends in medical treatment, a damning assessment considering such planning was key to the government's reforming rhetoric and the zeitgeist in public administration throughout the UK.[69] The Ministry of Finance stressed the need for the Authority to incorporate enhanced financial management, including improved budgetary oversight and greater consideration of the financial implications of building proposals.[70] These findings also resonated with wider attempts by civil servants in the late 1950s and early 1960s in Britain to move the NHS towards a more management-focused organisation.[71] The Authority was born in 1948 out of a compromise between the government and powerful hospital stakeholders, which ultimately undermined its potential to meet the modernisation agenda of the 1960s. These failings became increasingly apparent to the apparatus of a newly engaged central government looking to modernise public administration.

The Hospitals Authority grossly underestimated the cost of projects in the 1961 and 1963 hospital building programmes. For example, by 1966, it was envisaged that Belfast City Hospital would cost twelve million pounds compared to the four million cited three years previously.[72] The Authority's original estimate failed to account for increased building costs, the growing complexity of hospital design and medical equipment, and changing concepts of hospital care.[73]

Although the Hospital Plan in Britain experienced similar problems, leading government officials placed much of the blame at the door of the Authority. Since 1963 leading officials in the Ministry of Health and Social Services including Norman Dugdale and S. E. Taylor, the Assistant Secretary, had many reservations about the running of the Authority.[74] In 1965, Dugdale wrote to Ronald Green, Permanent Secretary of the Ministry of Health and Social Services, criticising a Hospitals Authority proposal regarding clinical areas, which was a nascent concept in health planning aimed at aligning clinical staffing and hospital organisation. Dugdale, who examined the proposal with other Ministry officials, including Dr Kidd (now the Chief Medical Officer) and Taylor, vilified the Authority for failing to consider the building programme in the plans. He stated:

> the result is veritable hotchpotch; no logical plan or progression, good points and bad all mixed up together, serious issues dodged, and others met head-on (unnecessarily in our opinion), and confusion between ends and means: the whole more likely to baffle, bewilder and enrage rather than to persuade or assuage.

Instead of the Authority's proposal, Dugdale wanted the Ministry to undertake a Northern Irish version of the Hospital Plan that would incorporate the building programme and clinical staffing. He firmly believed that it was the responsibility of the Ministry and not the Authority to draw up and implement the proposed new Hospital Plan. He contended that while they were 'not rushing into this with cries of enthusiasm ... They fe[lt] deeply that this is the Ministry's job and that there is no real alternative but to turn our hands to it'.[75] The Ministry's confidence in the Authority to develop complex, coherent and effective plans had eroded to the point that its civil servants increasingly assumed responsibility for hospital planning.

Much of the impetus behind the Northern Ireland Hospital Plan came from the reforming zeal of some civil servants. In particular, Dugdale, who enjoyed swift promotion in the Ministry, ultimately becoming permanent secretary in 1970 after positions as assistant secretary (1955), senior assistant secretary (1964) and second secretary (1968), was a key driver of reform.[76] Dugdale would also become well respected across the political divide, and Paddy Devlin of the Social Democratic Labour Party praised him as 'a most compassionate and civilised man' during his short reign as the first non-unionist Minister of Health and Social Services in the ephemeral power-sharing Executive of the Northern Ireland Assembly between January and May 1974.[77] During the mid- to late 1960s, a cohort of civil servants in the Ministry was at the forefront of the government's attempt to modernise and rationalise the administration of health services while sidelining the Hospitals Authority.

This was a major policy change for Northern Ireland's central government. Initiated by the Ministry, the Hospital Plan's terms were dictated to the Hospitals Authority. For example, the Ministry, led by Dugdale, dismissed the Authority's plans to revise its 1963 Building Programme, drew up the first draft and ultimately decided where to locate four large area hospitals outside Belfast.[78] In a departure from the Authority's earlier plans, the Ministry now proposed to concentrate resources on fewer but larger hospitals. Concerns from the Authority that concentration on 'a few large schemes' was inimical to other essential works fell on deaf ears. Ministry officials imperiously informed the Authority that they were pioneering a 'radical new approach' and should proceed 'quickly' with two major projects – Craigavon and Belfast City Hospital – which 'deserved maximum priority'.[79] The Ministry also intended to take over many of the responsibilities, previously the remit of the Authority, of building the new hospitals. Dugdale informed the Ministry of Finance that his Ministry needed greater resources 'to enable us to exercise more effective supervision of the hospital building programme as whole and of the planning and execution of the really big schemes in particular'.[80] The Ministry now had a far greater role in the planning and building of hospitals, leading to its growth in personnel, expertise and funding.

The obsolescence of the Hospitals Authority's role in hospital planning was apparent at a March 1966 cabinet meeting when W. J. Morgan, appointed Minister of Health and Social Services in 1965, acknowledged that his Ministry had informally defenestrated the Authority for responsibility for the building programme. Morgan lambasted the Authority's earlier programmes which, he claimed, 'did not seem to be based on any clear and consistent principles'.[81]

He further censured the Authority for funding too many initiatives in an attempt to 'please every area', leading to the spreading of resources too 'thinly' and slow completion of projects.[82] He replaced the Authority's plans with a revised ten-year scheme. Morgan justified the Ministry's assumption of responsibility for health policy and management through notions of scientific rationale. Although such rhetoric also pervaded the Authority, the advent of O'Neill's government led to a renewed planning ethos which promised the modernisation and rationalisation of public administration.

The 1966 Hospital Plan concentrated resources on a smaller number of large schemes. The Plan proposed to establish five clinical areas in Northern Ireland. Outside Belfast, a new layer of large facilities called area hospitals were to provide comprehensive services and specialities such as pathology, orthopaedics, geriatrics, dermatology, ENT and ophthalmology that were still predominantly offered in Belfast. The Plan was to build the newly termed area hospitals in 'carefully chosen centres', which would provide the needs of the immediate neighbourhood and a more expansive and surrounding clinical area. The services and staff of area hospitals would then support lower tiers of general and local hospitals.[83] Each area hospital would serve a catchment population of two to three hundred thousand.[84] The Plan aimed to group consultants in teams centred in area hospitals rather than disperse specialists in isolated single-handed units. The growth in consultancy services outside Belfast since 1948 brought medical staffing issues to the fore, including shortages in certain specialties like radiology and psychiatry and some grades of junior medical staff.[85] In many peripheral areas, consultants complained of the lack of career progression and in places there was an incapacity to get locum staff to cover consultants' leave.[86] Overall, the Plan was purportedly based on the deployment of 'human resources, buildings and equipment to the best advantage'.[87] Planners believed that efficiencies and rationalisation would be achieved by the concentration of resources in a small number of large hospitals that would have large catchment areas.

The 1966 Hospital Plan also reversed earlier commitments made by the Hospitals Authority. Funding previously earmarked for the building of a new hospital in Downpatrick was abandoned while funds committed to the extension of Altnagelvin, development of long-stay patients in Gransha and building of a new general hospital in Coleraine were all deferred until after 1975.[88] Altnagelvin in Derry, Ballymena, Ulster Hospital in Dundonald and Craigavon were all selected as area hospitals – the building of the proposed area hospital in Ballymena was also deferred. The development of the new Craigavon Area Hospital was the key project of the Plan. It was based on population predictions of the planned new city, controversially named Craigavon in 1965, which arose from the 1963 *Matthew Plan* and sought to 'de-magnetise' Belfast's economic and social pull and was endorsed by O'Neill's government.[89] In Belfast, the Hospital Plan committed to funding the development of Belfast City Hospital at the expense of the Royal Victoria rebuild, as promised under the previous programme, which was also postponed until after 1975. The Hospital Plan deferred, abandoned or reduced funding for numerous other planned projects.

The locations of the area hospitals were purportedly based on non-political criteria such as the geographical distribution of services and population growth. Morgan, however, was fully aware of the political implications of the whittling down of projects promised to hospitals and localities. He justified not seeking extra funding from Westminster – a common panacea for Northern Ireland's financial difficulties – on the grounds that Northern Ireland had

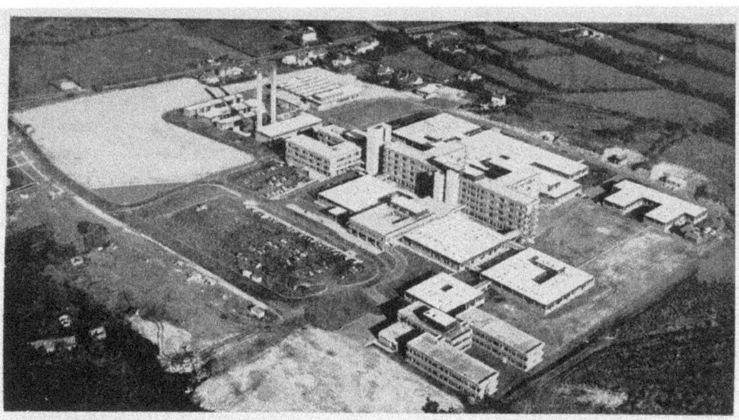
An aerial view of Craigavon Area Hospital—one of the major developments in the provision of area hospital facilities where none existed before. Craigavon Hospital was opened in September 1972.

Figure 6.4 Aerial view of Craigavon Area Hospital, 1972. *Source: NIHA Annual Report for… 31 Sept. 1973* (Belfast: NIHA, 1973), n.p.

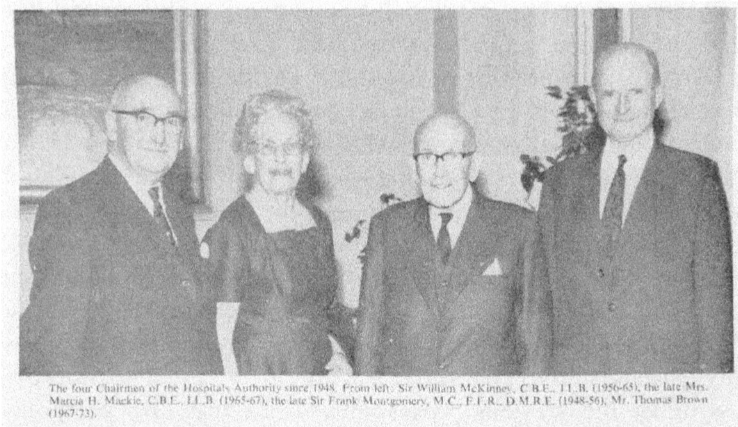
The four Chairmen of the Hospitals Authority since 1948. From left: Sir William McKinney, C.B.E., LL.B. (1956-65), the late Mrs. Marcia H. Mackie, C.B.E., LL.B. (1965-67), the late Sir Frank Montgomery, M.C., F.F.R., D.M.R.E. (1948-56), Mr. Thomas Brown (1967-73).

Figure 6.5 The four chairpersons of the Northern Ireland Hospitals Authority, 1948–73. *Source: NIHA Annual Report for… 31 Sept. 1973* (Belfast: NIHA, 1973), n.p.

already exceeded parity of hospital provision with Britain, which created 'obvious difficulties' in pressing for higher standards. Amazingly, the investment in Northern Ireland's hospital services was so significant since 1948 that parity in health services with Great Britain had been reached; any extra investment from London threatened to breach the parity principle by creating better services. Morgan also turned to the lexicon of modernisation, stating that the Plan would 'reshape' the hospital service on the 'basis of well-defined principles and priorities'.[90] This supposed scientific approach to the location of hospitals invoked ideas of planning, technocracy and apolitical expertise that the O'Neill modernising and rationalising government propagated. Similar rhetoric was evident in other areas of government intervention, such as tertiary education, urban planning and communications, including the building of railways and motorways and economic investment. Indeed, the location of the area hospitals stemmed partly from these other facets of government action. Projected population growth in the new town of Craigavon prompted the need for an area hospital. Also, new transport infrastructure in the form of motorways allowed greater access to many of the proposed area hospitals.[91]

Nationalist opposition and unionist division

Despite the apolitical and value-free technocratic veneer of modernism, the practical implementation of many of these schemes in Northern Ireland further alienated the Catholic and nationalist population from the Northern Irish state. While Craigavon was originally planned to allow social and religious mixing in innovative urban living, the government ultimately ensured that the town would have a Protestant majority, leading to unionist political gain.[92] Located in the strongly unionist North Armagh area between Portadown and Lurgan, the new city's naming after Northern Ireland's founder further provoked nationalists. The development drew political criticism from across the divide, and by the outbreak of the Troubles in the late 1960s it had been confined to a few disconnected housing estates, polarised on sectarian lines, and vandalised and dilapidated.[93] It is no wonder that Craigavon is viewed as perhaps the greatest failure of the post-war new towns experiment in the UK.[94] Other areas of government planning gave nationalists reason for suspicion and resentment of modernisation, including the location of the new university in Coleraine and not in Derry/Londonderry, a Catholic-majority city with a tradition of tertiary education. The drive for investment brought new business, but largely to the eastern part of Northern Ireland where the unionist population predominated.[95] The political implications of 1960s planning and state intervention are viewed as having helped to reignite centuries-old animosities that escalated into a deep and lasting crisis that became the Troubles.

The extent to which political motivations determined hospital funding, however, is far from clear. Significant Hospitals Authority funding for capital projects did go to unionist and Protestant areas. For example, by 1963, County Antrim's four hospital management committees outside Belfast, with a combined population of 204,000, the majority of whom were unionist and Protestant, had spent £1,181,195 on capital projects since 1948. This was somewhat higher than the £810,126 that five HMCs with large Catholic populations – Fermanagh, Tyrone and Fermanagh, South Tyrone, South Armagh and South Down – and with a higher combined population of 388,000 received in the same period.[96] Such funding further embedded interwar trends in hospital development, whereby the more advanced hospitals in the east received greater resources compared to the less well-developed western and southern regions. Strongly unionist areas continued to receive substantial funding in the early years of the Hospitals Authority.

Nationalist grievances, however, about the hospital services focused more on the alienation of the Mater Hospital, the lack of Catholics in management structures and discriminatory employment practices (described in Chapter 5) than the capital programme. Catholics and nationalists also benefited from the free-at-the-point-of-contact and universalist health services, which guaranteed eligibility and accessibility to all the population to increasingly advanced hospitals. During a Stormont debate in 1960, the benefits of the post-war welfare state were recognised by the Nationalist Party MP for West Tyrone, R. H. O'Connor, who highlighted the 'vastly improved conditions for the citizens of Northern Ireland' brought about by high expenditure on social and health services.[97]

The completion of key hospital projects in predominantly nationalist parts of Northern Ireland further garnered support for the services and also helped to address regional imbalances in provision. The opening of Altnagelvin in Derry/Londonderry brought a comprehensive range of general and specialist medical services to the north-west for the first time. Other peripheral areas with large Catholic and nationalist populations that were not overly unionist in outlook, such as County Tyrone and County Fermanagh, also enjoyed significant hospital development.[98] In Enniskillen, a new general hospital opened in 1964, replacing the former workhouse.[99] Similarly, the South Tyrone Hospital in Dungannon was modernised by the mid-1960s.[100] In this regard, the Hospitals Authority's independence helped to insulate medical planning from the extremities of unionism, often evident in local government and Stormont. The Northern Ireland Housing Trust was a similar statutory body that was independent of the impulses of central and local government and demonstrated much impartiality.[101] The revised 1963 building programme also assuaged nationalist fears of geographical biases in hospital development. In the nationalist majority town of Downpatrick, a new hospital was planned at an estimated cost of over £1.6 million to replace the existing Downe and Downshire hospitals.[102] In Derry/Londonderry, close to one million pounds was earmarked to develop the Gransha Hospital into a modern facility with geriatric and convalescent provision. A £600,000 extension was planned for Altnagelvin.[103] Under the auspices of the Tyrone and Fermanagh HMC, a new general hospital in Omagh was proposed to be built at a cost of four and a half million pounds.[104] Such plans helped the Hospitals Authority to avoid accusations that political and religious factors overly influenced its building programme. While the hospital building programme up to the early 1960s often succumbed to local pressures, it was less focused on rewarding predominantly unionist regions and more aimed at spreading hospital services across Northern Ireland.

The 1966 Hospital Plan's shelving of hospital projects, some in nationalist areas, provoked much criticism and, in some cases, fuelled suspicions of political motivations which had already enveloped nationalist opinion towards other aspects of state planning. The failure to include further funding for the Omagh Hospital redevelopment led to the Western Hospital Management Committee complaining that the Plan was 'another instance of the way in which the north-west [was] being neglected'.[105] Similar fears were evident in Downpatrick in County Down after the downgrading of its hospital under the Plan. Instead, the Ulster Hospital at Dundonald was to act as the area hospital for much of County Down. Dundonald was located between the largely unionist areas of the eastern part of Belfast and the northern region of County Down. At a meeting to protest against the Plan, the Catholic parish priest of Castlewellan, Rev. McNabb, articulated nationalist frustrations and declared: 'I believe there is discrimination in the location of industries in this country, and now, still worse, it looks as though there is discrimination in the location of hospitals'.[106] The Nationalist Party MP for Mourne, James O'Reilly, specified that he would fight the Plan 'tooth and nail' in Stormont.[107] A petition of 12,000 signatures was presented to O'Neill, and plans were in place to hold a motorcade protest at Stormont (a tactic that nationalists also used to protest against the location of the new university in Coleraine), although this later fell through.[108] The form and rhetoric of protest against the Downpatrick decision resonated with nationalism's recalibrated engagement with Northern Irish politics, which increasingly challenged unionism on social and economic issues and not just the constitutional question.[109]

Yet hospital services impacted the whole population, and protest often transcended traditional nationalist and unionist divisions. Local reaction was not confined to nationalist outcry and encompassed widespread criticism of the Plan from across the nationalist and unionist population. In a coordinated protest, the Hospitals Authority received letters condemning the Downpatrick decision from a wide range of civic, religious, sporting and political organisations. Bodies associated with nationalists, including the local branch of the Ancient Order of Hibernians, the Downpatrick Gaelic Athletic Association club (named Thomas Russell Gaelic Union), and the all-island Irish National Teachers' Organisation (under its Irish language title, Cumann Múinteoirí Éireann), all wrote to the Hospitals Authority in protest. Unionist bodies, including the Dunmore Loyal Orange Lodge and the East Down Unionist Association, sent similar letters. All the major local religious bodies also complained to the Authority. This was an organised protest, and the letters contained common language, citing 'medical, social and humanitarian reasons' for their opposition.[110] Numerous public meetings were held, and the Downpatrick HMC chairman, Colonel M. C. Perceval-Price, a unionist who unsuccessfully ran in the 1962 general election for the Mourne constituency, resigned in protest.[111]

These protests appeared to have had some impact on policy. The Plan initially committed to only developing geriatric and maternity beds in Downpatrick. By the Stormont vote on the Plan in June 1966, Morgan conceded that this scaled-down development could be regarded as the first phase of a new hospital, which would be fully built if the long-term need became apparent over the following years. Morgan's 'strong assurances' led to James Reilly's withdrawal of an amendment that opposed the Plan.[112] The threat to local hospital services galvanised the local nationalist and unionist community to jointly protest central government decision-making, indicating that social protest was not solely demarcated across the political and sectarian divide, despite the widening polarisation of Northern Irish society during the years leading up to the Troubles. Centralised, technocratic decision-making which negatively impacted on local health services could provoke community-wide protest. While the Hospital Plan generated much negative reaction, it is not overly evident that this fuelled the political and sectarian divisions of the Troubles.

The ramifications of the Hospital Plan did, however, fragment unionist health policy, further destabilising the unionist government during a period of developing political crisis. Largely unionist areas were vociferous in opposition to the perceived loss of services which the Plan entailed. For example, W. J. Gillingham, secretary of the Hospitals Authority, had a tumultuous meeting with the Coleraine and Portrush HMC, during which the chairman, J. W. Stewart, resigned in protest at the decision to delay the building of a new hospital in Coleraine, and the whole membership threatened to resign *en masse*. The HMC was especially provoked by the fact that it had postponed the development and renovation of the existing facilities because of a 'pathetic reliance' on the Authority's prior commitment to a new hospital.[113] Central government's measures to rationalise the building programme led to much backlash from local hospital powers. In areas such as Coleraine, these were predominantly from a unionist middle-class and elite background, which illustrated how increased state intervention in health policy fractured political unionism.

Fissures within unionism brought about by Morgan's reorganisation of hospital services were further evident in the Hospital Plan's deferment of the Royal Victoria's redevelopment. The reneging on previous promises to the hospital was met with dismay by the hospital's representatives and some unionists. In an open letter to the *Belfast Telegraph*, Ian McClure, gynaecologist and Unionist Party MP, and J. S. Loughridge, chairman of the Royal Victoria medical staff and sitting president of the Ulster Medical Society, chastised the Plan.[114] They derided 'planners' for their lack of 'front-line' experience of the day-to-day 'difficulties of actually running the hospital service'. Loughridge and McClure claimed that the Plan would deprive the Royal Victoria of its status and 'undo the vast amount of good work and careful management of the past hundred years'.[115] Other medical figures were equally aghast. In late 1966, Dr W. H. T. Shepherd of the Royal Victoria deplored the Minister's decision as 'inexplicable' and highlighted the hospital's deficiencies, such as large open wards, meagre toilet facilities and lack of provision for the isolation of infected or noisy patients.[116] In 1967, the Belfast HMC reported that, despite making 'vigorous appeals' for a change of policy, there was 'very little hope' that the Royal Victoria's capital development plan would commence before 1976.[117] However, the Ministry appointed a standing medical advisory committee in 1967, chaired by Prof. J. H. Biggart, Dean of Queen's Medical School, which recommended the redevelopment of the Royal Victoria's specialist services including neurosurgery, cardiac surgery and a regional accident centre which were approved by the Ministry.[118] While this was welcome, it was not the major redevelopment of the hospital originally envisaged. The significant dilution of the Royal Victoria plans and the granting of twelve million pounds to Belfast City Hospital's redevelopment represented a significant shift in Belfast's medical and hospital power base. The Royal Victoria could no longer claim to be the most influential medical institution in Belfast or Northern Ireland, as resources were directed towards City Hospital. In some ways, central government appeared to be rewarding City Hospital for its greater acquiescence with post-1948 hospital structures, especially compared to the recalcitrant Royal Victoria which resisted, often bitterly, increased oversight under the NHS. Somewhat ironically, the building of the City Hospital was beset with problems, and it did not open its doors until 1986, ten years after the hospital's initial projected completion and far over budget.[119]

O'Neill's reform agenda brought divisions within unionism to the fore, which sabotaged his premiership during a period of increasing political and social unravelling. Historians and political scientists have long understood such unionist political fragmentation as emanating from radical right-wing populist unionism and Protestantism, embodied by Ian Paisley's religious and political extremism in reaction to perceived threats to Northern Ireland from O'Neill's conciliatory policies towards nationalism and Catholicism. This also took the form of Protestant working-class anti-establishment politics, which challenged the moral authority of the unionist elite to lead.[120] Yet the outcry brought about by O'Neill's hospital policy led to divisions within the very elite that historically led unionism and were supposedly the very proponents and supporters of the reformist unionist agenda. The unsteady coalition of leading medics, hospitals and unionism, which shaped health policy in Northern Ireland up to this point, threatened to dissolve over the government's modernisation policies, leading to fissures in not just medical policy but unionism generally.

Shifting power in Northern Irish hospitals

The Hospital Plan represented the central government's most extensive involvement in health and hospital planning since the introduction of the health services in 1948. Influenced by prevailing notions of administrative rationalisation, the Minister and his civil servants articulated a faith in centralised planning and expertise which sought to move decision-making away from the interests of stakeholders such as former voluntary hospitals, local interest groups and strands within Ulster unionism. This represented a shift in the power balance in Northern Irish hospital management and the direction of policy. While a modernising central government was important in this transformation, other factors such as the growth of consultants and emergence of new specialisms also attenuated the long-standing medical powers in Northern Ireland.

The expansion of consultancy services ensured that expertise was no longer predominantly concentrated in the former Belfast voluntary hospitals but spread more evenly across Northern Ireland. The growth in the number of consultants and specialists – more than doubling from 154 in 1948 to 385 by 1964 – significantly altered the makeup of the medical profession in Northern Ireland.[121] Many of these consultants were from outside the well-established Belfast medical elite. The Nuffield surveyors in the 1940s warned that a predominance of Queen's University graduates on the staff of the Medical School would lead to parochialism and, in turn, 'restrict outlook, retard progress and react adversely upon its reputation'.[122] Such concerns were somewhat accurate, and in 1948, the clinical professorships were dominated by local medical men, invariably unionist in outlook.[123] Reform of clinical academic appointments was introduced through joint appointments by the Hospitals Authority and Queen's University. By 1963, the Ministry reported that the canvassing for senior medical appointments had been largely eradicated.[124] This was unique to Northern Ireland and contrasted with England and Wales, where appointments were made solely by the university or RHB and individual hospitals.[125] The growth of consultants and greater impartiality in appointments to the Medical School lessened the influence of former voluntary teaching hospitals such as the Royal Victoria.

The emergence of new medical specialities also partly led to the gravitational pull of medical influence away from Northern Ireland's medical power base around the Grosvenor Road medical site. Increased resources were directed to the Cinderella fields – psychiatry and geriatrics – which were often concentrated in the former local authority sector. The care of older people was an emerging field of medicine which the Hospitals Authority embraced. It inherited the former local authority and poor law institutions, which had a long history of caring for older, long-stay patients whom the more prestigious and curative previous voluntary sector mostly ignored. The 1950s and 1960s ushered in a new age of geriatric care focused on deinstitutionalisation and community provision. Focus shifted from the pauperising institutionalism of the poor law to active treatment, rehabilitation and domiciliary care along with peripheral hospitals and residential accommodation specialising in long-stay care.[126]

In 1948, Belfast City Hospital set up one of the first purpose-built units for older care, expressly designed for the treatment and rehabilitation of older people in a hospital setting in the UK. This unit became known as Wakehurst House and was spearheaded by Dr George Adams, Northern Ireland's first consultant in geriatrics, who led a multidisciplinary team that included a physiotherapist, occupational therapist and almoner. Adams succeeded in significantly reducing the number of long-stay patients in the hospital through a combination of medical treatment and social work.[127] A second older care unit was established in 1951 in Braid Valley Hospital, the former workhouse which had developed into an auxiliary facility to Waveney Hospital in Ballymena.[128] Braid Valley helped to address the problem of chronic patients in Waveney Hospital, where by 1950 the hospital authorities complained that large numbers of long-stay patients made it impossible to 'separate surgical and medical wards'.[129] Opened in 1951 under the aegis of the Mid-Antrim Hospital Management Committee, Braid Valley became the first hospital solely for older care in Northern Ireland.[130] At its opening, the Minister of Health and Local Government Dehra Parker highlighted that the government and Hospitals Authority 'were very conscious of the necessity of providing special hospitals for old people'. Parker described how older patients were too often regarded as chronic long-stay patients with little hope of ultimate cure, but that new treatments could restore patients' health, with the possibility of rehabilitation.[131] Growth in geriatrics led to a new medical specialism which was independent of the deep-rooted medical elite in Northern Ireland and lay in older traditions of local authority care.

The nascent academic field of social medicine was also influential in Northern Ireland. A product of the socially radical atmosphere of 1940s Britain, the field drew on social science and aimed to provide health services that took account of the social dimensions of ill health.[132] Social medicine's focus on primary care and the combining of health and welfare services offered a potential counter to the dominance of hospitals and specialisms under the NHS. In 1947, Queen's University created a Chair and Department of Social and Preventive Medicine.[133] In 1948, Prof. Alan Stevenson and Dr Cheeseman were appointed as the Department's first chair and lecturer, respectively. Both had experience from Britain – Stevenson trained in Glasgow – and were previously in the London School of Hygiene and Tropical Medicine, illustrating the shifting strands in Northern Irish medicine that a parochial medical elite had long dominated.[134] After Stevenson left for the Medical Research Unit in Oxford University in 1958, the chair was filled by Prof. John Pemberton, who came from the University of Sheffield, after holding a one-year Rockefeller Travelling Fellowship at the Harvard School of Public Health. Pemberton was an influential figure in the field internationally, having established the Society of Social Medicine two years previously.[135] Social medicine had a positive impact on medical education in the region. In 1954, the Hospitals Authority believed that Queen's Medical School devoted more time to social medicine than many other schools in the UK.[136] Other new fields also heralded the arrival of senior medics from outside Northern Ireland. In 1957, the jointly funded new University chair in mental health was filled by Prof. John G. Gibson. Although a Belfast graduate, Gibson had developed his career in London.[137]

These new medical fields and medics diluted the prominence of local medical men in Northern Ireland's healthcare. In medicine fields like cardiology and neurosurgery have remained at the top of the medical stratification order and offer consultants higher social status, better pay, power and influence. In contrast, those in the Cinderella fields, such as geriatrics, remained lower down the ladder of the medical profession.[138] In Northern Ireland, however, social medicine and the Cinderella specialisms appeared to be stronger than elsewhere, which further weakened the influence of the traditional medical elite.

Hawnt Report and creeping managerialism

These transformations in medical power were aligned with the modernisation emphasis of the O'Neill government and zealous civil servants committed to the planning spirit of the 1960s. The ground was now laid for the attempted reform of the fragmentation of hospital management, which had plagued the services since their inception in 1948. The reforming pulses of central government were further evidenced by the publication of the Hawnt Report in 1966. In 1965, the Ministry and Hospitals Authority, partly in response to the Royal Maternity scandal, jointly appointed a working party to examine the administrative structure of the hospital service, including the relationship between the Authority and hospital management committees. Although a joint committee, the inquiry was primarily driven by the Ministry. In 1964, Dugdale wrote to A. A. Hughes in the Scottish Home and Health Department (SHHD), seeking input on the reform of hospital management committees. He stated how the lower tier of management was previously the Authority's concern, but that the Ministry now believed that the multitude of committees led to an 'unnecessarily complicated' and fragmented scheme and proclaimed that '[a] thorough shake-up and rationalisation of the lower structure is probably long overdue'.[139] Similar to the introduction of the Hospital Plan, government officials were influenced by prevailing ideas relating to efficiencies and sought the committee to consider reforms that brought the 'most effective distribution and discharge of management duties'.[140] Such reforms were not new, and the 1955 Tanner Report called for HMC amalgamations. Still, neither the Authority nor the government of that time were willing to tackle such a contentious issue. O'Neill's quest for the rationalisation of public administration, however, brought renewed focus on HMCs.

The inquiry was influenced by developing managerialist ideas that emanated from business and industry. The Ministry appointed Dr Stuart Hawnt, an experienced education administrator, as chairman. The Minister, Morgan, recommended Hawnt because he was a 'non-political figure with real knowledge and experience of public administration' and was independent of existing hospital management and politics.[141] Other appointees to the inquiry foretold the Ministry's motivations. Increasingly, the government looked to Scotland, rather than England, as a framework for reshaping the health services. Robert Moore, secretary of the Scottish Hospital Staff Advisory Committee, was also appointed to the Working Party. In 1966, the Farquharson-Lang Report, which examined the administration of hospital boards in Scotland, was published. Significantly, this drew an analogy with industry, arguing that the Scottish Hospital Boards were akin to a board of directors, in which the chairman and members should concentrate on policymaking, with day-to-day management delegated to a chief executive with an administrative, rather than medical, background.[142] Such an approach, adopted by the SHHD, focused extensively on a managerial quest for greater efficiency and effectiveness, which emerged across the NHS, notably after the 1974 reorganisation.[143] This was a departure from the technocratic spirit, which focused on expertise, that pervaded much thinking in the NHS since its inception; instead, managerialism sought to implement corporate management approaches adopted from the private sector. Both technocracy and managerialism had the same goal in mind – a more rational, efficient and cost-effective delivery of services – but different rhetoric, approaches and, overtime, ideological underpinnings.

In an example of policy learning across the UK's different NHS systems, the Northern Irish Ministry was also interested in applying managerial techniques to healthcare. It sought an expert with a business background to join the Hawnt Committee, preferably from a large organisation that faced similar challenges to the Hospitals Authority, such as reconciling 'central control of policy with local initiative and the exercise[ing] of responsibility at dispersed units'. In turn, Reginald Garnsey, general manager of the Courtaulds – the UK business which was the world's largest textile manufacturer at this time – factory in Carrickfergus, was appointed to the Hawnt Committee.[144] The composition of the Working Party ensured that new techniques and modes of organisation, adapted from outside Northern Irish hospital policymaking, would shape the recommendations.

Business-oriented management ideas permeated the findings of what became known as the Hawnt Report, which was published in 1966. With a workforce of eighteen thousand and an annual budget of twenty-seven million pounds, the Hawnt Report compared the hospital services to a major industry. At the same time, it asserted that the recommended reforms would achieve a better financial economy and efficiency in the use of staff and facilities.[145] A business-orientated recommendation was the proposed appointment of a chief executive who would be responsible for the overall administration of the group and management duties. Medical superintendents – medics who were responsible for many administrative duties in hospitals – were to be phased out, and their tasks were to be shared among lay administrators.[146] Although in decline in England and Wales since 1948, medical superintendents historically managed hospitals whereby their medical status facilitated clear authority over lay and nursing administrations.[147] Non-medical staff traditionally had a lower status in hospitals, often considered as 'kindly technicians' who ensured the running of laundries, kitchens, accounts and medical records departments.[148] The Hawnt Report sought to enhance the authority of non-clinical staff with an emphasis on recruitment and training, which included management courses and promotion opportunities. Career opportunities for lay staff had progressed in Britain but were underdeveloped in Northern Ireland.[149] The Hawnt Report sought to reconfigure the relationship between lay and clinical staff by providing the former with enhanced professional status and adopting managerial structures and approaches.

The Hawnt Report's recommendations were the early beginnings of new public management techniques in Northern Ireland. It is commonly assumed that it was not until the 1980s that managers were introduced into the NHS, whereas previously, administrators were viewed as doctors' support staff with little independence.[150] New public management is generally considered to have emerged after the 1979 election of Margaret Thatcher's Conservative government and the subsequent implementation of policies overly influenced by free market principles, think tanks and management consultancies. These evolved with the election of New Labour in

1997 and the evolution of measurement methods of clinical and financial performance, ultimately aimed at cost management. This managerial revolution has been the focus of much criticism and seen by many academics as the root of many of the modern-day failures of the NHS.[151] Recent research, however, has argued that the shift from administration to management gradually took place over a more extended period and can be traced back to 1950s initiatives, such as the emergence of the NHS's national administrative training scheme.[152] By the 1960s, the Ministry of Health and Social Services in Northern Ireland began to promote managerial techniques, partly evident in the Hospital Plan, but most clearly articulated in the Hawnt Report. Such business-influenced managerialism sought greater power for professional managers to bring about better organisational performance.[153] This represented a new factor in hospital relations, very much reflective of the financial objectives of government, which challenged the older power structures in healthcare.

Inevitably, medical opposition emerged. Sensing a shift in authority to lay administrators and managers, medical interests felt the Hawnt Report threatened their power. The BMA favoured the maintenance of medical superintendents, emphasising that they were 'medically qualified' and key to maintaining 'close liaison between medical staff, lay administrators and the management committees'.[154] The consultant staff in the Royal Belfast Hospital for Sick Children informed the Ministry that the Report was 'completely erroneous' to conclude that lay administrators could take over the functions of medical administration. Medical superintendents, according to the consultants, provided 'impartial medical advice' and often assisted medics. At the same time, the reforms would result in more lay administrators whose lack of medical qualifications would impede hospitals.[155] Similarly, the Northern Ireland Hospital Junior Staff Group informed the Ministry that it had an 'unease' with the 'shift away from medical staff', believing that the proposed reforms would 'aggravate, if anything, the uncertainty and occasional misunderstandings between medical staff and administration'.[156] Some publicly aired these fears. Drs James Blundell and J. Lowry from the North Armagh HMC chastised the report's proposed new management structures in the *BMJ*, writing that the medical profession was heavily opposed to 'super managers', who would reduce the status of medical staff to mere 'hospital workers', undermine 'professional freedom' and jeopardise the doctor-patient relationship, ultimately leading to hospital practice becoming 'an unattractive and unrewarding career'.[157] More powerful administrators and managers threatened doctors' authority and status in hospital administration and such a proposed reform was inevitably opposed by the profession.

Government officials recognised the difficulties of implementing the Hawnt recommendations. Dugdale acknowledged that the BMA's concerns could not be brushed aside, although he believed they were overstated and 'partly misconceived'. Dugdale maintained that the inefficient and irrational use of medical resources would persist without reform.[158] There was also disagreement between the Ministry and the Hospitals Authority about the proposed reforms. Although the Authority approved of a chief executive, it refused to accept the cessation of medical superintendents in general hospitals, instead believing that more should be appointed.[159] Dugdale was far from happy with the Authority's position, informing Morgan that existing medical administration in HMCs led to the inefficient management of clinical resources.[160] Despite Dugdale's concerns, the proposals were shelved in a clear indication of the medical profession's continued power and influence over government policymaking. In the realpolitik of 1960s health politics, the potential of a new class of professional lay managers to run hospitals along managerial and business-inspired methods was limited by traditional medical stakeholder resistance.

One of the Hawnt Report's most controversial recommendations was the reduction of the existing twenty-nine hospital management committees to fifteen groupings and the disbandment of individual hospital committees. As outlined in the previous chapter, the Tanner Committee sought a reduction of hospital management committees, but by the mid-1960s, only three amalgamations were brought about.[161] Similarly to the proposals for managers in hospitals, the plans for further regrouping were met with much resistance. Medics feared the loss of power in their institutions if they were forced to come together with other hospitals.[162] Ian McClure agreed that greater coherence was necessary but did 'not like the shot-gun marriage in the grouping of certain hospitals'.[163] Politicians were quick to counter any perceived threat to local medical services. During a

Stormont debate, MPs criticised the proposals. Joseph Burns, the Ulster Unionist Party MP for the North Londonderry Constituency, argued that it should be left to individual committees to decide whether they wanted amalgamation.[164]

Local and parochial opposition also came to the fore. For example, the chairman of Mid-Antrim HMC, Dr Brian McHenry, claimed one hospital committee for three hospitals would be unwieldly and adversely affect the patients. Another committee member, A. A. K. Lewis, complained that 'local contacts, interests and sympathies' would be lost.[165] The Lisnaskea Rural Council in County Fermanagh objected to forced mergers, and one councillor, Thomas McPhillips, sought cross-political support, stating: 'orange and green should join together and fight for their rights on the green grassy slopes of the Erne'.[166] Reform and rationalisation of hospital management committees threatened local political power bases, influence and patronage. This generated much opposition to not just the immediate reforms but also to the wider programme of modernisation and rationalisation of public life inherent to the O'Neill premiership. Much opposition came from within Ulster unionism, often when unionist clientelism was in danger, although the Lisnaskea example illustrated that local protest could have a cross-political hue.[167]

Hawnt's recommended groupings had also become outdated in the context of nascent ideas on clinical areas which informed the 1966 Hospital Plan. As already highlighted, under the Plan, clinical services were to be organised around hospitals in the area. The Plan emphasised the need for the 'rational and harmonious ordering' of the administrative and clinical structures of the hospital services. However, it did not make any recommendations, waiting on the Hawnt Report, which hitherto was not completed.[168] The fifteen HMCs subsequently recommended by Hawnt were not aligned with the area hospitals envisaged under the Hospital Plan. This was seized on by opponents to Hawnt, such as McClure, who informed Stormont that there 'should be integration of administrative and of clinical effort'.[169] The lack of crossover between the Hawnt Report and Hospital Plan weakened the case for the implementation of the former's recommendations.

The Ministry now sought new groupings which would align hospital management committee restructuring with the area hospital concept. In 1968, Morgan informed the cabinet these were the 'key units of the future' and proposed new groupings which would align with area hospital catchment regions and emphasised that 'administration and clinical organisation will go hand in hand'. He chastised the existing large number of hospital management committees as inefficient and generating 'pressure' for nonviable piecemeal local developments. These new groupings were to have responsibility for one of the new area hospitals, access to well-qualified professional and technical staff and the ability to undertake 'far more important functions than most existing groups'. Morgan also believed that the new structure would facilitate the eventual reform of the existing tripartite division of health – hospitals, GPs and local authority – into a single service administered by area boards. Such an emphasis on fusing the various branches of the health services was reflective of emerging policy debates in Britain, ultimately leading to the NHS reorganisation in 1974. Morgan's plans in 1968 were ambitious and far exceeded Hawnt's recommendations.

Morgan was wary of the difficulties of implementing such radical administrative reforms. He advised against an elongated piecemeal approach which would only indicate 'deference to powerful vested interests' and optimistically sought the hastened completion of the regroupings by 1970. At the same time, Morgan recognised the 'drastic' nature of the proposals and the dangers of acting too quickly if the 'preponderance of opinion [was] heavily against them', recommending that they be initially trialled in the catchment area of the planned Craigavon Hospital.[170] Acute to the potential alienation of local, invariably unionist, interests, Morgan informed a meeting with the Association of Hospital Management Committees that any proposals were not 'a cut and dried scheme' but the basis of further consultation in which local committees would be given every opportunity to put forward their viewpoint. Morgan wrote to Thomas Brown, the chairman of Hospitals Authority, stating that 'detailed consultations' were to be undertaken with each HMC.[171] Morgan sought reform but was also apprehensive about the political backlash. He attempted to bring about change through consultation, which contrasted with his bullish and top-down introduction of the 1966 Hospital Plan.

Regrouping was trialled in the proposed Central Hospital Management Committee which intended to amalgamate six hospital management committees (Banbridge and Dromore, North

Armagh, South Armagh, St Luke's, South Tyrone and South Down) in the catchment of the soon to be built Craigavon Area Hospital under the management of a chief executive officer. Unsurprisingly, resistance emerged. The chairman of the South Tyrone HMC, T. G. Eakins, ridiculed the trialled regrouping because 'it centred on a hospital [Craigavon] which did not exist and quite frankly they thought that they were being asked to consider something which meant absolutely nothing at all'.[172] Other HMCs in the proposed trial grouping were equally incongruous.[173] The Hospitals Authority and Ministry's attempt to bring about consolidation through consultation with individual committees brought little success.

The O'Neill government's capacity to implement its rationalising and modernising agenda was restricted. Hawnt's recommendations offered the rationalisation of public administration, which was one of the government's key objectives. Greater managerial power and techniques, along with large, merged hospital management committees, were policies that promised to deliver the ever-elusive efficient use of resources to squeeze the greatest possible healthcare outcomes out of inevitably finite resources.[174] Yet the government was unable to implement these reforms successfully for much of the late 1960s, and it succumbed to localism, individual hospital loyalty and the medical profession. These dynamics marked the development of hospitals since the establishment of Northern Ireland. Although the modernistic emphasis on rationality, efficiency and expertise capitulated central government to the fore of hospital planning and administration, the long-standing stakeholders continued to have much influence over hospital policy. The weakness of the Ministry also pointed to a wider fragmentation of Ulster unionism during O'Neill's modernisation era.

Integration and the outbreak of the Troubles

The policymaking arena in Northern Ireland was drastically changed with the outbreak of the Troubles and the widespread civil unrest, political instability and violence which engulfed the region. The Troubles had an unprecedented impact on the delivery of health services, chiefly emergency care. Many had difficulty accessing hospitals that were in areas that were the focus of upheaval, such as doctors in the Royal Victoria in republican west Belfast who reported being caught in gun battles on their way from work in the late 1960s.[175] This monograph does not overly concentrate on the impact of the Troubles on the delivery of health services. While traditionally under-researched in the historiography of Northern Ireland, the work of the historian Ruth Duffy provides a highly original and in-depth exploration of the impact of the Troubles on healthcare and medical professionals.[176]

Instead, the remainder of this chapter analyses health policy developments in the early 1970s. The Troubles compelled the Northern Irish government, under much pressure from Westminster, to introduce radical reforms to address many of the inequalities suffered by nationalists and Catholics under unionist rule since 1921. Much of the nationalist discontent with the health services lay in the failure of the state to support the Mater Hospital. The appointment of Terence O'Neill as Prime Minister helped relations, although in 1964, backbench unionist opposition to funding the institution delayed action. Morgan and the Mater entered negotiations, which lasted several years, and a meeting of the parliamentary Unionist Party in 1967 finally agreed to provide state aid to the hospital based on protection for its religious character.[177] There was no easy solution, and it was not until January 1971 that the cabinet, largely overwhelmed with the disorder of the period, approved an agreement for the hospital to enter the health services.[178]

The need for reform of local government, long the source of discrimination against Catholics, was highlighted by the Cameron Commission (established by the Governor of Northern Ireland on behalf of the British government in 1969 to examine the worsening political and civil conditions), which forced the Northern Irish government to act finally. This also led to a greater focus on the administration of health services. In June 1969, the cabinet agreed to publish a Green Paper on plans to reform the health services in line with local government change. The newly appointed Minister of Health and Social Services, W. K. Fitzsimmons, informed the cabinet that the likelihood of local government reform, including the disbandment of county councils and bodies with health and welfare responsibilities, necessitated health reforms.[179]

The winds of health reform also blew from Britain where policy developments were moving towards the integration of health services. At its worst, the tripartite system led to a multitude of entities that nearly surpassed pre-NHS dysfunctionality and was viewed as having ineffective and overly complicated management structures. As the NHS historian Charles Webster has argued, it was inevitable that at some stage the longer-term viability of the tripartite system of administration would come into question.[180] For specific categories of patients, specifically older people with complex care plans, difficulties persisted in providing comprehensive and coordinated care across hospital authorities, GPs and local authorities.[181] Reorganisation of the NHS in Britain came to the fore of debates after the Porritt Report in 1962. Potential reorganisation was delineated in Westminster Green Papers in 1968 and 1970. Multiple consultative papers ultimately led to the 1973 NHS Reorganisation Act for England and Wales, while similar legislation was introduced for Scotland. The focus of reform in Britain influenced Northern Ireland. In 1969 Fitzsimmons acknowledged that 'widespread public discussion' in Britain led to 'growing pressure to make known the Government's views on these matters locally'.[182]

Fitzsimmons' Green Paper went further than Morgan's 1967 plans and proposed the replacement of the existing structures – Hospitals Authority, twenty-nine HMCs, Special Care Management Committees, General Health Services Board and eight local authority Health Committees – with three to five boards. It was envisaged that there would be a single-tier system working directly under the central government in a structure in which the role of the latter would be significantly enlarged; this also proposed the removal of an intermediary body such as the Hospitals Authority. The Green Paper also focused on the potential alignment of health services with relevant social services provided by local authorities, such as care for the elderly, home assistance and child welfare.[183] Although the Green Paper merely sought 'consultation' on the potential to align health and social services, it indicated that the government was considering significant reform.[184] By 1970, the Minister, Fitzsimmons, proposed an even more radical measure, the complete consolidation of social and medical personal services under five area boards, which went further than similar reforms in Britain, where the focus was solely on medical services. Fitzsimmons and the Ministry were emboldened by the Macrory Report, published in 1970, which recommended widespread reform of local government.[185] With the reorganisation of local government social services inevitable, Fitzsimmons maintained the proposed merger would ensure that health and social services were 'planned together and integrat[ed] in their day-to-day' management, allowing for their 'coordinated development' and 'efficient economy'.[186] This was ultimately agreed to and formed the basis of the 1972 Health and Social Services Act Order, which uniquely merged social and medical services in Northern Ireland.

The convergence of health and social services is now viewed as the ultimate goal of health organisation and has been at the heart of health reforms throughout the late twentieth and early twenty-first centuries. Northern Ireland's introduction of a combined health and social services predated similar reforms in Britain by decades. The changes took the logic of rationalisation further than in Britain in the early 1970s, where there was no real debate over local government social services in health reform. The Northern Irish reform has been viewed as allowing for better and more efficient, cost-effective and comprehensive provision.[187] Hospital planners in the 1940s, post-war technocracy and O'Neill's ill-fated hospital reform agenda all sought to rationalise services but were hampered by stakeholder resistance. The reform of the early 1970s, however, achieved a degree of rationalisation which was unprecedented not just in Northern Ireland but across the UK.

The Ministry hired the management consultancy firm Booz, Allen and Hamilton to design the new services in Northern Ireland. Policymakers increasingly turned to management consultants to fill gaps in capacity or manpower and to bring expertise that was believed not to be available in government.[188] The leading American management consultancy firm McKinsey advised the Irish Republic's government in 1971 on the management of its recently established health board system.[189] McKinsey was also heavily involved in the 1973 NHS reorganisation in Britain and became synonymous with the reform's subsequent failures.[190] In Northern Ireland, since the 1960s, the government increasingly turned to management consultants to deliver key projects for the welfare state. The NBA management services firm project managed the Craigavon Development Commission and was charged with the synchronisation of the planning and development of the new town. In 1966, the Hospitals Authority also turned to the NBA to project manage the design and construction of the new five million pounds Craigavon Hospital. The management consultants oversaw its design, pricing, selection of building contractors and 'commissioning of the hospital' with equipment, staff and transfer of services. The on-site NBA consultant reviewed progress daily while weekly meetings were held with the architect. The NBA's methods appeared successful when the hospital opened in 1972, less than six years since their appointment. Hospitals of that scale usually took ten years to build.[191] The use of professional consultants further illustrated the early tentacles of new public management, previously highlighted by the Hawnt Report, in health administration in Northern Ireland.

Booz, Allen and Hamilton provided the structure for the new service. Four area boards (Belfast and South-Eastern Area, North-Eastern Area, Western Area and Southern Area) were established. Members were appointed by the Ministry and were to be representative of a broad range of interests, including 30 per cent from professional backgrounds, 30 per cent from the lower tier, district councils, while the remainder would be appointed after consultation with other interests such as universities, industry, trade unions and voluntary bodies. Each board had three principal officers, including a chief administrative medical officer, director of social services, and secretary. The chief medical officer had general oversight of the health of the population and responsibility for organising the professional aspects of all the health services.[192] The creation of the National Health Service in Northern Ireland resulted from negotiations, political tensions and concessions, leading to piecemeal measures which ultimately undermined the coherent organisation of services. In contrast, the shaping of the new structure in the early 1970s by external management consultants reflected the emphasis on management principles, supposedly free from political and stakeholder influence.

Why did Northern Ireland reform?

It is widely considered that the Northern Irish reforms of the early 1970s had more to do with circumstance than any forward-looking health policy or planning on the part of Northern Irish officials or politicians of an ultimately failed political entity. It is believed that the merging of medical and social services was brought about by a reaction to the critical necessity to reorganise local government, in which social services were politicised, marked by sectarianism and a significant source of Catholic grievance. For example, Deirdre Heenan, a public administration and social policy scholar, argues that

> the original decision was not informed by theoretical models of healthcare, but by an urgent need to reorganise the system of local government, which had become widely discredited. There was little awareness that this model of reorganisation, which was given a cautious, lukewarm welcome by healthcare professionals, would become viewed by many policymakers, politicians and academics as the holy grail.[193]

Similarly, political scientist Scott Greer views the reforms as an attempt to address systematic discrimination by local government, which was introduced by a Stormont regime that was desperate to modernise and less concerned with developing enhanced health and social services.[194]

Within the context of Northern Ireland's descent into political and civil unrest and the government's belated efforts to address the deep-rooted causes of the conflict, the perspective that the reforms were the floundering attempts of a discredited regime to save itself is understandable. This analysis, however, fails to fully account for the significant changes in health, especially hospital care, in Northern Ireland since the introduction of the National Health Service in 1948; these, it is argued here, paved the way for the reforms of the early 1970s. For much of the early post-war decades Northern Ireland's hospital policies were shaped by slow and gradual reform, which challenged social conservatism and traditional stakeholder power. The central state's attempts at reform, often couched in the rhetoric of modernisation and planning, sought to bring about greater collaboration, efficiency and rationalisation. While this monograph has described how many efforts at reform by central government policymakers ultimately failed, the outbreak of the Troubles created a policy environment in which radical change was possible, and stakeholder resistance overcome. In this sense, the reforms of the early 1970s have had a longer trajectory than previously understood by historians and political and social scientists, dating back to at least the 1940s and reenergised in the early 1960s by O'Neill's reformist unionism.

The joining of health and social services had also been a policy concern in Northern Ireland long before the crisis of the late 1960s. This was evident in geriatric care. As already highlighted, the Belfast and Ballymena older care units worked closely with local welfare authorities to ensure that rehabilitated patients continued to receive provision after treatment, when needed, demonstrating an early, localised approach to systemised social and medical care.[195] In 1956, the hospitals jointly acquired a convalescent home which acted as a half-way house for cases that no longer needed medical attention.[196] Belfast and Ballymena's efforts reflected the BMA's 1940s reports that called for the diagnosis and classification of older sick people in hospitals, and their subsequent discharge, depending on need and sickness, to long-stay annexes, residential homes and domiciles.[197] As already explained in this chapter, the Hospitals Authority, spearheaded by George Adams, made progress in aligning medical and social services for older people. The Authority wanted to align hospital reform with geriatric care, and in 1964 Adams undertook a review of 'geriatric services', which mapped existing provision and needs against notional clinical areas.[198] A subsequent review in 1969, also conducted by Adams, asserted that social and medical services were 'closely interdependent' for the care of older people and needed to be aligned.[199] Ideas about integrating medical and social care for older people were well developed in Northern Ireland by a strong and innovative gerontology field which had developed since the 1940s.

Early focus on the harmonisation of medical and social services was not solely on unifying older care. The emergence of new medical fields and academic disciplines, including gerontology, psychiatry and preventive and social medicine, had brought many patient groups in need of complex and holistic medical and social care to the fore in the post-war years. Since the 1950s, the Hospitals Authority was concerned about consolidating primary and secondary care, and in 1954, it recommended greater communication between hospitals and GPs in the post-hospital treatment of patients.[200] The 1966 Hospital Plan focused on the importance of harmonisation between welfare authorities, GPs and hospitals. The

Plan's establishment of the Northern Ireland Health and Welfare Services Liaison Committee – chaired by the minister and including representatives from all medical and welfare services – sought to streamline services in the short and long term.[201] Policymakers in Northern Ireland had long been interested in developing such care, a focus that predated the outbreak of the Troubles.

Influential figures supported a more systematic approach when it was proposed in the early 1970s. John Pemberton, chair of social and preventive medicine in Queen's University, championed the combination of medical and social services, believing that the medical profession understood that social action was key to preventing much illness. Pemberton valued collaboration, stating that the joint administration will make 'each service more fully aware of [what] the other can do in the prevention, treatment and management of diseases'.[202] Integration was, at one level, a victory for social and preventive medicine, which was well-developed in Northern Ireland. Leading members of the Hospitals Authority also tended to connect medical and social services. Thomas Brown became the Hospitals Authority's chairman in 1967; he had a strong background in social care and was previously the chairman of Belfast Council of Social Welfare.[203] Individuals such as Pemberton and Brown were strong advocates for a joined-up system. They were well positioned to support the opportunity to implement the radical reforms that the turmoil of the era presented.

Yet, what was different in the late 1960s and early 1970s was the capacity of policymakers to force through reforms previously out of the grasp of a modernising officialdom. Periods of crisis, whether political, social or medical, have often created propitious circumstances for reform which would otherwise be difficult to introduce. Indeed, the creation of the NHS in the UK in 1948 owed much to the Emergency Medical Service, established to respond to air attacks during the Second World War, which succeeded in rapidly overcoming decades of policy inertia and provided a blueprint for the new service. One study of eleven countries identified upheavals (financial crises, pandemics and post-Second World War reconstruction) as creating favourable policy conditions to establish universal healthcare systems and overcome interest group resistance.[204] The crisis of the Troubles provided what the comparative healthcare political scientist Carolyn Tuohy describes as a 'window of opportunity' to bring about significant reforms.[205] The Troubles created circumstances in which the balance of power between stakeholders and the state was realigned. This allowed the government, mainly its civil service, to introduce radical administrative reform, which previously proved difficult to bring about, such as when the Hawnt recommendations faltered.

The state's newfound capacity to overcome traditional stakeholder resistance to reform was evident on multiple occasions. The Northern Ireland Association of Hospital Management Committees, often one of the most recalcitrant stakeholders to centralisation, attempted to lobby the Ministry to protect 'peripheral management', a euphemism for individual hospital power, but was ineffective.[206] Similarly, the BMA pressed the government to alter the proposed structure of four area boards directly under the Ministry. Echoing the medical profession's stance during the negotiations over the 1948 Health Services Act, the BMA wanted to create a single central authority, like the Hospitals Authority. Although the BMA claimed that area boards would lead to geographical fragmentation in health services and competition between 'rival bureaucracies', its major fear was the medical profession's potential loss of independence. In discussions with the Ministry, the BMA believed that a central authority would act as a 'buffer' between the Ministry and the profession, helping to avoid power resting with civil servants and preventing health services becoming politicised.[207] The Ministry rejected these assertions, informing the BMA that the proposed area board system avoided the duplication of function and responsibility between the Ministry and Hospitals Authority, which became more evident as the former assumed greater power since the early 1960s.

The Ministry defended its proposals in the context of the ongoing political and civil upheaval of the Troubles. It claimed that the reforms were aligned with the ongoing Macrory inquiry and maintained, somewhat meretriciously, that the health proposals were part of the wider reform of the Northern Irish government, which was key to the 'future political stability of the province as a whole'.[208] The Ministry was quick to use the ongoing Troubles as a reason for reform. Still, the new health structures had more to do with the government looking to centralise authority than the alleviation of communal tensions by aligning health and local government reform. The decisions to reject the BMA's demands to create a buffer authority between central government and boards had nothing to do with addressing Catholic inequality. Instead, it aimed to consolidate control in the Ministry and diminish the influence of medical professionals and hospitals. In 1971, Fitzsimmons, the Minister for Health and Social Services, rejected the BMA's calls for a single central authority. While stressing that he was 'anxious' that the 'cooperative relationship' between the Ministry and BMA would continue, the rebuttal of the latter's requests represented central government's newfound capacity to resist stakeholder influence.

Conclusion

The appointment of Terence O'Neill brought a reforming zeal to central government, which increasingly targeted the power of the Hospitals Authority and sought to enhance the government's role in health policymaking and management. Spearheaded by the newly established Ministry of Health and Social Services, with leading O'Neill loyalists like Morgan and supported by dedicated and energised civil servants, above all Norman Dugdale, attempts at reform were initiated. Couched in the lexicon of modernisation and rationalisation and influenced by nascent managerial techniques, central government attempted to bring about efficiencies in administration, budgets and hospital building. The Hawnt Report and 1966 Hospital Plan sought to restructure hospital services in Northern Ireland. Some of these measures provoked a hostile reaction. Hawnt's proposals to restructure hospital management committees were obstructed by long-standing medical power brokers, including the medical profession, particularly elite consultants. Furthermore, individual hospitals and hospital management committees, supported by local political activity, further curtailed these central government-led measures. The reforms also generated much political opposition, especially from local unionists fearful of the loss of local services and patronage. Such a political reaction was not confined to reform of hospital management; attempts to rationalise other areas of public administration, notably local government, generated much opposition to the modernising O'Neill-led government from within unionism.

Yet, the O'Neill premiership was successful in implementing other reforms of the hospital services. The Hospital Plan revised the Hospitals Authority's building programme, which laid the bedrock of the area hospital concept and shaped the hospital services for years to come. The Plan's initial focus on two major developments – Craigavon and Belfast City Hospital – led to the abandonment and/or postponement of several other high-profile building projects, which also provoked much hostility. Although Northern Ireland's political divisions were increasingly embittered, local reaction to central government health policies often led to cross-party social protest; this was the case in Downpatrick where the Ministry's decision not to develop the local hospital led to widespread nationalist and unionist protest. In other areas, such as Coleraine, cracks emerged within unionism and reneged promises to build new hospitals led to much local and political opposition. Politics continued to shape the debate on health reform.

The Hospital Plan's decision to invest in Belfast City Hospital and the deferment of the RVH's redevelopment represented a significant shift in power in Belfast and Northern Ireland's medical power base. The emergence of new specialisms, greater diversity in the background of consultants and the development of services outside Belfast diluted the prominence of the Royal Victoria and the Grosvenor Road medical site. Central government was now able to challenge the power of the former medical voluntary hospitals, which initially won major concessions from the government at the establishment of the health services in 1948. The political project of the O'Neill government's modernisation agenda brought central government to the fore of health and hospital policy.

The outbreak of the Northern Irish Troubles created circumstances which allowed central government to introduce radical reforms which exceeded similar NHS reorganisation in Britain. Integration under the 1972 Health and Social Services Order has been viewed as resulting from the unrest and need for reform brought about by the Troubles. Little credit is given to Northern Irish policymakers. Yet the trajectory of consolidation policies predated the Troubles. It can be traced to developments in the 1950s and 1960s emanating from the Hospitals Authority's focus on care for older people and the emergence of preventive and social medicine in Queen's University's Medical School. Modernity, the zeitgeist of public administration of the 1950s and 1960s, increasingly sought a rationalised, planned and efficient hospital system and became influential in Northern Ireland. While Altnagelvin and Nuffield House were flagship projects of the Hospitals Authority, which projected the supposed rationality of the new age, the reforming O'Neill government increasingly viewed the body as ineffective and sought to centralise power. This was evidenced in the 1966 Hospital Plan, which essentially removed the Authority's responsibility for the hospital building programme and placed the Ministry at the forefront of hospital planning and policy. Other administrative reforms proved elusive, and O'Neill's government was incapable of overcoming many of the stakeholders in hospitals. It was not until the outbreak of the Troubles that the equilibrium swung favourably to central government, providing the window of opportunity to create a joined-up system based on perceived administrative efficiency and rationality. The Ministry and its civil servants now had an unprecedented degree of power in health policy, service delivery and management. The 1972 reforms effectively reversed the settlement between the state, medical profession and hospitals achieved in 1948, which limited the role of central government. The reforms were the embodiment of a new managerialism promoted by the Ministry, its civil service and policymakers aligned with an emerging class of managers. This new alliance was strengthened by the newfound faith in public administration of methods and rhetoric from business, embodied by the appointment of the consultancy firm Booz, Allen and Hamilton to design the new system. Ironically, the proroguing of the Northern Ireland parliament in 1972, followed by its ultimate dissolution in 1973, meant that the unionist government never got to administer the reformed service.

Notes

1 MHLG, *Report on Health and Local Government Administration in Northern Ireland for the Year 1951*, p. 16.

2 For a biography of Abel-Smith, see S. Sheard, *The Passionate Economist: How Brian Abel-Smith Shaped Global Health and Social Welfare* (Bristol: Policy Press, 2013).

3 C. Ham, *Health Policy in Britain: The Politics and Organisation of the National Health Services* (5th ed. Basingstoke, Palgrave Macmillan, 2004), pp. 16–17.

4 Webster, *The National Health Service*, p. 57; also see Lowe, *Welfare State*, p. 193.

5 Elder, 'The Health Services of Northern Ireland', 106.

6 P. Buckland, *A History of Northern Ireland* (Dublin: Gill and Macmillan, 1981), pp. 162–3.

7 Lawrence, 'The health services', 302, 308.

8 PRONI, HOS/1/1/184, NIHA records, Appointment of HMCs, Extract of the minutes of the Coleraine and Portrush HMC meeting, 17 April 1950.

9 MHLG, *Report on Health and Local Government Administration in Northern Ireland, 1947–49*, pp. 73–4.

10 Tanner Report, p. 19.

11 *NIHA Annual Report for 1955*, p. 13.

12 NIHA, *Report of the Special Committee on the Hospital and Specialist Services with the Authority's Observations thereon* (Belfast: HMSO, 1954), p. 23.

13 A. Gilig, *Planning in Britain: Understanding and Evaluating the Post-War System* (London: Sage, 2005), p. 2.

14 V. Bates, *Making Noise in the Hospital* (Cambridge: Cambridge University Press, 2021).

15 NPHT, *Studies in the Functions and Designs of Hospitals: The Report of an Investigation sponsored by the NPHT and the University of Bristol* (Oxford: Oxford University Press, 1955), pp. 143–4.

16 NIHA, *NIHA Annual Report for the Year Ending 1952* (Belfast, 1953), p. 38.

17 P. Harron, *Architects of Ulster: Young & Mackenzie – A Transformational Provincial Practice, 1850–1960* (Belfast: Ulster Architectural Heritage Society, 2016).

18 S. V. Ward, *Planning and Urban Change* (London: Sage, 2nd edn., 2004), p. 93.

19 Gilg, *Planning in Britain*, p. 2.

20 J. Hughes, 'The "Matchboxes on a Muffin": The design of hospitals in the early NHS', *Medical History*, 44 (2000), 33, 41.

21 C. W. Kidd, 'Medical aspects of hospital planning', *UMJ*, 25:2 (November 1956), 81; for an outline of Kidd's career, see 'C. W. Kidd: Obituary', *BMJ*, 290:6472 (23 March 1985), 938.

22 N. T. J. Bailey, 'Operation research in medicine', *Operational Research Quarterly*, 3:2 (1952), 24; for the historical development of operational research see M. W. Kirby, *Operational Research in War*

and Peace: The British Experience from the 1930s to 1970s (London: Imperial College Press, 2003).

23 S. Davis, 'Promoting productivity in the National Health Service, 1950 to 1966', *Contemporary British History*, 31:1 (2017), 51–3.

24 NPHT, *Studies*.

25 S. Francis, R. Glanville, A. Noble and P. Scher, *50 Years of Ideas in Health Care Buildings* (London: Nuffield Trust, 1999), p. 15.

26 D. Theodore, 'Treating architectural research: The Nuffield Trust and the post-war hospital', *Journal of Architecture*, 24:7 (2019), 987–8.

27 NPHT, *Studies*, p. xix.

28 NIHA, *NIHA Annual Report for Year ending March 1950* (Belfast: NIHA, 1951), p. 71.

29 Kidd, 'Medical aspects of hospital planning', 83.

30 Kidd, 'Medical aspects of hospital planning', 96.

31 NPHT, *Studies*, p. viii.

32 Kidd, 'Medical aspects of hospital planning', 81; NPHT, *Studies*, p. xix.

33 V. D. Allison, 'Hospital central sterile supply departments', *BMJ*, 2:5201 (10 September 1960), 772–8.

34 *BT*, 27 January 1959.

35 McLachlan, *A History of the NPHT*, p. 110.

36 Hughes, 'The "matchbox on a muffin"', pp. 43, 55.

37 For example, McKinney and J. H. Jones, chair and secretary of the NIHA respectively, presented a paper entitled 'Mental well-being of the patient in the General Hospital' at the Ninth International Hospital Congress, while Jones presented another paper called 'The management of the Hospital; duties of the Chief Administrative Officer to the patient; and the effects on the patient of economic and financial stringency', see *NIHA Annual Report for 1955*, p. 75.

38 PRONI, CAB/4/1328/11, Cabinet Secretariat/Cabinet Conclusions, Third draft Hospital Plan for Northern Ireland, 1966–75, p. 33.

39 NIHA, *The Development of Hospital and Specialist Services*, p. 36.

40 MHLG and NIHA, *Summary of the Hospital Building Programme of the NIHA, March 1963* (Belfast: HMSO, 1963), foreword; NIHA, *The Development of Hospital and Specialist Services*, p. 44.

41 NIHA, *The Development of Hospital and Specialist Services*, p. 80.

42 NIHA, *The Development of Hospital and Specialist Services*, p. 67.

43 *BT*, 8 October 1963.

44 P. Bew and J. Bew, 'War and peace in Northern Ireland: 1965–2016', in T. Bartlett (ed.), *The Cambridge History of Ireland: Volume 4, 1800 to the Present* (Cambridge: Cambridge University Press, 2018), p. 445; M. Mullholand, 'O'Neill, Terence Marne', in *DIB*, https://www.

dib.ie/biography/oneill-terence-marne-a6940 (accessed 20 November 2024).

45 M. Mulholland, *Northern Ireland at the Crossroads: Ulster Unionism in the O'Neill Years 1960–69* (Basingstoke: Macmillan Press, 2000), p. 34.

46 F. Cochrane, '"Meddling at the crossroads": The decline and fall of Terence O'Neill within the Unionist community', in R. English and G. Walker (eds), *Unionism in Modern Ireland: New Perspectives on Politics and Culture* (Basingstoke: Palgrave, 1996), p. 160.

47 M. Glendinning, '"The Forgotten Revolution": Northern Ireland's heritage of modern reconstruction', *The Journal of Architecture*, 15:5 (2010), 621–36.

48 A. Grant, '"Everything was concrete": The everyday impacts of planning and urban development policy before and during the Troubles', in L. McAtackney and M. Ó Catháin, *The Routledge Handbook of the Northern Ireland Conflict and Peace* (London: Routledge, 2023), p. 147.

49 *BT*, 30 October 1964.

50 PRONI, HSS/11/43/28, Ministry of Health and Social Services [hereafter MHSS], Royal Maternity Hospital: Allegations made by H. I. McClure, J. Gillingham, Sec of MHLG, 9 November 1964; *BT*, 10 November 1964.

51 *BT*, 13 November 1964.

52 PRONI, CAB/4/1278, Cabinet Secretariat/Cabinet Conclusions, Northern Ireland Hospitals Authority and Royal Maternity Hospital – notice of motion, 18 November 1964.

53 Gray, 'Government and the administration of hospital services in Northern Ireland', 230.

54 *Ibid.*

55 PRONI, HSS/11/43/32, MHSS, Hawnt Committee [Joint Working Party on Relationships between the NIHA and MHCs], Norman Dugdale, Senior Assistant Secretary, HSS, to A. A. Hughes, Scottish Home and Health Department, 15 December 1964.

56 *BT*, 25 November 1964.

57 O'Leary, *A Treatise on Northern Ireland; Volume* 2, p. 165.

58 Klein, *The New Politics of the NHS*, p. 48.

59 H. Patterson, 'Craig, William', in *DIB*, www.dib.ie/biography/craig-william-bill-a9999 (accessed 20 November 2024).

60 For a positive account of these administrative reforms from a leading civil servant, see J. A., Oliver, *Working at Stormont: Memories by John Andrew Oliver* (Dublin: Irish Public Administration, 1978), pp. 84–90.

61 G. O'Hara, *From Dreams to Disillusionment: Economic and Social Planning in 1960s Britain* (Basingstoke: Palgrave Macmillan, 2007), p. 25.
62 O'Hara, *From Dreams to Disillusionment*, p. 92.
63 Mohan, *Planning*, p. 123.
64 Davis, 'Promoting productivity in the NHS', 51; O'Hara, *From Dreams to Disillusionment*, p. 184.
65 Webster, *The National Health Service*, p. 45.
66 Mohan, *Planning*, p. 120.
67 NIHA, *NIHA Annual Report for the Year Ending 1965* (Belfast: NIHA, 1966), p. 10.
68 *BT*, 8 October 1965.
69 Ministry of Finance, *Report by Organisation and Methods Branch Ministry of Finance: NIHA, Review of Headquarters Administration* (Belfast: HMSO, 1965), p. 3.
70 *Report by Organisation and Methods Branch*, p. 2.
71 N. Robson, 'Adapting not adopting: 1958–74: Accounting and managerial "reform" in the early NHS', *Accounting, Business and Financial History*, 17:3 (2007), 455.
72 PRONI, CAB/4/1328/11, Cabinet Secretariat/Cabinet Conclusions, Third draft hospital plan for Northern Ireland, 1966–75, p. 3.
73 *Ibid.*, p. 4.
74 Gray, 'Government and the administration of hospital services in Northern Ireland', 292.
75 PRONI, HSS/13/22/15, 'Hospital plan', Dugdale to HSS Secretary, 22 July 1965.
76 Dugdale was also a poet of much acclaim, see N. Allen, 'Dugdale, Norman', in *DIB*, www.dib.ie/biography/dugdale-norman-a2819 (accessed 20 November 2024).
77 P. Devlin, *Straight Left: An Autobiography* (Belfast: Blackstaff Press, 1993), p. 215
78 PRONI, HOS/1/1/776, NIHA Records, The Hospital Plan for Northern Ireland, Dugdale to W. J. Gillingham, NIHA 31 August 1965; Dugdale to Gillingham, 3 November 1965.
79 PRONI, HOS/1/1/776, NIHA Records, Meeting between representatives of the NIHA and MHSS, 3 December 1965.
80 PRONI, HSS/13/22/15, MHSS, Hospital Plan, Dugdale to R. H. Kidd, Ministry of Finance, 7 February 1966.
81 PRONI, CAB/4/1328/12, Cabinet Secretariat/Cabinet Conclusions, Hospital Plan 1966–1975: Memorandum by the Minister of Health and Social Services. J Morgan, 31 March 1966.

82 PRONI, CAB/4/1328/14, Cabinet Secretariat, Cabinet Conclusions, Notes.
83 PRONI, CAB/4/1328/11, Cabinet Secretariat, Cabinet Conclusions, third draft hospital plan for Northern Ireland, 1966–75.
84 MHSS, *Hospital Plan for Northern Ireland 1966–75* (Belfast: HSMO, 1966) p. 18.
85 MHSS, *Hospital Plan*, pp. 19–20.
86 PRONI, HOS1/1/474, NIHA Records, Sub-Committee on Social and Preventive Medicine, 4 May 1954.
87 MHSS, *Hospital Plan*, p. 20.
88 MHSS, *Hospital Plan*, pp. 28, 35.
89 R. H. Matthew, *Belfast Regional Survey and Plan 1962: A Report Prepared for the Government of Northern Ireland* (Belfast: HMSO, 1964); B. Morrison, 'Planning the city; planning the region', in F. W. Boal and S. A. Royle (eds), *Enduring City: Belfast in the Twentieth Century* (Belfast: Blackstaff Press, 2006), pp. 141–54; A. G. McClelland, 'A "ghastly interregnum": The struggle for architectural heritage conservation in Belfast before 1972', *Urban History*, 41:1 (2018), 157.
90 PRONI, CAB/4/1328/12, Cabinet Secretariat/Cabinet Conclusions, Hospital Plan 1966–75: Memorandum by the Minister of Health and Social Services, 31 March 1966.
91 MHSS, *Hospital Plan*, pp. 10, 17.
92 Mulholland, *Northern Ireland at the Crossroads*, p. 52; G. Legg, 'Contradictory capitalism, geographical inertia and the New City of Craigavon', *The Irish Review*, 52 (2016), 4.
93 Glendinning, 'The Forgotten Revolution', p. 633.
94 A. Alexander, *Britain's New Towns: Garden Cities to Sustainable Communities* (Abingdon: Routledge, 2009), p. 48.
95 A. Jackson, *Ireland 1798–1998: War, Peace and Beyond* (Oxford: Wiley-Blackwell, 2nd ed., 2010), p. 359; O'Leary, *A Treatise on Northern Ireland: Volume 2*, p. 167.
96 MHLG, *Summary of the Hospital Building Programme*, pp. 65–100.
97 Norton, *The Politics of Constitutional Nationalism*, p. 143.
98 MHLG, *Summary of the Hospital Building Programme*, pp. 36–7.
99 MHLG, *Summary of the Hospital Building Programme*, p. 12.
100 MHLG, *Summary of the Hospital Building Programme*, p. 21.
101 For an account of the policies of the Northern Ireland Housing Trust, see M. Elliott, *Heartlands: A Memoir of the White City Housing Estate in Belfast* (Belfast: Blackstaff Press, 2018).
102 MHLG, *Summary of the Hospital Building Programme*, p. 10.
103 MHLG, *Summary of the Hospital Building Programme*, p. 13.

104 MHLG, *Summary of the Hospital Building Programme*, p. 23.
105 *SC*, 9 July 1966.
106 *BT*, 31 May 1966.
107 *BT*, 31 May 1966.
108 Mulholland, *Northern Ireland at a Crossroads*, p. 53; *BT*, 23 June 1966.
109 S. Campbell, 'New Nationalism? The SDLP and the creation of a socialist and labour party in Northern Ireland, 1969–75', *IHS*, 38:151 (May 2013), 425.
110 PRONI, HOS1/1/776, NIHA Records, Hospital Plan for Northern Ireland – papers, minutes and correspondence [this file has a series of letters to the NIHA protesting the Downpatrick decision].
111 *BT*, 14 June 1966; for Perceval-Price's election result, see *BT*, 26 May 1962.
112 *BT*, 30 June 1966.
113 PRONI, HOS/1/1/776, NIHA Records, Coleraine and Portrush HMC to NIHA, 13 May 1966; *BT*, 12 May 1966.
114 For Loughridge as president of the Ulster Medical Society see J. S. Loughridge, 'What of the future? Presidential address to the Ulster Medical Society', *UMJ*, 34:2 (December 1965), 53–65.
115 *BT*, 13 June 1966.
116 Shepherd, 'Hospital relationships', 16.
117 *BT*, 11 August 1967.
118 Gray, 'Government and the administration of hospital services in Northern Ireland', pp. 315–16.
119 Ibid, pp. 342–9.
120 J. Greer, 'The Paisleyites: from protest movement to electoral breakthrough', *The Sixties: A Journal of History, Politics and Culture* (2:2), 187–205.
121 PRONI, CAB/4/1328/11, Cabinet Secretariat/Cabinet Conclusions, Third draft hospital plan for Northern Ireland, 1966–75, p. 2.
122 NPHT, *Survey of the Hospital Services of Northern Ireland*, p. 48.
123 B. M. Walker, *A Political History of the Two Irelands: From Partition to Peace* (Basingstoke: Palgrave Macmillan, 2012), p. 69.
124 MHLG, *Summary of the Hospital Building Programme*, p. 10.
125 The National Archives, Kew, FD 9/707, Employment of consultants: comparison of joint appointments by the Queen's University, Belfast and the NIHA, 1963.
126 Gorsky, 'To regulate and confirm inequality?'; P. Thane, *Old Age in English History: Past Experience, Present Issues* (Oxford: Oxford University Press, 2002).

127 S. Burge, 'G. F. Adams: obituary', *BMJ*, 344:7855 (30 April 2012), e3047; 120 older patients were discharged over a twelve-month period in 1948, G. F. Adams, 'Geriatrics in Northern Ireland', *The Lancet*, 254:6589 (10 December 1949), 1095.
128 *BWT*, 14 October 1949.
129 *BO*, 7 July 1950.
130 *BO*, 15 June 1951.
131 *Mid-Ulster Mail*, 16 June 1951.
132 S. Murphy, 'The early days of the MRC Social Medicine Research Unit', *Social History of Medicine*, 12:3 (December 1999), 389–406.
133 *BN*, 26 May 1947.
134 *BT*, 27 July 1948, 6 November 1948.
135 'Northern Ireland', *BMJ*, 2:5096 (6 September 1958), 618; W. W. Holland, 'Appreciation: John Pemberton, 1912–2010', *International Journal of Epidemiology*, 39:3 (June 2010), 641–3.
136 PRONI, HOS 1/1/391, NIHA Sub-Committee on Preventive Medicine, 4 May 1954.
137 'Northern Ireland: Queen's University', *BMJ*, 2:5044 (7 September 1957), 576; J. G. Gibson, 'Psychological relationships', *UMJ*, 28:1 (1959), 1–10.
138 L. Ashley and I. McDonald, 'When the penny drops: understanding how social class influences speciality in the UK medical profession', *Social Science & Medicine*, 348 (2024), 116747; C. Olsson, H. Järnbert-Pettersson, S. Ponzer, M. Dahlin and T. Bexelius, 'Swedish doctors choice of medical speciality and associations with cultural capital and perceived status: A cross-sectional study', *BMC Medical Education* 19:244 (2019), 2.
139 PRONI, HSS/11/43/32, MHSS, Hawnt Committee, Dugdale to Hughes, 15 December 1964.
140 PRONI, HSS/11/43/32, MHSS, Hawnt Committee, J. H. Copeland, MHSS to G. P. Darling, MoF, 1 February 1965.
141 PRONI, HSS/11/43/32, MHSS, Hawnt Committee, Morgan to Prime Minister O'Neill, December 1964.
142 C. Ham, *Policymaking in the NHS: A Case Study of the Leeds Regional Hospital Board* (London: The Macmillan Press, 1981), p. 42; A. E. Weiss, *Management Consultancy and the British State: A Historical Analysis Since 1960* (Basingstoke: Palgrave Macmillan, 2019), p. 110.
143 D. J. Hunter, 'Organising for health: The NHS in the UK', *Journal of Public Policy*, 2:3 (August 1982), 285.
144 PRONI, HSS/11/43/32, MHSS, Ministry to Hawnt, 15 January 1965.

145 MHSS and HINA, *Administrative Structure of Hospital Management Committees and Hospital Committees: Report by a Joint Working Party appointed by the Minister of Health and Social Services and the Chairman of the Northern Ireland Hospitals Authority* (Belfast: HMSO, 1966) p. 5 [hereafter Hawnt Report].
146 Hawnt Report, p. 33.
147 S. J. Snow, '"I've never found doctors to be a difficult bunch": Doctors, managers and the NHS reorganisations in Manchester and Salford, 1948–2007', *Medical History*, 57:1 (2013), 69–70.
148 P. Begley, '"The type of person needed is one possessing a wide humanity": The development of the NHS national administrative training scheme', *Contemporary British History*, 34:2 (2020), 232; M. Learmonth, 'Kindly technicians: Hospital administrators immediately before the NHS', *Journal of Management in Medicine*, 12:6 (1998), 325.
149 Hawnt Report, p. 36.
150 M. Learmonth, 'Doing things with words: The case of "management" and "administration"', *Public Administration*, 83:3 (2005), 626.
151 P. Regan and E. Ball, 'A critical commentary on management science in relation to reforms after institutional National Health Service failures', *Journal of Nursing Management*, 25:2 (March 2017), 149–56.
152 Begley, 'The type of person needed is one possessing a wide humanity', 244.
153 C. Wood, 'A public management for all seasons?', *Public Administration*, 69:1 (1991), 8.
154 Hawnt Report, p. 32.
155 PRONI, HSS/13/24/18, MHSS, Hawnt Committee – Consultants etc. following issues of Report, Royal Belfast Hospital for Sick Children: Memorandum on the Report of Joint Working Party on the Administrative Structure of Hospital Management Committees and Medical Committees.
156 PRONI, HSS/13/24/18, MHSS, Hawnt Committee – Consultants etc. following issues of Report, A. E. S. Rainey, Joint Honorary Sec. Hospital Junior Staffs Group (Northern Ireland) to BMA, 11 January 1967.
157 J. Blundell and J. Lowry, 'Managing the hospitals', *BMJ*, 4:5579 (December 1967), 617.
158 PRONI, HSS/13/24/18, MHSS, Hawnt Committee – Consultants etc. following issues of Report, Dugdale to S. E. Taylor, 23 March 1967.
159 PRONI, HSS/13/24/18, MHSS, Hawnt Committee – Consultants etc. following issues of Report, NIHA to HMCs, 29 September 1967.

160 PRONI, HSS/13/24/18, MHSS, Hawnt Committee – Consultants etc. following issues of Report, Dugdale to Morgan, 4 July 1967.
161 Hawnt Report, p. 18.
162 For example, see the Mid-Antrim HMC opposition to regrouping, *BT*, 25 January 1967.
163 *BT*, 15 March 1967.
164 *Ibid.*
165 *BN*, 7 December 1967.
166 *BT*, 9 January 1967.
167 O'Leary, *A Treatise on Northern Ireland: vol. 2*, p. 169.
168 MHSS, *Hospital Plan*, p. 20.
169 *BT*, 15 March 1967.
170 PRONI, CAB/4/1393/7, Cabinet Secretariat, Cabinet conclusions, grouping of hospitals: memorandum by the Minister of Health and Social Services, 28 March 1968.
171 PRONI, HOS/1/1/816, NIHA Records, Working party on regrouping of hospitals in central area, Morgan to T. Brown, NIHA Chairman, 30 May 1968.
172 PRONI, HOS/1/1/816, NIHA Records, Working party on regrouping of hospitals in central area, Report of meeting of representative of the NIHA and South Tyrone HMC, 11 March 1969.
173 *Ibid.*, North Armagh HMC to NIHA, 17 April 1969.
174 Klein, *The New Politics of the NHS*, p. 47.
175 McKenna *et al.*, *Candles in the Dark*, p. 4.
176 Duffy, *Health Care and the Troubles.*
177 Mulholland, *Northern Ireland at the Crossroads*, p. 150.
178 Martin, 'Why have a Catholic Hospital at all?', p. 114.
179 PRONI, CAB/4/1446, Administrative structure of health and personal social services, 3 June 1969.
180 Webster, *The National Health Service*, p. 61.
181 Ham, *Health Policy in Britain*, p. 21.
182 PRONI, CAB/4/1446, Administrative structure of health and personal social services: Memorandum by the Minister of HSS, Annex 1, 3 June 1969.
183 *BT*, 3 July 1969.
184 PRONI, CAB/4/1446, Administrative structure of health and personal social services: Memorandum by the Minister of Health and Social Services, Annex 1, 3 June 1969.
185 For an outline of the Macrory Report, see J. P. Mackintosh, 'The Report of the Review Body on Local Government in Northern Ireland: The Macrory Report', *Public Administration*, 49:1 (March 1971), 13–24.

186 HSS/13/27/31, MHSS Policy Files, Administrative structure of health and personal social services – review body on local government – general, January 1970, p. 12.
187 R. A. W. Rhodes, P. Carmichael, J. McMillan and A. Massey, *Decentralising the Civil Service: From Unitary State to Differentiated Polity in the United Kingdom* (Buckingham: Open University Press, 2003), p. 61.
188 P. Begley and S. Sheard, 'From "Honeymoon Period" to "Stable Marriage": The rise of management consultants in British health policymaking', *Bulletin of the History of Medicine*, 95:2 (2021), 238–54.
189 McKinsey and Company, *Towards Better Health Care: Management in the Health Boards [A Report prepared for the Department of Health]* (Publisher and place of publication not available, 1970).
190 P. Begley and S. Sheard, 'McKinsey and the "Tripartite Monster": The role of management consultants in the 1974 NHS reorganisation', *Medical History*, 63:4 (2019), 390–410; *ibid.*, 'From "Honeymoon Period" to "Stable Marriage"', 238–54; Weiss, *Management Consultancy and the British State*, pp. 110–46.
191 'NBA in Northern Ireland: management services', *Official Architecture and Planning*, 31:11 (1968), 1497; 'Project coordination', *Official Architecture and Planning,* 31:11 (1968), 1486.
192 'NHS reorganisation in Northern Ireland', *BMJ*, 1:5801 (11 March 1972), 68–9.
193 D. Heenan, 'Northern Ireland', in C. Ham, D. Heenan, M. Longley and D. R. Steel (eds), *Integrated Care in Northern Ireland, Scotland and Wales: Lessons for England* (London: The King's Fund, 2013), p. 1.
194 Greer, *Territorial Politics and Health Policy*, p. 165.
195 PRONI, HOS/1/1/303, NIHA Records, Care of the elderly, 'Who cares for old people?', paper presented to NIHA Planning and General Purposes Committee.
196 *BT*, 10 July 1956.
197 M. Martin, 'Medical knowledge and medical practice: Geriatric medicine in the 1950s', *Social History of Medicine*, 8:3 (1995), 447.
198 G. F. Adams, *Review of Geriatric Services in Northern Ireland Hospitals, 1964: A Report to the NIHA* (Belfast: NIHA, 1964).
199 *Ibid.*, *Review of Geriatric Services in Northern Ireland Hospitals, 1969: A Report to the NIHA* (Belfast: NIHA, 1969), pp. 7–9.
200 NIHA, *Special Committee on the Hospital and Specialist Services*, pp. 15–16.
201 MHSS, *Hospital Plan*, p. 9.
202 *BT*, 19 February 1971.

203 *BT*, 18 August 1967.

204 M. R. Reich, J. H. Harris, N. Ikegami, A. Maeda, C. Cashin, E. C. Araujo, K. Takemi and T. G. Evans, 'Moving towards universal health coverage: Lessons from eleven country studies, *The Lancet*, 387:10020 (February 2016), 811–16.

205 C. H. Tuohy, *Accidental Logics: The Dynamics of Change in the Health Care Arena in the United States, Britain, and Canada* (Oxford: Oxford University Press, 1999), pp. 6–7.

206 *Northern Ireland Association of the Hospital Management Committees 15th Annual Report* (No date or place of publication), p. 4 [this pamphlet is held in QUB's Medical Library, Belfast].

207 PRONI, HSS/13/27/23, MHSS Policy Files, Administrative structure of health and personal social services, Ministry-BMA Discussion Group, 4 November 1970.

208 *Ibid.*, 25 November 1970.

Conclusion

The new structures set out in 1972 and introduced in 1973 finally placed central government firmly at the top of the health services, leading to an unprecedented level of state control. Since the 1920 Public Health Report on the eve of Irish partition and creation of Northern Ireland, medical reformers, planners and government officials had, to varying degrees, sought transformation in the management of healthcare services through increased centralisation, greater coordination and rationalisation. Yet, for the lifespan of the Stormont government, Northern Ireland had the weakest centralised health administration in any part of the United Kingdom.

The incapacity of Northern Ireland's government to challenge stakeholder power stemmed from multiple factors. The interwar period witnessed significant developments in Northern Ireland's mixed economy of healthcare. Leading voluntary hospitals, in collaboration with Queen's University, developed an early integrated health system situated around the Grosvenor Road medical site in Belfast. This system emerged as the most prestigious, advanced and powerful stakeholder in Northern Irish healthcare. Outside Belfast, local authorities developed increasingly modernised and sophisticated district hospitals. These developments indicate that interwar healthcare in Northern Ireland was more advanced than historians have previously understood and reflected wider trends in healthcare across Britain and Ireland. This expansion also ingrained powerful forces and influential stakeholders in the healthcare system, including an entrenched localism, loyalty to individual hospitals and a form of medical voluntarism that was intertwined with the political and social elite of Northern Ireland. These dynamics greatly shaped the direction of policy and management of healthcare. They filled the void created by a weak central government, which was marked by a social and political conservatism that discouraged government action as it grappled with the challenges of its recent establishment. This era was marked by limited centralisation of services, in which the power of individual hospitals, the medical profession and an embedded localism prevailed.

The 1940s, however, forced the restructuring of healthcare and the emergence of the central state. This was evident in the Emergency Hospital Service, which led to new regional structures of healthcare that central government created, funded and managed. This, in many ways, provided the basis for the NHS. Yet, the 1940s was far from an era marked by a prevailing consensus about health organisation. Instead, conflict emerged between the medical stakeholders, who solidified their position during the interwar era, and a central state apparatus, whose role and responsibility in health policy and management was expanding. This resulted in significant concessions ceded by the government to these stakeholders, which, in many ways, baked into the new NHS the fragmentation and inequalities that the health reforms sought to eradicate. The establishment of the Hospitals Authority was key to the settlement reached between the central government and the voluntary hospitals and medical profession. In an apparent concession to the interests of these groups who feared state management, the Authority had much independence from the Ministry; this effectively represented the government's surrendering of power over health policy and delivery of services. Notwithstanding this, the Authority represented a major, if somewhat curtailed, step towards greater coordination and was the biggest transformation in health management in Northern Ireland to that point.

The post-war decades were, in many ways, a story of further conflict between the deep-rooted sectional powers and a reforming centre in the form of the Hospitals Authority, initially, followed by a newly engaged central government in the 1960s. The power structures inherited from the interwar period continued to shape and play a key role in healthcare. Much of the leadership of the former voluntary hospital system transitioned into the Authority, and the lower tier of hospital management committees protected the interests of localism and individual hospitals. Post-war ideas around modernisation, initially evident in technocratic faith in expertise and scientific knowledge, followed by the emergence of business principles and management in public administration, became increasingly prevalent in Northern Ireland. These approaches sought to rationalise health services through coordination, which many reformers believed would bring about greater efficiencies. Yet this modernisation process was bitterly resisted by traditional stakeholders, whose position was now threatened by a reforming and expanding central government. The capacity of local interests, medical professionals and hospitals to curtail reform was illustrated during Terence O'Neill's reformist term as Prime Minister, when the government sought to modernise Northern Ireland's society, including hospital administration. Stakeholder resistance to modernisation policies, such as attempts to introduce non-clinical managers into hospital management, amalgamate hospital management committees and implement the 1966 Hospital Plan, led to much hostility, further fracturing not just unionist health policy but unionism generally in an era of collapsing social, political and religious relations. It was not until the outbreak of the Northern Irish Troubles, and the last attempts of the beleaguered Stormont administration to quell political and sectarian unrest, that the power of medical stakeholders was finally weakened. This allowed reformers a policy window of opportunity to create a highly integrated and centrally governed medical and personal social services system.

Select bibliography

Primary sources

Government archives

The National Archives of the United Kingdom (TNA)

Dominions Office	DO
Housing and Local Government	HLG
Home Office	HO
Medical Research Council	FD

Public Record Office of Northern Ireland (PRONI)

Belfast Corporation/County Borough Council	LA/7
Benn Ulster Eye, Ear and Throat Hospital	HOS/3
Board of Guardians, Belfast	BG/7
Board of Guardians, Lisnaskea	BG/20
Board of Guardians, Magherafelt	BG/23
Cabinet Secretariat, Records of	CAB
Development, Department of	DEV
East Antrim Hospital Records	HOS/5
Health and Local Government, Ministry of	HLG
Health and Social Services, Ministry of	HSS
North Antrim Hospital Records	HOS/9
Finance, Ministry of	FIN
Northern Ireland Hospitals Authority	HOS
Royal Victoria Hospital Records	HOS/2/1 & MIC514 [microfilm]
Royal Maternity Hospital Records	HOS/2/2

Down & Connor Diocesan Archives (DCDA)

Mater Infirmorum Records (Uncatalogued Archives)

McClay Library, Queen's University Belfast

Queen's University, Belfast Senate minute books, 1920–32

Newspapers

Ballymena Observer
Ballymena Weekly Telegraph
Ballymoney Free Press and Northern Counties Advertiser
Belfast Telegraph
Belfast News-Letter
Derry Journal
Frontier Sentinel
Irish News
Larne Times
Londonderry Sentinel
Mid-Ulster Mail
Northern Whig
Portadown Times
Strabane Chronicle
Witness

Official publications

Pre-1921

Annual Reports of the Local Government Board for Ireland, 1900–21.

Report of the Irish Public Health Council on the Public Health and Medical Services in Ireland [cmd. 761], xvii (1075), 1920.

Poor Law Reform Commission (Ireland). Appendix to the Report of the Vice-Regal Commission on Poor Law Reform in Ireland, *vol. 2*, HC [Cd. 3203], 1906.

Poor Law Reform Commission (Ireland): Minutes of evidence taken before the Vice-Regal Commission on Poor Law Reform in Ireland, *vol. 3*, HC [Cd. 3204], 1906.

Post-1921 Northern Ireland Government

Blake, J. M., *Northern Ireland in the Second World War* (London: HMSO, 1956).

Committee on the Health Services in Northern Ireland, *Report of the Committee on the Health Services in Northern Ireland* (Belfast: HMSO, 1955).

Departmental Commission on Local Government Administration in Northern Ireland, *Report of the Departmental Commission on Local Government Administration in Northern Ireland* (Belfast: HMSO, 1927).

Dunn, C. L. (ed.), *The Emergency Medical Services, Volume 2: Scotland, Northern Ireland and Principal Air Raids on Industrial Centres in Great Britain* (London: HMSO, 1953).

Health Advisory Council, *First Annual Report of the Health Advisory Council* (Belfast: HMSO, 1946).

Matthew, R. H., Belfast Regional Survey and Plan 1962: A Report Prepared for the Government of Northern Ireland (Belfast: HMSO, 1964).

Ministry of Finance, *Report by Organisation and Methods Branch Ministry of Finance: NIHA, Review of Headquarters Administration* (Belfast: HMSO, 1965).

Ministry of Health and Local Government, *Report on Health and Local Government Administration in Northern Ireland*, 1938–65.

Ministry of Health and Local Government and NIHA, *Summary of the Hospital Building Programme of the NIHA* (Belfast: HMSO, 1963).

Ministry of Health and Social Services, *Hospital Plan for Northern Ireland 1966–75* (Belfast: HSMO, 1966).

Ministry of Health and Social Services and NIHA, *Administrative Structure of Hospital Management Committees and Hospital Committees* (Belfast: HMSO, 1966).

Ministry of Home Affairs, *Report on the Administration of Local Government Services in Northern Ireland, 1921/3–37/8* (Belfast: HMSO).

Ministry of Home Affairs, *Local Taxation Returns, 1921–39* (Belfast: HMSO).

Ministry of Home Affairs, *Report of Maternity Services. Committee on Maternal Mortality and Morbidity in Northern Ireland* (Belfast: HMSO, 1943).

MacNalty, A. S. (ed.), *The Civilian Health and Medical Services: vol. II* (London: HMSO, 1955).

Northern Ireland Hospitals Authority, *Annual Reports*, 1948–72 (Belfast: HMSO).

Northern Ireland Hospitals Authority, *Report of the Special Committee on the Hospital and Specialist Services with the Authority's Observations thereon* (Belfast: HMSO, 1954).

Northern Ireland Hospitals Authority, *The Development of Hospital and Specialist Services / A Memorandum Prepared by The Authority, June 1961 and Revised in November 1963* (Belfast: HMSO, 1964).

Northern Ireland House of Commons Select Committee on Health Services, *Special Interim & Final Reports of the Select Committee on Health Services in Northern Ireland together with Proceedings of the Committee and Minutes of Evidence and Appendix* (Belfast: HMSO, 1944).

Titmuss, R., *History of the Second World War: Problems of Social Policy* (London: HMSO, 1950).

Webster, C., *The Health Services Since the War. Vol. 1: Problems of Health Care. The National Health Service before 1957* (London: HMSO, 1988).

Post-1921 Ireland, Oireachtas, Dáil Éireann

North-Eastern Boundary Bureau, *Handbook of the Ulster Question* (Dublin: Stationary Office, 1923).

Contemporary publications

Adams, G. F., 'Geriatrics in Northern Ireland', *The Lancet*, 254:6589 (10 December 1949), 1095–97.

Adams, G. F., *Review of Geriatric Services in Northern Ireland Hospitals, 1964: A Report to the NIHA* (Belfast: Northern Ireland Hospitals Authority, 1964).

Adams, G. F., *Review of Geriatric Services in Northern Ireland Hospitals, 1969: A Report to the NIHA* (Belfast: Northern Ireland Hospitals Authority, 1969).

Bailey, N. T. J., 'Operation research in medicine', *Operational Research Quarterly*, 3:2 (June 1952), 24–30.

Blundell, J. and J. Lowry, 'Managing the hospitals', *BMJ*, 4:5579 (December 1967), 617.

Burdett, H., *Burdett's Hospitals and Charities: Being the Yearbook of Philanthropy and the Hospital Annual* (London: Scientific Press, 1930).

Burge, S., 'G. F. Adams: Obituary', *BMJ*, 344:7855 (30 April 2012), e3047.

Campbell Young, J., 'A plan for the reorientation of the social services', *UMJ*, 6:3 (July 1937), 187–202.

Donaldson, G. A., 'Group medical practice', *UMJ*, 33:1 (June 1964), 17–27.

Elder, A. T., 'The health services of Northern Ireland', *British Journal of Preventive and Social Medicine*, 7 (1953), 105–11.

Freer, L. G. P., 'Recent tendencies in Northern Ireland administration', in F. H. Newark (ed.), *Devolution of Government: The Experiment in Northern Ireland* (London: Institute of Public Administration, 1953).

Gibson, J. G., 'Psychological relationships', *UMJ*, 28:1 (May 1959), 1–10.

Hickey, E. M., 'The problem of the aged in Northern Ireland', *UMJ*, 15:2 (November 1946), 150–2.

Kelly, M. P., *The Northern Ireland Hospitals Authority and Catholics* (Belfast: P. Quinn & Co Ltd, 1961).

Kidd, C. W., 'Medical aspects of hospital planning', *UMJ* 25:2 (November 1956), 80–97.

Kidd, L., 'A Ministry of Health for Northern Ireland', *UMJ*, 7:4 (October 1938), 229–40.

Lawrence, R. J., 'The health services in Northern Ireland', *Public Administration*, 34:3 (Autumn 1956), 289–308.

Leman, R. M., 'Fifty years – a radiographic retrospect', *UMJ*, 35:1 (January 1966), 1–11.

Loughridge, J. S., 'What of the future? Presidential address to the Ulster Medical Society', *UMJ*, 35:2 (December 1965), 53–65.

MaCafee, C. H. G., 'The history of the Chair of Midwifery and Gynaecology in the Queen's University of Belfast', *UMJ*, 44:2 (1975), 93–115.

MaCafee, D., 'Three Ulster surgical gentlemen', *UMJ*, 281:2 (2012), 91–6.

Main, F. F., *Our Health Services* (Belfast: NA, 1959).

Marshall, R. and R. W. M. Strain, 'Belfast', *BMJ*, 1:5284 (14 April 1962), 131–4.

McComb, S. and J. S. Peatt, 'National Health Insurance notes – Belfast and county areas', *UMJ*, 1:1 (January 1932), 65–6.

Montgomery, F. P., 'The Future of the Hospitals': Presidential address delivered before the Northern Ireland branch of the BMA', *UMJ*, 11:2 (November 1942), 114–34.

Neely, M. R., 'Some aspects of hospital planning', *UMJ*, 34:1 (1965), 1–7.

Neill, D. G., 'Some problems of integration in the hospital service of Northern Ireland', *Journal of the Statistical and Social Inquiry Society of Ireland*, 19 (1955–6), 169–83.

N. A., 'Queen's University Institute of Pathology', *UMJ*, 2:3 (July 1933), 151–2.

N. A., 'Emergency Hospital Service for Northern Ireland', *BMJ*, 2:4170 (23 September 1939), 189.

N. A., 'Regionalisation of Scottish hospitals', *BMJ*, 2:4166 (9 November 1940), 653.
N. A., 'Surveys of hospital services', *BMJ*, 2:4310 (14 August 1943), 209.
N. A., 'BMA Annual Representative', *BMJ*, 2:S147 (16 December 1944), 149.
N. A., 'Thomas Carnwath: obituary', *BMJ*, 1:4869 (17 August 1954), 938.
N. A., 'Stanley Barnes: obituary', *BMJ* 2:4938 (17 August 1955), 567.
N. A., 'Health services in Northern Ireland', *BMJ*, 1:4924 (21 May 1955), 1266.
N. A., 'Northern Ireland: Queen's University', *BMJ*, 2:5044 (7 September 1957), 576.
N. A., 'Northern Ireland', *BMJ*, 2:5096 (6 September 1958), 618.
N. A., 'Hospitals at home and abroad', *BMJ*, 2:5201 (10 September 1960), 1–12.
N. A., 'Lieut.-General William P. MacArthur: Obituary', *BMJ*, 2:5405 (8 August 1964), 389.
N. A., 'C. W. Kidd: Obituary', *BMJ*, 290:6472 (23 March 1985), 938.
Nuffield Provincial Hospitals Trust, *Survey of the Hospital Services of Northern Ireland* (Belfast: Privately Printed for the Northern Ireland Regional Hospital Committee, 1944).
Nuffield Provincial Hospitals Trust, *Studies in the Functions and Designs of Hospitals: The Report of an Investigation sponsored by the NPHT and the University of Bristol* (Oxford: Oxford University Press, 1955).
Shepherd, W. H. T., 'Hospital relationships', *UMJ*, 36:1 (1967), 13–22.
Thomson, C. S., 'Small-pox and vaccination', *BMJ*, 1:43 (6 January 1923), 43.
Thomson, C. S., 'Administrative problems connected with puerperal fever and puerperal pyrexia', *Journal of the Royal Society of Promotion of Health*, 48:5 (1 January 1927), 236–44.

Secondary readings

Thesis

Gray, A. M., 'Government and the administration of hospital services in Northern Ireland: The Northern Ireland Hospitals Authority, 1948–73' (Coleraine: University of Ulster, D Phil Thesis, 1993).

Books

Abel-Smith, B., *The Hospitals 1800–1948: A Study in Social Administration in England and Wales* (Cambridge, MA: Harvard University Press, 1964).

Anderson, M., H. Alderwick, E. Pitchforth, A. McGuire, N. Edwards and E. Mossialos, *Health Systems in Transition: United Kingdon: Health System Review,* 2022, vol. 1 (Copenhagen: World Health Organization, 2022).

Baldwin, P., *The Politics of Social Solidarity; Class Bases of the European Welfare State, 1875–1975* (Cambridge: Cambridge University Press, 1990).

Barrington, R., *Health, Medicine and Politics in Ireland, 1900–1970* (Dublin: Institute of Public Administration, 1987).

Barton, B., *The Blitz: Belfast in the War Years* (Belfast: Blackstaff Press, 1989).

Berridge, V., *Health and Society in Britain since 1939* (Cambridge: Cambridge University Press, 1999).

Bevan, G., M. Karanikolos, J. Exley, E. Nolte, S. Connolly and N. Mays, *The four health systems of the United Kingdom: how do they compare?* (London: The Nuffield Trust, 2014).

Bew, P., P. Gibbons and H. Patterson, *Northern Ireland, 1921–2001: Political Forces and Social Classes* (London: Serif, 3rd ed., 2002).

Bielenberg, A., *Ireland and the Industrial Revolution: The Impact of the Industrial Revolution on Irish Industry, 1801–1922* (London: Routledge, 2009).

Birrell, D., *Direct Rule and the Governance of Northern Ireland* (Manchester: Manchester University Press, 2009).

Birrell, D., *The Impact of Devolution on Social Policy* (Bristol: Policy Press, 2009).

Buckland, P., *The Factory of Grievances: Devolved Government in Northern Ireland, 1921–39* (Dublin: Gill & Macmillan, 1979).

Budge, I. and C. O'Leary, *Belfast: Approach to Crisis: A Study of Belfast Politics, 1613–1970* (London: Macmillan, 1973).

Clarke, R. S. J., *The Royal Victoria Hospital, Belfast: A History, 1797–1997* (Belfast: Blackstaff Press, 1997).

Crossman, V., *Poverty and the Poor Law in Ireland, 1850–1914* (Liverpool: Liverpool University Press, 2013).

Crossman, V. and P. Gray (eds), *Poverty and Welfare in Ireland, 1838–1948* (Dublin: Irish Academic Press, 2011).

Dallat, C., *Altnagelvin's Thirty Glorious Years: Two Hundred Years of Medical Care in Londonderry* (Derry: Altnagelvin Area Hospital, 1992).

Daly, M. E., *The Buffer State: The Historical Roots of the Department of Environment* (Dublin: Institute of Public Administration, 1997).

Bates, V., *Making Noise in the Hospital* (Cambridge: Cambridge University Press, 2021).

Devlin, P., *Straight Left: An Autobiography* (Belfast: Blackstaff Press, 1993).

Ditch, J., *Social Policy in Northern Ireland between 1939–50* (Aldershot: Avebury, 1988).
Dixon, P., *Northern Ireland: The Politics of War and Peace* (Basingstoke: Palgrave Macmillan, 2001).
Douds, S., *The Belfast Blitz: The People's Story* (Belfast: Blackstaff Press, 2011).
Doyle, B. M., *The Politics of Hospital Provision in Early Twentieth-Century Britain* (London: Pickering and Chatto, 2014).
Duffy, R., *Health Care and the Troubles: The Conflict Experience of the Northern Ireland Health Service, 1968–1998* (Liverpool: Liverpool University Press, 2024).
Dunn, C. L. (ed.), *The Emergency Medical Services, Volume 2: Scotland, Northern Ireland and Principal Air Raids on Industrial Centres in Great Britain* (London: HMSO, 1953).
Edwards, A., *A History of the Northern Ireland Labour Party: Democratic Socialism and Sectarianism* (Manchester: Manchester University Press, 2009).
Elliot, M., *The Catholics of Ulster: A History* (London: Penguin, 2001).
Fields, R. M., *Society under Siege: A Psychology of Northern Ireland* (Philadelphia, PA: Temple University Press, 1977).
Finlayson, G., *Citizen, State and Welfare in Britain, 1830–1990* (Oxford: Oxford University Press, 1994).
Fox, D. M., *Health Policies, Health Politics: The British and American Experience, 1911–65* (Princeton, NJ: Princeton University Press, 1985).
Francis, S., R. Glanville, A. Noble and P. Scher, *50 Years of Ideas in Health Care Buildings* (London: Nuffield Trust, 1999).
Fraser, D., *The Evolution of the British Welfare State* (Basingstoke: Palgrave Macmillan, 3rd ed., 2003).
Froggatt, P. and B. Bridges, *The Belfast Medical School, 1835–1985* (Belfast: Ulster Medical Journal, 1986).
Gilig, A. W., *Planning in Britain: Understanding and Evaluating the Post-War System* (London: Sage, 2005).
Gorsky, M. and S. Sheard (eds), *Financing Medicine: The British Experience Since 1750* (London: Routledge, 2006).
Gorsky, M., J. Mohan and T. Willis, *Mutualism and Health Care: British Hospital Contributory Schemes in the Twentieth Century* (Manchester: Manchester University Press, 2006).
Gosling, G. C., *Payment and Philanthropy in British Health Care, 1918–49* (Manchester: Manchester University Press, 2017).
Gould, M. H., *The Workhouses of Ulster* (Belfast: Ulster Architectural Heritage Society, 1983).

Grant, A., *Derry: The Irish Revolution, 1912–23* (Dublin: Four Courts Press, 2018).

Gray, P., *William Sharman Crawford and Ulster Radicalism* (Dublin: University College Dublin Press, 2023).

Greer, S. L., *Territorial Politics and Health Policy: UK Health Policy in Comparative Perspective* (Manchester: Manchester University Press, 2004).

Green, E. H. H., *Ideologies of Conservatism: Conservative Political Ideas in the Twentieth Century* (Oxford: Oxford University Press, 2002).

Ham, C., *Health Policy in Britain* (Basingstoke: Palgrave Macmillan, 5th ed., 2004).

Ham, C., *Policymaking in the NHS: A Case Study of the Leeds Regional Hospital Board* (London: The Macmillan Press, 1981).

Harkness, D., *Northern Ireland since 1920* (Dublin: Helicon, 1983).

Harris, B., *The Origins of the British Welfare State: State and Social Welfare in England and Wales, 1800–1945* (Basingstoke: Palgrave Macmillan, 2004).

Hennock, E. P., *The Origin of the Welfare State in England and Germany, 1850–1914: Social Policies Compared* (Cambridge: Cambridge University Press, 2007).

Howell, D., *MacDonald's Party: Labour Identities and Crisis, 1922–31* (Oxford: Oxford University Press, 2002).

Hughes, A. M., *Gender and Political Identities in Scotland, 1919–39* (Edinburgh: Edinburgh University Press, 2010).

Jackson, A., *Ireland 1798–1998: War, Peace and Beyond* (Oxford: Wiley-Blackwell, 2nd ed., 2010).

Jenkinson, J., *Scotland's Health, 1919–48* (Oxford: Peter Lang, 2001).

Jones, G., *'Captain of all these Men of Death': The History of Tuberculosis in Nineteenth and Twentieth Century Ireland* (Amsterdam: Rodopi, 2001).

Jones, G. and E. Malcolm (eds), *Medicine, Disease and the State in Ireland, 1650–1940* (Cork: Cork University Press, 1999).

Jordan, A., *Who Cared? Charity in Victorian and Edwardian Belfast* (Antrim: W. G. Baird, 1993).

Katz, M. and C. Sachsse (eds), *The Mixed Economy of Social Welfare: Public/Private Relations in England, Germany and the United States, the 1870s to the 1930s* (Baden-Baden: Nomos, 1996).

Kelly, L., *Irish Women in Medicine* c.*1880s–1920s: Origins, Education and Careers* (Manchester: Manchester University Press, 2012).

King, S. and J. Stewart (eds), *Welfare Peripheries: The Development of Welfare States in Nineteenth and Twentieth Century Europe* (Oxford: Peter Lang, 2007).

Kirby, M. W., *Operational Research in War and Peace: The British Experience from the 1930s to 1970s* (London: Imperial College Press, 2003).

Klein, R., *The New Politics of the NHS: From Creation to Reinvention* (London: CRC Press, 7th ed., 2013).

Lawrence, R. J., *The Government of Northern Ireland. Public Finances and Public Services, 1921–64* (Oxford: Oxford University Press, 1965).

Levene, A., M. Powell, J. Stewart and B. Taylor, *Cradle to Grave: Municipal Medicine in Interwar England and Wales* (Oxford: Peter Lang, 2011).

Lewis. J., *What Price Community Medicine? The Philosophy, Politics and Practice of Public Health since 1919* (Brighton: Wheatsheaf Books, 1986).

Lowe, R., *The Welfare State in Britain since 1945* (Basingstoke: Macmillan Press, 2nd ed., 1999).

Lucey, D. S., *The End of the Irish Poor Law? Welfare and Health Care Reform in Revolutionary and Independent Ireland* (Manchester: Manchester University Press, 2015).

Lucey, D. S. and V. Crossman (eds), *Healthcare in Ireland and Britain from 1850: Voluntary, Regional and Comparative Perspectives* (London: Institute of Historical Research, 2014).

Milne, I., *Stacking* the *Coffins: Influenza, War and Revolution in Ireland, 1918–19* (Manchester: Manchester University Press, 2018).

Mohan, J., *Planning, Markets and Hospitals* (Abingdon: Routledge, 2002).

Mulholland, M., *Northern Ireland at the Crossroads: Ulster Unionism in the O'Neill Years 1960–69* (Basingstoke: Macmillan Press, 2000).

Marks, L. V., *Metropolitan Maternity: Maternal and Infant Welfare Services in Early Twentieth-Century London* (Amsterdam: Clio Medica, 1996).

McCormick, L., *Regulating Sexuality: Women in Twentieth-Century Northern Ireland* (Manchester: Manchester University Press, 2009).

McCrae, M., *The National Health Service in Scotland: Origins and Ideals, 1900–50* (East Lothian: Tuckwell Press, 2003).

McKenna, J., F. Manzoor and G. Jones, *Candles in the Dark: Medical Ethical Issues in Northern Ireland During the Troubles* (London: The Nuffield Trust, 2009).

Michael, P. and S. Thompson, *Public Health in Wales (c.1800–2012): A Brief History* (Cardiff: Welsh Government, 2012).

Norton, C., *The Politics of Constitutional Nationalism in Northern Ireland, 1932–1970: Between Grievance and Reconciliation* (Manchester: Manchester University Press, 2014).

O'Hara, G., *From Dreams to Disillusionment: Economic and Social Planning in 1960s Britain* (Basingstoke: Palgrave Macmillan, 2007).

Ollerenshaw, P., *Northern Ireland in the Second World War: Politics, Economic Mobilisation and Society, 1939–45* (Manchester: Manchester University Press, 2013).

Pérez, P. F., *The Emergence of Modern Hospital Management in the World, 1880s–1930s* (Leeds: Emerald Publishing, 2021).

Pickstone, J. V., *Medicine and Industrial Society: A History of Hospital Development in Manchester and its Regions, 1752–1946* (Manchester: Manchester University Press, 1985).

Pierson, P., *Politics in Time: History, Institutions and Social Analysis* (Princeton, NJ: Princeton University Press, 2004).

Potter, M., *Municipal Revolution in Ireland: Local Government in Cities and Towns since 1800* (Dublin: Irish Academic Press, 2011).

Powell, M. (ed.), *Understanding the Mixed Economy of Welfare* (Bristol: Policy Press, 2007).

Prochaska, F. K., *Christianity and Social Service in Modern Britain: The Disinherited Spirit* (Oxford: Oxford University Press, 2008).

Purdue, O., *The Big House in the North of Ireland: Land, Power and Social Elites* (Dublin: University College Dublin, 2009).

Purdue, O. and G. Laragy, *Poverty, Children and the Poor Law in Industrial Belfast, 1880–1918* (Liverpool: Liverpool University Press, 2024).

Reinarz, J., *Health Care in Birmingham: The Birmingham Teaching Hospitals 1779–1939* (Woodbridge: Boydell Press, 2009).

Reinarz, J. and L. Schwarz (eds), *Medicine and the Workhouse* (Rochester, NY: University of Rochester Press, 2013).

Rintala, M., *Creating the NHS: Aneurin Bevan and the Medical Lords* (London: Frank Cass Publishing, 2003).

Rivett, G., *From Cradle to Grave: Fifty Years of the NHS* (London: Kings Fund Publishing, 1986).

Sheard, S., *The Passionate Economist: How Brian Abel-Smith Shaped Global Health and Social Welfare* (Bristol: Policy Press, 2013).

Thompson, S., *Unemployment, Poverty and Health in Interwar South Wales* (Cardiff: Cardiff University Press, 2006).

Urquhart, D., *Women in Ulster Politics, 1890–1940: A History Not Yet Told* (Dublin: Irish Academic Press, 2000).

Walker, B. M., *A Political History of the Two Irelands: From Partition to Peace* (Basingstoke: Palgrave Macmillan, 2012).

Walker, G., *The Politics of Frustration: Harry Midgley and the Failure of Labour in Northern Ireland* (Manchester: Manchester University Press, 1985).

Ward, S. V., *Planning and Urban Change* (London: Sage, 2nd ed., 2004).

Webster, C., *The National Health Service: A Political History* (Oxford: Oxford University Press, 2nd ed., 2002).

Weiss, A. E., *Management Consultancy and the British State: A Historical Analysis Since 1960* (Basingstoke: Palgrave Macmillan, 2019).
Welshman, J., *Municipal Medicine: Public Health in Twentieth Century Britain* (Oxford: Peter Lang, 2000).
Wright, J., *The 'Natural Leaders' and their World: Politics, Culture and Society in Belfast, c. 1801–1832* (Liverpool: Liverpool University Press, 2012).

Journal articles and book chapters

Ashley, L. and I. McDonald, 'When the penny drops: Understanding how social class influences speciality in the UK medical profession', *Social Science & Medicine*, 348 (2024), 116747.
Begley, P., '"The type of person needed is one possessing a wide humanity": the development of the NHS national administrative training scheme', *Contemporary British History*, 34:2 (2020), 228–50.
Begley, P. and S. Sheard, 'McKinsey and the "Tripartite Monster": The role of management consultants in the 1974 NHS reorganisation', *Medical History*, 63:4 (2019), 390–410.
Begley, P. and S. Sheard, 'From "Honeymoon Period" to "Stable Marriage": The rise of management consultants in British health policymaking', *Bulletin of the History of Medicine*, 95 (2021), 227–55.
Bew, P. and J. Bew, 'War and peace in Northern Ireland: 1965–2016', in T. Bartlett (ed.), *The Cambridge History of Ireland: Volume 4, 1800 to the Present* (Cambridge: Cambridge University Press, 2018), pp. 441–75.
Bridgen, P., 'Voluntary failure, the middle classes, and the nationalisation of the British voluntary hospitals, 1900–46', in B. Harris and P. Bridgen (eds), *Charity and Mutual Aid in Europe and North America since 1800* (New York: Routledge, 2007), pp. 212–34.
Campbell, S., 'New Nationalism? The SDLP and the creation of a socialist and labour party in Northern Ireland, 1969–75', *IHS*, 38:151 (May 2013), 422–38.
Casey, B., 'The Franciscan Missionaries of the Divine Motherhood and the Provision of Healthcare in Provincial Ireland, 1942–1970', *The Historical Journal* (December 2024), 1–21.
Cherry, S., 'Before the National Health Service: Financing the voluntary hospitals, 1900–1939', *Economic History Review*, 50:2 (1997), 305–26.
Cherry, S., 'Accountability, entitlement, and control issues and voluntary hospital funding, *c*1860–1939', *Social History of Medicine*, 9:2 (1996), 215–33.

Cochrane, F., '"Meddling at the Crossroads": The decline and fall of Terence O'Neill within the Unionist community', in R. English and G. Walker (eds), *Unionism in Modern Ireland: New Perspectives on Politics and Culture* (Basingstoke: Palgrave, 1996), pp. 148–69.

Cox, C., 'Health and welfare, 1750–2000', in E. F. Biagini and M. E. Daly (eds), *The Cambridge Social History of Modern Ireland* (Cambridge: Cambridge University Press, 2017), pp. 261–81.

Daly, M. E., '"An atmosphere of sturdy independence": the state and the Dublin hospitals in the 1930s', in E. Malcolm and G. Jones (eds), *Medicine, Disease and the State in Ireland, 1650–1940* (Cork: Cork University Press, 1999), pp. 234–52.

Darwin, J. 'A third British Empire?: The dominion idea in imperial politics', in J. Brown and W. R. Louis (eds), *The Oxford History of the British Empire: Volume IV: The Twentieth Century* (Oxford: Oxford University Press, 1999), pp. 64–87.

Davis, S., 'Promoting productivity in the National Health Service, 1950 to 1966', *Contemporary British History*, 31:1 (2017), 47–68.

Doyle, B. M., 'The economics, culture and politics of hospital contributory schemes: The case of interwar Leeds', *Labour History Review*, 77:3 (2012), 289–315.

Doyle, B. M. and A. McElligott, 'The rise and fall of European municipal power since 1800', *International Journal of Regional and Local Studies*, 7:1/2 (2011), 8–35.

Doyle, B. M. 'Labour and Hospitals in urban Yorkshire: Middlesbrough, Leeds, and Sheffield, 1919–38', *Social History of Medicine*, 23:2 (2010), 374–92.

Doyle, B. M. 'Power and accountability in the voluntary hospitals of Middlesbrough, 1900–48,' in A. Borsay and P. Shapely (eds), *Medicine, Charity and Mutual Aid: The Consumption of Health and Welfare, c. 1550–1950* (Aldershot: Ashgate, 2007), pp. 207–24.

Doyle, B. M. and N. Hayes, 'Eggs, rags and whist drives: popular munificence and the development of provincial medical voluntarism between the wars', *Historical Research*, 86:234 (2013), 712–40.

Fleming, N. C., '"Incorrigibly Plural": Recent Histories of Ulster and Northern Ireland', *Twentieth Century British History*, 21:1 (2010), 110–17.

Froggatt, P., 'The "Connexion" between the Royal and Queen's 1849–1949: Alliance or special relationship?', *UMJ*, 67:1 (1998), 108–23.

Fox, D. M., 'The National Health Service and the Second World War: The elaboration of consensus', in H. L. Smith (ed.), *War and Social Change: British Society in the Second World War* (Manchester: Manchester University Press, 1986), pp. 32–57.

Glendinning, M., '"The Forgotten Revolution": Northern Ireland's heritage of modern reconstruction', *The Journal of Architecture*, 15:5 (2010), 621–36.

Gorsky, M., J. Mohan and M. Powell, 'The financial health of voluntary hospitals in interwar Britain', *Economic History Review*, 4:3 (2002), 533–57.

Gorsky, M., '"To regulate and confirm inequality"? A regional history of geriatric hospitals under the English National Health Service, c. 1948–c. 1975', *Ageing and Society*, 33:4 (2013), 598–625.

Gorsky, M., 'Hospitals, finance, and health system reform in Britain and the United Kingdom, c. 1910–50: Historical revisions and cross-national comparison', *Journal of Health Politics, Policy and Law*, 37:2 (June 2012), 365–404.

Gorsky, M., 'Local government health services in interwar England: Problems of quantification and interpretation', *Bulletin of the History of Medicine*, 85:3 (autumn 2011), 384–412.

Gorsky, M., 'The British National Health Service 1948–2008: A review of the historiography', *Social History of Medicine*, 21:3 (December 2008), 437–60.

Gorsky, M., 'Public health in interwar England and Wales: Did it fail?', *Dynamis*, 28 (2008), 175–98.

Gorsky, M., 'The Gloucestershire extension of medical services scheme: An experiment in the integration of health services in Britain before the National Health Service', *Medical History*, 50:4 (2006), 491–512.

Gorsky, M., '"Threshold of a new era": The development of an integrated hospital system in Northeast Scotland, 1900–39', *Social History of Medicine*, 17:2 (2004), 248–67.

Gosling, G. C., '"Open the Other Eye"': Payment, civic duty and hospital contributory schemes in Bristol, *c.*1927–1948', *Medical History*, 54:4 (October 2010), 475–94.

Gray, A. M. and D. Birrell, 'The structures of the NHS in Northern Ireland: Divergence, policy copying and policy deficiency', *Public Policy and Administration*, 28:3 (2013), 274–89.

Gray, P., 'Conceiving and constructing the Irish workhouse, 1836–54', *IHS*, 38:149 (2012), 22–35.

Gudgin, G., 'Discrimination in housing and employment under the Stormont Administration', in P. J. Roche and B. Barton (eds), *The Northern Ireland Question: Nationalism, Unionism and Partition* (Aldershot: Ashgate, 1999), pp. 97–121.

Harris, B., 'Social security, full employment and voluntary action: The three pillars of William Beveridge's welfare society', *Social Policy & Administration*, 56 (2022), 203–16.

Harris, B. and R. Cresswell, 'The legacy of voluntarism: Charitable funding in the early NHS', *The Economic History* Review, 77:2 (May 2024), 554–83.

Hayes, N., 'Do we really want a National Health Service? Hospitals, patients and public opinions before 1948', *English Historical Review*, cxxvii:526 (2012), 625–61.

Heenan, D. and A. M. Gray, 'Administration in Ireland: The significance of public bodies', *Studies: An Irish Quarterly Review*, 89:356 (winter 2000), 372–9.

Hughes, J., 'The "Matchboxes on a Muffin": The design of hospitals in the early NHS', *Medical History*, 44 (2000), 21–56.

Hull, A., 'Hector's house: Sir Hector Hetherington and the academicization of Glasgow Hospital medicine before the NHS', *Medical History*, 45:2 (2011), 207–42.

Hunter, D. J., 'Organising for health: The NHS in the UK', *Journal of Public Policy*, 2:3 (1982), 263–300.

Jackson, A., 'Ireland, the union, and Empire, 1800–1960', in K. Kenny (ed.), *Ireland and the British Empire: The Oxford History of the British Empire Companion* (Oxford: Oxford University Press, 2000), pp. 123–53.

Jackson, A., 'Local government in Northern Ireland, 1920–73', in M. E. Daly (ed.), *County and Town: One Hundred Years of Local Government in Ireland* (Dublin: Institute of Public Administration, 2001), 56–66.

Jenkinson, J., 'Scottish health policy 1918–49 – paving the way to a National Health Service?', in C. Nottingham, *The NHS in Scotland: The Legacy of the Past and Prospect of the Future* (Aldershot: Ashgate, 2000), pp. 1–19.

Johnson, D. S., 'The Northern Ireland economy, 1914–39', in L. Kennedy and P. Ollerenshaw (eds), *An Economic History of Ulster, 1820–1939* (Manchester: Manchester University Press, 1985), pp. 184–223.

Jones, E., 'Nothing too good for the people: Local Labour and London's interwar health centre movement', *Social History of Medicine*, 25:1 (February 2012), 84–102.

Jones, G., 'The Rockefeller Foundation and medical education in Ireland in the 1920s', *IHS*, 30:120 (November 1997), 564–80.

Jones, G., 'Marie Stopes in Ireland – The Mother's Clinic in Belfast, 1938–47', *Social History of Medicine*, 5:2 (August 1992), 255–77.

Jones, G., 'Eugenics in Ireland: The Belfast Eugenics Society, 1911–15', *IHS*, 28:109 (May 1992), 81–95.

Kelly, S., 'Education of tubercular children in Northern Ireland, 1921 to 1955', *Social History of Medicine*, 24:2 (August 2011), 407–25.

Kenny, K., 'Ireland and the British Empire: An introduction', in K. Kenny (ed.), *Ireland and the British Empire: The Oxford History of the British Empire Companion* (Oxford: Oxford University Press, 2004), pp. 1–25.

Laragy, G., 'Poor relief in the south of Ireland, 1850–1921', in V. Crossman and P. Gray (eds), *Poverty and Welfare in Ireland, 1838–1948* (Dublin: Irish Academic Press, 2011), pp. 53–68.

Levene, A., 'Between less eligibility and the NHS: The changing place of Poor Law hospitals in England and Wales, 1929–39', *Twentieth Century British History*, 20:3 (2009), 322–45.

Levene, A., M. Powell and J. Stewart, 'The development of municipal general hospitals in English County Boroughs in the 1930s', *Medical History*, 50:1 (January 2006), 3–28.

Lucey, D. S. and V. Crossman, 'Introduction', in D. S. Lucey and V. Crossman (eds), *Healthcare in Ireland and Britain from 1850: Voluntary, Regional and Comparative Perspectives* (London: Institute of Historical Research, 2014), pp. 1–28.

Lucey, D. S. and G. Gosling, 'Paying for health: Comparative perspectives on patient payment and contributions for hospital provision in Ireland', in D. S. Lucey and V. Crossman (eds), *Healthcare in Ireland and Britain from 1850: Voluntary, Regional and Comparative Perspectives* (London: Institute of Historical Research, 2014), pp. 81–100.

Lucey, D. S., '"These schemes will win for themselves the confidence of the people": Irish independence, poor law reform and hospital provision', *Medical History*, 58:1 (2014), 46–66.

Lyons, J. B., 'Irish medicine's appeal to Rockefeller, 1920s', *Irish Journal of Medical Science*, 166:1 (1997), 50–6.

McTavish, D., 'The NHS – is Scotland different? A case study of the management of health care in the hospital service in the West of Scotland, 1947–87', *Scottish Medical Journal*, 45 (October 2000), 155–8.

Marks, L., '"The Luckless Waifs and Strays of Humanity": Irish and Jewish immigrant unwed mothers in London, 1870–1929', *Twentieth Century British History*, 3 (1992), 113–37.

Martin, M., 'Medical knowledge and medical practice: Geriatric medicine in the 1950s', *Social History of Medicine*, 8:3 (December 1995), 443–61.

Martin, P., '"Why have a Catholic Hospital at all?": The Mater Infirmorum Hospital Belfast and the state, 1883–1972', in D. S. Lucey and V. Crossman (eds), *Healthcare in Ireland and Britain from 1850*, pp. 101–17.

Martin, P., 'Social policy and social change since 1914', in L. Kennedy and P. Ollerenshaw (eds), *Ulster Since 1600: Politics, Economy, and Society* (Oxford: Oxford University Press, 2013), pp. 308–24.

Martin, P., 'Ending the pauper taint: Medical benefit and welfare reform in Northern Ireland, 1921–39', in V. Crossman and P. Gray (eds), *Poverty and Welfare in Ireland, 1838–1948* (Dublin: Irish Academic Press, 2011), pp. 223–36.

McClelland, A. G., 'A "ghastly interregnum": The struggle for architectural heritage conservation in Belfast before 1972', *Urban History*, 41:1 (2018), 150–72.

McCormick, L., 'Venereal disease in interwar Northern Ireland', in C. Cox and M. Luddy (eds), *Cultures of Care in Irish Medical History* (Basingstoke: Palgrave, 2010), pp. 191–207.

McCormick, L., 'Venereal diseases in Northern Ireland during the Second World War', in M. H. Preston and M. Ó hÓgartaigh (eds), *Gender, Medicine and the State in Ireland, 1700–1950* (New York: Syracuse University Press, 2012), pp. 221–35.

McIntosh, G., '"Who's looking after the baby?" Nursery school care in Northern Ireland during the Second World War', in G. McIntosh and D. Urquhart (eds), *Irish Women at War* (Dublin: Irish Academic Press, 2010), pp. 69–86.

Mitchell, J., 'Undignified and inefficient: Financial relations between London and Stormont', *Contemporary British History*, 20:1 (2006), 55–71.

Murphy, S., 'The early days of the MRC Social Medicine Research Unit', *Social History of Medicine*, 12:3 (December 1999), 389–406.

Neill, E. 'Conservative thinkers and the post-war state', in Lawrence Goldman (ed.), *Welfare and Social Policy in Britain Since 1870: Essays in Honour of Jose Harris* (Oxford: Oxford University Press, 2019), pp. 162–77.

Neville, J., 'Explaining local authority choices on public hospital provision in the 1930s: A public policy hypothesis', *Medical History, 56:01* (2012), 48–71.

Nolan, C., 'Creating jobs, manufacturing unity: Ulster unionism and mass unemployment 1922–34', *Contemporary British History*, 15:2 (2001), 1–44.

O'Connell, S., 'An age of conservative modernity, 1914–68', in S. Connolly (ed.), *Belfast 400: People, Place and History* (Liverpool: Liverpool University Press, 2012), pp. 271–316.

Ollerenshaw, P., 'Northern Ireland and the British Empire-Commonwealth, 1923–61', *IHS*, 36:142 (November 2008), 227–42.

Powell, M., 'Hospital provision before the NHS: A geographical study of the 1945 hospital survey', *Social History of Medicine*, 5:3 (1992), 483–504.

Powell, M., 'An expanding service: Municipal acute medicine in the 1930s', *Twentieth Century British History*, 8:3 (1997), 334–57.

Powell, M., 'Socialism and the British National Health Service', *Health Care Analysis*, 5:3 (1997), 187–94.

Privilege, J., 'The Northern Ireland government and the welfare state, 1942–8: The case of health provision', *IHS*, 39:155 (May 2015), 439–59.

Privilege, J. and G. Jones, 'Crisis and scandal: Government, local government and health reform in Northern Ireland, 1939–44', *Irish Economic and Social History*, 42 (2015), 33–52.

Purdue, O., 'Poor relief in the north of Ireland, 1850–1921', in V. Crossman and P. Gray (eds), *Poverty and Welfare in Ireland 1838–1948* (Dublin: Irish Academic Press, 2011), pp. 23–36.

Purdue, O., 'Poverty and power: The Irish Poor Law in a north Antrim town, 1861–1921', *IHS*, 37:148 (November 2011), 567–83.

Snow, S. J., '"I've never found doctors to be a difficult bunch": Doctors, managers and the NHS reorganisations in Manchester and Salford, 1948–2007', *Medical History*, 57:1 (2013), 65–86.

Stewart, J., 'Health care systems in Britain and Ireland in the nineteenth and twentieth centuries: The national, international and sub-national contexts', in D. S. Lucey and V. Crossman (eds), *Healthcare in Ireland and Britain from 1850*, pp. 31–60.

Stewart, J., '"The Finest Municipal Hospital Service in the World?": Contemporary perceptions of the London County Council's hospital provision, 1929–39', *Urban History*, 32:2 (August 2005), 327–44.

Sheard, S., 'Space, place and (waiting) time: Reflections on health policy and politics', *Health Economics, Policy and Law*, 13 (July 2018), 226–50.

Stewart, J., 'The National Health Service in Scotland, 1947–74: Scottish or British', *Historical Research*, 76:193 (July 2003), 389–410.

Sturdy, S. and R. Cooter, 'Science, scientific management and the transformation of medicine in Britain, c. 1870–1950', *History of Science*, 36:4 (1998), 421–66.

Taylor, B., J. Stewart and M. Powell, 'Central and Local Government and the Provision of Municipal Medicine, 1919–39', *English Historical Review*, 122:496 (April 2007), 397–426.

Thane, P., 'Voluntary action in Britain since Beveridge', in M. Oppenheimer and N. Deakin (eds), *Beveridge and Voluntary Action in Britain and the Wider World* (Manchester: Manchester University Press, 2011), pp. 121–34.

Theodore, D., 'Treating architectural research: The Nuffield Trust and the post-war hospital', *The Journal of Architecture*, 24:7 (2019), 982–98.

Thomas, L., 'Manifestations of institutional reform and resistance to reform in Ulster Workhouses, Ireland, 1838–1855', *International Journal of Historical Archaeological*, 21:4 (2017), 867–900.

Thompson, J. H., 'Canada and the "Third British Empire", 1901–39', in P. Buckner (ed.), *Canada and the British Empire* (Oxford: Oxford University Press, 2008), pp. 87–106.

Thompson, S., 'The mixed economy of care in the south Wales coalfield, *c.* 1850–1950', in D. S. Lucey and V. Crossman (eds), *Healthcare in Ireland and Britain from 1850: Voluntary, Regional and Comparative Perspectives* (London: Institute of Historical Research, 2015), pp. 141–60.

Thompson, S., 'To relieve the sufferings of humanity, irrespective of party, politics or creed: Conflict, consensus and voluntary hospital provision in Edwardian south Wales', *Social History of Medicine*, 16:2 (August 2003), 247–62.

Robson, N., 'Adapting not adopting: 1958–74. Accounting and managerial "reform" in the early NHS', *Accounting, Business and Financial History*, 17:3 (2007), 445–67.

Walker, G., 'Northern Ireland: The United Kingdom's first example of devolution', in C. Nic Dháibhéid, M. Coleman and P. Bew (eds), *Northern Ireland 1921–2021: Centenary Historical Perspectives* (Belfast: Ulster Historical Foundation, 2022), pp. 92–113.

Walker, G., 'Scotland, Northern Ireland and devolution, 1945–79', *Journal of British Studies*, 49:1 (2010), 117–42.

Webster, C., 'Devolution and the health service in Wales, 1919–69', in P. Michael and C. Webster (eds), *Health and Society in Twentieth Century Wales* (Cardiff: University of Wales Press, 2006), pp. 240–69.

Webster, C., 'Conflict and consensus: explaining the British health service', *Twentieth Century British History*, 1:2 (1990), 115–51.

Webster, C., 'Healthy or hungry thirties?', *History Workshop Journal*, 13 (1982), 110–29.

Welshman, J., 'Inequalities, regions and hospitals: The Resource Allocation Working Party', in M. Gorsky and S. Sheard (eds), *Financing Medicine: The British Experience Since 1750* (London: Routledge, 2006), pp. 221–41.

Whyte, J., 'How much discrimination was there under the Unionist regime, 1921–68?', in T. Gallagher and J. O'Connell (eds), *Contemporary Irish Studies* (Liverpool: Liverpool University Press, 1983), 1–35.

Internet sources

Dictionary of Irish Biography: https://www.dib.ie/

Voluntary Hospital Database: http:/hospitalsdatabase.lshtm.ac.uk

Index

Note: Page numbers in *italics* refer to figures; page numbers in **bold** refer to table; page numbers followed by 'n' indicate note numbers.

EU authorised representative for GPSR:
Easy Access System Europe, Mustamäe tee 50,
10621 Tallinn, Estonia
gpsr.requests@easproject.com

www.ingramcontent.com/pod-product-compliance
Ingram Content Group UK Ltd.
Pitfield, Milton Keynes, MK11 3LW, UK
UKHW021834100926
8556IPUK00004B/336
9781526119803